Behavioral Consultation and Primary Care: A Guide to Integrating Services

Behavioral Consultation and Primary Care: A Guide to Integrating Services

Patricia J. Robinson, PhD
Zillah, WA

and

Jeffrey T. Reiter, PhD, ABPP
Seattle, WA

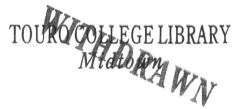
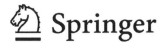 Springer

Library of Congress Control Number: 2006924589

ISBN-13: 978-0-387-32971-0   e-ISBN-13: 978-0-387-32973-4
ISBN-10: 0-387-32971-4   e-ISBN-10: 0-387-32973-0

Printed on acid-free paper.

9 8 7 6 5 4 3 2 1

springer.com

4/11/07

To Kirk Strosahl, my partner for 1000 lifetimes, and to our children, Regan, Frances, and Joanna, who provide daily doses of joy

P. R.

To the dedicated teachers who have believed in, mentored and challenged me throughout the years, especially Hayden, James, Mom, and Dad (in no particular order!)

J. R.

PREFACE

There exists a very large and growing demand for behavioral health care, and all too often the responsibility for such care falls not on mental health clinics but on primary care clinics. The mental health professions have been slow to respond to this problem, but an emerging and promising strategy has been to improve collaboration between mental health and primary care by integrating the two services. These efforts have taken a number of forms, but they all share the common goal of better meeting the health care needs of the population. As with any new endeavor, however, confusion about how to proceed is widespread. Individuals and clinics attempting to integrate primary care and behavioral health can easily feel as if they are in a boat adrift without a rudder (and sometimes it can feel as if that boat is alone in the middle of a very large sea!). Imagine being the medical director of a primary care clinic wanting to develop an integrated service, or the mental health provider hired to do that. Where would you start? With whom would you consult? This being a relatively new field, few people have training, and this means that finding guidance for establishing a service can be challenging. Even when knowledgeable consultants are found, the advice given is likely to be discrepant from one consultant to another.

In this book we provide practical advice to those interested in integrating primary care and behavioral health services. We describe a specific model, the Primary Care Behavioral Health (PCBH) model, that we believe offers a great deal of promise for improving both mental and physical health outcomes. In doing so, we hope to contribute to the standardization of primary care behavioral health integration efforts. The PCBH model is in widespread use around the USA, but has never before been detailed in a book. The model represents a radically different approach to treating behavioral problems, relative to the traditional specialty mental health model. It is also dramatically different from other approaches to integration.

Hopefully this book will help the reader understand both the need for a different model and the basics of how to apply it. We write from a strong scientist–practitioner perspective, and also inject plenty of anecdotal advice based on our experiences in the primary care behavioral health arena. Our goal was to create a book that is readable and friendly, yet also full of substance. Scientific literature is reviewed in some parts and cited as needed, but this work is first and foremost a "nuts and bolts" guide for behavioral health providers who want to work in primary care and for the administrators who seek to hire them.

In the PCBH model, the behavioral health provider is a consultant (termed "Behavioral Health Consultant" or "BHC") to primary care colleagues. We both work as BHCs in federally qualified health centers (also knows as community health centers), one in a relatively small clinic and the other in a large one. One of us (PR) also worked as a BHC in a large health maintenance organization for eight years prior to moving into the community health sector. In our experience the PCBH model is a durable one that works well in various clinic settings and with patients from diverse socio-economic, racial, and ethnic backgrounds. Further, the model allows for delivery of behavioral health services to a much larger group of patients than is possible in specialty mental health care or with other models of integration.

One of us is newer to this field (JR) and one has more experience (PR). We believe the combination of a neophyte and a seasoned provider is a good one for this type of book. There are aspects of transitioning from specialty mental health to primary care that one forgets about after doing this work for a while, hence the benefit of a neophyte's perspective. But there is also knowledge one can only acquire from experience, hence the benefit of the seasoned veteran. The blend of the two will hopefully provide the reader with a solid feel for how to both get started in primary care and how to maintain momentum.

The book is organized into six parts and four appendices, including a CD that has reproducible patient education handouts and other tools. Part one of the book gives readers an overview of the rationale for integrating primary care and behavioral health, including the most common approaches to integration. A chapter in this part also provides an introduction to the mission of primary care and the people who work there. Part two defines the mission of the PCBH model and describes six domains of competence for the BHC. Ideas for recruiting, training, and evaluating the performance of a BHC are also discussed. Other operational issues in this part include where to locate a BHC service, what items to budget, specific types of BHC services, recruiting for a Behavioral Health Assistant (BHA), and billing issues.

Beginning with the third part of the book the focus becomes more clinical. We review the theoretical models, therapeutic approaches and measurement practices that match well with the PCBH model. Though these will not be new to many readers, the application of them in primary care may be. Part four provides practice tools for the BHC, such as interview and dictation templates, and describes charting practices. In this section, readers with less background in behavior therapy can learn more about conducting a functional analysis, which is a core part of BHC patient visits. This part also provides a Start-Up Checklist for new BHCs and ideas for overcoming potential barriers to referrals from primary care providers (PCPs). Part five is perhaps the heart of the book, as it provides examples of BHC consultations, including common clinical interventions. One chapter is devoted to each of three populations, including children/teenagers and their families, adults, and older adults. Through consultations with patients, the BHC can have a significant effect on PCPs and their ongoing management of patients. Part five also includes a chapter on providing group services, which may range from seeing families to seeing large groups of patients for classes, workshops, and group medical visits.

In part six, we share the lessons from some of our more challenging moments in primary care and give examples of common ethical issues for a BHC to be mindful of. This section ends with a chapter offering strategies for evaluating services provided by the BHC. Because ongoing efforts are needed to evaluate, refine, and further develop the PCBH model, we consider this to be an important chapter. The appendices include recommended readings on theoretical and therapeutic approaches to expand a BHC's base of preparedness, as well as clinical readings to aid one's work with children and adults. To help jumpstart a new BHC service, a compact disc with patient education handouts and other tools is also included. Materials on the disc are completely reproducible.

We wrote this book to appeal to a wide audience. The book is not only for behavioral health providers starting a primary care service, but also for the primary care clinic administrators, medical staff members, and medical directors who will partner with them. We also hope this work will be helpful to graduate students in psychology, social work, counseling, and nursing, who plan to work in the primary care setting or collaborate with PCPs. Primary care and psychiatry residents interested in behavioral approaches to common health problems should also find much of relevance here. Even school psychologists and counselors, who in many ways face similar problems to PCPs (i.e., they work in an environment that requires them to address many behavioral issues with limited resources), might benefit from understanding the PCBH model and the clinical strategies described here. Finally, one of our greatest hopes is that this book might offer a foundation for the development of more training programs in primary care behavioral health. There is a great need for more training opportunities, but up until now not much guidance has existed for interested training directors.

Before ending this introduction, a couple of qualifiers are needed. The first is that we haven't done everything in this book in our own clinics, and readers needn't think they have to in order to develop a successful BHC service. The services we provide in our own clinics are dynamic and grow and change as the larger healthcare environment changes. Though remaining true to the basic PCBH model is important, within the model there is plenty of room for creativity and innovation. Consider this book a toolbox from which you hopefully can create a product that meets both your needs and the needs of your clinic. Our second qualifier is that we both are psychologists, and though we have attempted to write the book in fairly generic language there are bound to be places where we could have done better. One challenge of writing for a variety of disciplines is that each discipline seems to use different words to refer to the same or similar concepts. Where we use language or concepts less likely to be understood outside of psychology, we do our best to note that and explain it.

Finally, we must thank the many people who have inspired, helped, advised, encouraged, and—in some cases—fed us, throughout the course of writing this book. Patti wishes to thank Kirk Strosahl, Ph.D., for invaluable input at the time of need during the long days of writing and Regan Robinson for her support of relaxation time. She also expresses appreciation to her colleagues and friends who read parts of the book, including Joyce Strosahl, Julie Rikard, Ph.D., and David Brumbaugh, M.D.

Mark Sauerwein, M.D., Kyle Heisey, M.D., Kevin Walsh, M.D., Ivanna Iovino, M.D., Patricia Hernandez, M.D., Michael Chau, Janis Rue, M.D., Paul Monahan, M.D., Nic Oprescu, M.D., Julie Ricking, M.D., Mark Farley, M.D., Don Gargas, M.D., Natasha Leacock-Chau, Brian Ullom, M.D., and Myrna Ramos-Diaz, M.D. have provided exemplary models and inspiring ideas over the past four years at the Toppenish Clinic. Patti also respectfully acknowledges James Birge, M.D., and Corporate Medical Director, Janis Luvaas, MHA and Program Administrator, and Carlos Olivares, BA and CEO, for their pioneering efforts to bring BHC services to underserved populations. Finally, Patti thanks patients, providers, and nursing and support staff at Yakima Valley Farm Workers Clinic System (YVFWC) and Group Health Cooperative Clinics for teaching her, day after day, to be a better Behavioral Health Consultant.

For his part, Jeff wishes to thank Jim Berghuis, Ph.D., who has co-developed the BHC service at Community Health Centers of King County (CHCKC) in Washington along with Jeff for the last few years. Jim has been a valued friend and colleague, and his influence is seen in many places throughout this book. Judy Featherstone, M.D., deserves kudos for the bold vision and commitment to innovation that brought the BHC service to CHCKC, and Evan Oakes, M.D., has been simply invaluable to actually making the service work (while still managing to keep meetings fun). Kim McDermott, MD, was the original physician champion for behavioral health and is owed a heap of thanks for her collegiality and steadfast support of the service. Along with Evan and Jim, Wayne Dees, PsyD, Jeff Harvey, PsyD, and Mike Lee, PsyD, read parts of this manuscript and offered feedback that helped us tremendously. Thanks guys! Gratitude also goes to Kirk Strosahl, Ph.D., without whose generous mentoring Jeff would not be doing this work or this book. Few, if any, have the knowledge and passion Kirk has for this field, and we can only hope he will continue his work for many years to come. And finally, a big thank you to the patients and staff of Eastside Community Health Center, who teach, challenge, and inspire me on a daily basis. I know I am a better person for having worked with you.

Patricia Robinson
Zillah, WA

Jeffrey T. Reiter
Seattle, WA

ABBREVIATIONS USED IN THE BOOK

Abbreviation	Term
BH	behavioral health
BHA	behavioral health assistant
BHC	behavioral health consultant
EMR	electronic medical record
MH	mental health
MHP	mental health professional
PC	primary care
PCBH	primary care behavioral health (model)
PCP	primary care provider

LIST OF TABLES

LIST OF FIGURES

CONTENTS

PART I.
THE PERFECT STORM OF PRIMARY CARE

PART II.
YOUR MISSION, SHOULD YOU CHOOSE TO ACCEPT IT

PART III.   A HORIZON AND A COMPASS

PART VI.   UNCHARTED TERRITORY

PART I

THE PERFECT STORM OF PRIMARY CARE

The forces pressuring and buffeting primary and mental health care are like a series of interconnected weather conditions. Escalating rates of physical and mental health problems in the USA are combining with escalating health care costs to whip up a vortex of problems. Lifestyle and behavior issues are at the heart of the vortex, playing a major role in the escalation of health problems. Yet, while the pharmaceutical industry has grown in influence, attention to basic behavior change approaches has strayed. Our shelter, the mental health system, is collapsing, leaving many patients out in the cold and forcing many others into primary care for help. They join the growing ranks of patients seeking help in primary care for chronic medical problems, many of which have a significant behavioral component. As more people live with poor health, physicians are pressured to work faster and harder, and, not surprisingly, their patient relationships have suffered and their job satisfaction has declined. Patients have also become frustrated as they face the behavioral challenges of managing chronic diseases while fighting for access to their health care providers. We are no doubt in the midst of a violent storm and it is centered in primary care. Yet, there are emerging strategies for getting through it. Better integration of primary care and behavioral health services is one approach that may help see us through, and in Part I we provide the rationale for it. We introduce a specific approach to integration, the primary care behavioral health model

1

which we believe holds particular promise. Along the way we also introduce the reader to the structure, players, and milieu of the primary care world.

1

AN OVERVIEW OF PRIMARY CARE BEHAVIORAL HEALTH CONSULTATION

"Far better it is to dare mighty things, to win glorious triumphs, even though checkered by failure, than to take rank with those poor spirits who neither enjoy much nor suffer much, because they lie in the gray twilight that knows not victory nor defeat."

—Theodore Roosevelt (1858–1919)

For a number of years, we worked in traditional specialty mental health care (MH) settings. Like most MH providers, we worked hard, kept up on clinical innovations, and had the best interests of our clients at heart. We most certainly had clients who progressed and many who appreciated our assistance. However, we couldn't help but wonder what happened to clients who didn't show for follow-up appointments. On a typical day we and our co-workers would have seven clients scheduled, of which two or three wouldn't show. What happened to the no-shows? Were they still struggling? Why didn't they come in? Further, we felt frustrated that by the end of the day we might have only seen a handful of clients (many of whom were the same clients seen week after week). Thus, how many people were we really helping? First-time clients often failed to show as well, which was frustrating because the wait list was typically lengthy. We rationalized that a "no-show" meant the client probably wasn't ready for change. Yet, the questions also nagged of whether the wait might have deterred the client, and how the client was doing if he or she wasn't getting care from us.

Down the hall, but unbeknownst to us, our primary care (PC) colleagues also had some nagging questions. Why do so few of the patients referred to MH follow through on the referral? Why are so many "psych" patients coming in for care when an MH system exists to tend to their needs? How can we get patients with chronic conditions like diabetes to change the behaviors so crucial to managing their disease? How can a primary care provider (PCP) be expected to meet all of a patient's needs with 15-minute visits?

Unfortunately, as we have since learned, our experiences and questions were not unique. The MH system of the USA is simply not meeting the needs of the population, and the PC system is picking up the slack. Approximately 28 percent of Americans experience a diagnosable psychiatric disorder in any given year, but half of this group receives no care at all. Of those that do, only about half get the care from a specialty MH clinic. Instead, most rely on other health care providers, especially PCPs (Regier, Narrow, Rae, Manderscheid, Locke, & Goodwin, 1993). In keeping with these statistics, an overwhelming majority of prescriptions for psychotropic medications are written not by psychiatrists, but by nonpsychiatric physicians (Beardsley, Gardocki, Larson, & Hidalgo, 1988). Primary care providers end up delivering most of these prescriptions because, with 80 percent of the population visiting a PCP in the course of a year, they penetrate the population the deepest (Strosahl, 1998). These statistics begin to answer some of the questions we and our PC neighbors had. When clients didn't show for appointments, they probably eventually ended up in a PCP's office.

In this book we present readers a guide for providing health and MH care in a radically different fashion—one that begins to better meet the needs of the population. Called Primary Care Behavioral Health (PCBH), this model of care involves delivery of Behavioral Health Consultant (BHC) services in a PC clinic and differs in many respects from traditional MH care. It is also designed to change the way PC is conducted. As noted by Strosahl (1998), an early developer and proponent of the PCBH model, this model is best considered as a form of *health* care rather than *mental health* care. The goal is not to replace the specialty MH care system, but rather to improve the treatment of behavioral problems in PC. In doing so, the functioning of the PC system in general can improve, and attention to other health needs of the population can increase.

The model as well as the general rationale for integrating primary and behavioral health care have been discussed in other texts (e.g., Blount,

1998; Bray, Frank, McDaniel, & Heldring, 2004; Gatchel & Oordt, 2003). Rather than rehashing those writings, this book focuses on how to actually implement and practice the PCBH model. Although a BHC approach alone will not solve society's MH problems, it represents an important step toward improving overall population health. Before describing the PCBH model in more detail, some history and background information might help underscore the need for a change.

THE NATURE OF BEHAVIOR PROBLEMS IN PRIMARY CARE

Up to 70 percent of PC medical appointments are for problems stemming from psychosocial issues (Gatchel & Oordt, 2003). These concerns can take many forms, the most obvious being bona fide psychiatric disorders. For example, a survey of consecutively scheduled adult PC patients found that 19 percent met criteria for major depression, 15 percent for generalized anxiety, 8 percent for panic, and another 8 percent for substance use. Between 36 percent and 77 percent had more than one disorder (Olfson et al., 2000). The average PCP will see the full spectrum of MH disorders, from depression and anxiety to substance abuse to psychotic disorders within a week of practice. Primary care providers regularly handle care for chronic psychiatric problems as well as acute flare-ups (e.g., a suicidal patient). Because they provide care across the lifespan, many PCPs also treat child behavior problems (e.g., ADHD) in addition to the problems of adults and older adults. Keeping in mind that they do all of this while also tending to the medical needs of their patients, a PCP must truly be a generalist! Recalling our earlier comments that nonpsychiatric physicians treat the majority of psychiatric patients and prescribe the majority of psychotropic medications in the USA, it is no wonder that PC has been labeled the country's "de facto mental health care system" (Regier et al., 1993).

Activities of the prescription drug industry have played an important role in shifting psychiatric treatment from the MH specialist realm to the PCP realm. As described by Gray, Brody, and Johnson (2005), the delivery system for MH care changed dramatically over a 10-year period. Starting with the introduction of Prozac in 1986, there were increases in the number of people treated for depression, the percentage of depressed patients who received medication, and the percentage of patients receiving depression treatment by PCPs. At the same time, the percentage of patients receiving psychotherapy for depression dropped (Olfson, Marcus, & Druss, 2002). Specialty behavioral services accounted for about 6 percent of medical costs in 1988 and 3 percent in 2005, and this decrease is roughly equal to the costs of behavioral pharmaceuticals prescribed by PCPs (Gray et al., 2005). While MH clinics downsized, drug companies marketed additional SSRI medications to providers and, when the Federal Drug Administration lifted its ban on advertising directly to consumers, they marketed to patients.

Psychiatric disorders, though, are only the tip of the iceberg in primary care. Behavioral issues arise in many other forms as well. One oft-cited study tracked 1,000 PC patients over three years and found that 85% of their most common complaints could not be traced to any organic etiology (Kroenke & Mangelsdorff, 1989). Irritable bowel syndrome, tension headaches, insomnia, and chronic nonspecific pain are but a few examples of somatic complaints that can have a significant stress component. Most patients, however, view these as medical problems and seek help for them from a PCP rather than a MH provider. Kroenke et al. (1997) obtained a prevalence of 8 percent for primary care patients who struggle with somatization, and people in this group often use PC services excessively. They often do not need medications, but their distress level tends to be high and PCPs may not be able to offer them the time and skill training necessary to improve their functioning. Many patients also seek help from a PCP for "subthreshold syndromes," such as marital conflict, domestic violence, bereavement, and other life stressors.

Primary care providers also spend much time and energy counseling patients on behavior change issues important to health. According to the United States Department of Health & Human Services (2000), unhealthy lifestyles are responsible for most of the top ten causes of mortality and morbidity in the country. Behaviors such as smoking, poor diet, lack of exercise, and problematic alcohol and drug use are prime examples. Other behaviors such as the wearing of seat belts and bike helmets, the use of contraceptives, high-risk sexual behavior, and numerous others, also have implications for health. Almost any MH professional in a traditional MH setting would be surprised and perplexed if a client presented for help with one of these behavioral issues. However, PCPs confront and counsel patients regarding these issues everyday.

Behavioral issues also arise in PC when patients present with chronic medical problems. Primary care systems have historically been focused more on treating acute problems, but they increasingly must tend to chronic problems. Indeed, chronic conditions are the fastest growing part of PC (Patterson, Peek, Heinrich, Bischoff, & Scherger, 2002). This is due to several factors, including an aging population; an increase in conditions such as diabetes, lipid disorders, and obesity; and medical advances that allow people to live longer with diseases that would have been fatal in earlier years. The trend toward more chronic disease means that more patients must learn to cope with conditions that can disrupt lifestyle and relationships. Moreover, self-management practices such as complying with a medication regimen and maintaining a healthy lifestyle are often basic to good outcomes. Once again, PCPs are called upon to help patients navigate these issues. They must counsel patients on how to cope with a chronic condition, educate family members about it, and motivate patients to make the lifestyle changes needed to manage it. Unfortunately, estimates suggest that up to 60 percent of patients with chronic disorders adhere poorly to treatment (Dunbar-Jacob & Mortimer-Stephens, 2001).

BARRIERS TO RECOGNIZING AND TREATING BEHAVIORAL PROBLEMS IN PRIMARY CARE

At the same time PCPs are being inundated with these various behavioral needs of patients, other factors combine to make meeting these needs difficult. One often-cited factor is under-recognition of behavioral problems by both PCPs and patients. Given the chronic nature of many MH problems, they may persist and result in frequent PCP visits if not recognized and treated. Unfortunately, with 10 to 15 minutes per visit and on average three health concerns voiced by patients per visit (Kaplan, Gandek, Greenfield, Rogers, & Ware, 1995), PCPs have little time to explore problems in detail. Moreover, they may be reluctant to even ask about stressors, fearing the patient will become defensive or require a lot of extra time (Snugg & Inui, 1992). Patients often do not help this situation. They frequently fail to report emotional problems and are often more focused during physician visits on the physical manifestations of stress than on the stress itself (Bray et al., 2004; Patterson et al., 2002).

Stigma regarding MH care also makes it harder for PCPs to recognize and treat the behavioral needs of patients. Many patients and even many health care providers continue to be swayed by an obsolete mind–body distinction that separates mental health from physical health. Thus, rather than viewing a referral to MH as a routine part of health care, patients often interpret it as a sign that the PCP has given up on them or doesn't want to deal with their emotional health (Patterson et al., 2002; Strosahl, 1998). Many patients also are deterred from seeking treatment because of a fear that discrimination will result from it, or because of an internalized prejudice against mental illness (Corrigan, 2004). Other patients might simply refuse to trust anyone other than their PCP for care (Von Korff & Myers, 1987). Whatever the reason, when patients refuse to pursue specialty MH care, PCPs usually end up providing it.

Even when a problem is recognized and the patient is eager for treatment, poor access to MH care may frustrate the patient and the PCP. Under the current system, many patients who genuinely need and desire MH care simply cannot get it. The carving-out of MH care reimbursement (whereby it is considered separate from medical care) has allowed third-party payors to deny or restrict access to MH services, often severely. Additionally, most third-party payors only reimburse for DSM-IV-TR diagnoses, thereby stranding many patients with subthreshold syndromes. Mental health professionals have also not been able to bill for physical health diagnoses, making it difficult to help patients with diabetes, obesity, headaches, and other problems in that realm. The American Psychological Association (APA) has recently made some strides toward lessening this dilemma by successfully lobbying for new "health and behavior" reimbursement codes, but obtaining reimbursement with them has been difficult for many practitioners (Dittmann, 2004; Gray et al., 2005; Johnson, 2001). All of these issues and others, combined with the successful pharmaceutical marketing described earlier, have shrunk the MH funding stream to a muddy trickle. As resources have become sparser, so have services.

These problems, of course, are in addition to those posed by the growing ranks of the uninsured. Between 1990 and 2001, the number of uninsured persons in the USA grew 19 percent, from 34.7 million to 41.2 million (DeLeon, Giesting, & Kenkel, 2003). These uninsured do not have easy access to any type of health care, let alone MH care. If they do seek help for behavioral problems, they will most likely receive it not from a community *mental* health center, but from a community *health* center, i.e., a PC clinic (DeLeon et al., 2003).

THE EFFECTS ON PRIMARY CARE

One can easily imagine that PC clinics suffer many adverse effects from the deluge of behavioral issues and the lack of integrated behavioral services. Job satisfaction of clinic staff is a concern, and staffing shortages, particularly in rural areas, have led to concerted efforts to improve marketing and recruitment (Dickinson, Evans, Carter, & Burke, 2004). Primary care providers often do not feel that their training adequately prepared them for the daily barrage of psychosocial problems, and some are bitter about the lack of referral possibilities. Until PCPs feel better trained and prepared for the problems they face, as well as supported, they will likely continue to experience frustration on the job.

Given the team environment of medical settings, it is also true that if PCPs feel frustrated, ancillary clinic staff probably do as well. Medical assistants, nurses, and lab technicians are no more prepared to deal with behavioral problems than PCPs, yet they interact with patients sometimes even more frequently than do PCPs. Receptionists and other staff often must handle psychotic, depressed, or otherwise challenging patients, and referral coordinators must try (often in vain, due to the factors previously identified) to locate accessible MH services. All of this places additional strain on a PC system that is already very busy.

THE EFFECTS ON PATIENTS

Patients also suffer under the current system. The lack of access to therapy services means that most problems are treated solely with medications. Primary care providers have neither the time nor the training to provide therapy, so most rely heavily on medications. The use of psychotropic medications has gone up dramatically since the mid-1980s amongst all prescribers, and psychotropic medications are now among the most widely prescribed medications in the USA (Pincus et al., 1998). Given the wealth of data on the insufficiency of medication-only treatment and on the importance of a more comprehensive approach (see, for example, Badamgarav et al., 2003), one can easily argue that most patients receive inadequate treatment for psychiatric problems in PC.

More than being insufficient, this heavy reliance on medications may also make some problems worse. For example, when a PCP (desperate to help) is faced with a patient with chronic anxiety (desperate for a respite), the end result may be chronic use of a habit-forming anxiolytic. The patient and PCP may then end up with two problems: continuing anxiety plus dependence on a medication. Actually, they may end up with three or four problems, because without a behavior therapy component the anxiety will likely continue, and the frustrated patient may become depressed or begin to self-medicate with substances.

Even patients with no significant behavioral problems suffer under the current state of affairs. There is, of course, limited time in a day and PCPs are being asked to see, more patients than ever. Thus, a lengthy visit with a patient with multiple behavioral issues means a provider may need to recapture time from subsequent patients' visits to stay on schedule. In addition to more lengthy visits, patients with psychosocial problems utilize medical services more frequently (Simon, Von Korff, & Barlow, 1995; Unutzer, et al., 1997), which makes accessing services harder for other patients. One study of "high-utilizers," i.e., patients who utilize medical services the most, found that about half had significant problems with depression and anxiety (Katon at al., 1990). Not surprisingly, several studies have suggested that a significant cost offset can occur in the health care system if recognition and treatment of behavioral problems are improved (see for example, Friedman, Sobel, Myers, Caudill, & Benson, 1995). The inference from all of these findings is that without sufficient care for behavioral problems we all are paying the price.

CALMING THE STORM: THE MOVE TO INTEGRATE BEHAVIORAL HEALTH AND PRIMARY CARE

What hopefully becomes clear from our previous discussion is that the present health care system victimizes many people. Patients with behavioral problems are not getting the care they deserve; PC teams are overwhelmed and underprepared for dealing with behavioral problems, and health care for the entire population is thus compromised. Fortunately, as health care professionals have begun to recognize these problems, new models of care have emerged that aim to alleviate them. These models all attempt to bring MH services into PC in some fashion, in an effort to break down barriers to MH care and reduce the strain on PCPs.

The approaches developed to merge PC and MH care vary widely. One way to categorize them is by the degree of "co-location," "collaboration," and "integration" they possess. These are the three components Strosahl (1998) explains are crucial to the success of a PCBH service. "Co-location" refers to the actual placement of the behavioral health service. Placing it inside a PC clinic is ideal, as this will facilitate communication between providers and ease referrals. Additionally, this tactic may reduce stigma by linking physical and MH care in a tangible, visible fashion. "Collaboration" refers to the quality of the relationship between PC and MH providers. A collaborative relationship includes frequent sharing of information, joint treatment planning, and a truly biopsychosocial approach to care. It is entirely possible, though not desirable, for co-location to occur without collaboration. Such is the case with services that are in close physical proximity to each other yet rarely communicate. The third component, "integration," occurs when the MH provider is considered a regular part of the health care team. In an integrated service, a visit with the MH provider is as routine a part of care as a visit with the nurse. Truly integrated services require no special paperwork or processes to see the MH provider. Instead, behavioral health services are incorporated seamlessly into care, and both patients and staff view the MH provider as just another member of the PC team. Integration is important because without it many barriers to behavioral care will persist. There are plenty of examples of MH providers who co-locate with PC and collaborate closely with PCPs, but do not actually integrate. In this "house shrink" arrangement, the MH provider usually utilizes traditional lengthy assessment and therapy strategies, and as a result becomes quickly overwhelmed by the demand (Strosahl, 1998). Additionally, patients often continue to resist referrals in this situation, because of the stigma of going for MH services.

The various models developed to bring behavioral health into PC all attempt to co-locate, collaborate, and/or integrate to one extent or another. An excellent and concise review of the models can be found in a recently published text written by Gatchel and Oordt (2003). In their book, they review five types of PC behavioral health services and note that the decision of which to use will depend on several issues such as budgetary priorities, skills, and preferences of medical and MH staff, logistical considerations (e.g., office space), and buy-in from organizational leadership. We believe the PCBH model makes the most sense for the majority of PC clinics, because it is the only model that offers a MH provider (the Behavioral Health Consultant or BHC) who is co-located, collaborative, and fully integrated. The PCBH model is particularly suited to federally qualified health centers, which have the greatest behavioral health needs. However, before detailing the PCBH model and our partiality to it, we briefly review the others.

First of the models described by Gatchel and Oordt (2003) is the *co-located clinics* model. This approach consists of a MH service run as a specialty service (comprehensive intakes, hour-long appointments) but co-located with PC. The two clinics might share some space or staff but are run as separate services. As discussed, co-location *might* improve collaboration between providers and ease referrals, but running MH as a specialty service means the usual problems with accessibility will continue. In addition, the lack of integration increases the likelihood of patient resistance to MH care. When accessibility is limited by these or other factors, the perceived and actual usefulness of the service diminishes. A *primary care provider* model is a bit more integrated. It similarly uses a traditional MH approach, but the MH provider works out of PC and is considered a PC staff member rather than a specialty provider. Partial integration is obtained by linking MH care with regular health care, but it is not completely integrated because the traditional MH visits still have a very different feel from a PC visit. Additionally, the lengthy visits will continue to limit the accessibility of the MH provider. In a *staff adviser* model, the MH provider acts solely as a consultant to the PCP, perhaps seeing patients with the PCP or advising a PCP via phone. Gatchel and Oordt note this works well for training PCPs, but limits the assistance the MH provider can provide. A *stepped-care approach* may also be used, in which some aspects of each of the discussed approaches are combined. Psychological care begins at the lowest intensity possible (e.g., simple consultation to the PCP) and graduates upward (ultimately to more frequent, hour-long visits) as needed. This approach has been called the Med-Plus model by Pruitt, Klapow, Epping-Jordan, and Dresselhaus (1998). The flexibility afforded by this model improves accessibility, and the components of co-location, collaboration, and at least partial integration all exist. A disadvantage is that even a few lengthy (e.g., 50-min) appointments in a day quickly begin to limit accessibility.

THE PRIMARY CARE BEHAVIORAL HEALTH MODEL

We favor the PCBH model because its design allows it to have the largest effect possible on the population and to provide maximal help to PC patients and providers. This model is widely used, having been implemented in over 100 community health centers across the USA and in PC clinics throughout the United States Air Force and Army. A number of Veterans Administration clinics and many private health care organizations such as Group Health Cooperative of Puget Sound and Kaiser Permanente also utilize the PCBH model. Our description of the model comes largely from the work of Strosahl (Strosahl, 1996a,b, 1997, 1998; Strosahl, Baker, Braddick, Stuart, & Handley, 1997).

In the PCBH model, the BHC provides service side by side with PCPs, ideally sharing an office with them and/or seeing patients in exam rooms (co-location). The BHC may see 10 to 15 patients a day, but follow-up is usually limited to 1 to 4 visits. The goal is simply to develop a well-rounded treatment plan that the PCP then follows, thus ensuring the patient receives comprehensive biopsychosocial care and the PCP learns more about behavior change strategies (collaboration). The BHC operates as a member of the PC team whose role is to help PCPs manage the psychosocial needs of their patients (integration). The PCP retains control of the patient's care (hence the consultant title), which may feel more comfortable to both provider and patient and may reduce resistance to seeing the BHC. Given the close working relationship between PCP and BHC in this model, truly holistic care is enabled.

A key ingredient to the success of a BHC service is the easy access it affords to behavioral health care. This allows the BHC to meet the high demand for services to patients with acute, chronic, and preventive needs. Typically patients are seen immediately after a PCP visit, when a problem is identified, which means the BHC must maintain a very flexible schedule and avoid obstacles to referrals. Visits are brief, typically lasting 15 to 30 minutes, which requires a very different approach from that seen in traditional specialty MH. Instead of focusing on diagnosis, assessments focus on functional assessment, and treatment plans are geared toward functional restoration rather than symptom elimination. Brief, problem-focused notes are kept in the medical record, and no additional paperwork is required to see the BHC. Psychoeducation plays an important role in BHC visits and less time is devoted to development of therapeutic rapport (this is possible largely because of the close collaboration between the BHC and PCP, which allows the BHC to inherit the rapport between PCP and patient).

Another important component of the BHC model is the ability of the BHC to help with a wider variety of problems than he or she would see in specialty MH. Although a BHC will frequently help with MH problems such as depression and anxiety, a goal is to also see medical problems such as diabetes, chronic pain, headaches, obesity, hypertension, etc. The BHC may also assist with subthreshold problems, such as thumbsucking in a child or calming a patient who is overly anxious during a minor surgical procedure. A wealth of opportunity exists for BHCs to help with prevention efforts as well, especially secondary prevention activities such as smoking cessation, weight management, and stress management education. With the abundance of chronic diseases seen in PC, a BHC can also be readily incorporated into the routine care of these conditions. Algorithms can be developed that routinely and automatically include the BHC in the care of a given condition, rather than waiting for a PCP to refer a patient.

The consultant aspect of the BHC model denotes a significant difference between the services of a BHC compared to a specialty MH provider. As noted previously, the goal of a patient encounter in the BHC model is to develop a well-rounded treatment plan that the PCP can then follow. Thus, a BHC must learn to make clear, specific, evidence-based recommendations after seeing a patient. Feedback to the PCP regarding the plan can be accomplished either in person or via the chart note, but must occur promptly. Of course, the PCP may or may not choose to follow the recommendations, but it is through this feedback process that many PCPs will gain knowledge of behavioral treatment strategies. (The BHC will also find discussions with PCPs helpful for learning about the biomedical aspects of problems.) To the extent that the BHC follows up with a patient, the goal is primarily to get the patient started on the treatment plan. Once the patient begins to progress and feels comfortable with the plan, the goal is to turn follow-up over to the PCP. Of course, the patient may be referred back to the BHC if progress stagnates or reverses, or if a new problem develops.

The emphasis in a BHC model is on population management, which again is quite different from specialty MH. However, this approach blends well with family medicine, which is also based on population management strategies. A BHC service is designed to improve overall population health through truly comprehensive health care and by decreasing the MH load on the PC system. In contrast, specialty MH is designed to focus on the individual needs of a given client, providing in-depth and often extensive care. Of course individual patient care is important in a BHC service as well, but questions such as, "What can I do to save the PCP some time?" or "What systemic changes might make our care for this condition more effective?" or "How can we capture more people with this condition?" are at least as common as, "How can this patient be cured?" A basic point is that the work of a BHC should not be confused with therapy, which is practiced differently and has different goals. A BHC is much more appropriately considered a PCP than a MH provider.

Although the intensity of the patient contact may seem less in the BHC model (in terms of shorter and fewer visits for a given problem), an advantage of the model is that the BHC may consult intermittently with patients over their lifespan. As new problems develop, patients return to see the BHC, just as they would with a PCP. Similarly, for chronic problems, visits may be less frequent than a therapist would be comfortable with, but contact with the patient may extend over years. Numerous opportunities exist with this model to encourage small lifestyle changes or coping practices over time. This is very different from specialty MH, where patients and providers generally only meet for the duration of an acute problem and rarely develop a lifespan relationship. If possible, patients needing intensive MH care may still be referred out to a traditional specialty MH clinic. However, even patients seen in MH often return eventually to PC for the same or a different problem.

We recognize that many of the concepts in the BHC approach we are suggesting will leave those new to the model with a host of questions. Hopefully, as we expand on these concepts and provide specific examples of how to conduct BHC work, any confusion will begin to dissipate. We find that most people new to this field grow to embrace the PCBH model as their understanding of it grows. This is especially true of PCPs and staff, who typically welcome a BHC service with arms wide open. In subsequent chapters, we cover all aspects of developing and operating a BHC service, including the administrative, interpersonal, and ethical challenges one might encounter. Given the burgeoning demand for integrated services in community health centers (DeLeon et al., 2003), and given that we both work in such facilities, our suggestions will be especially geared toward those settings. However, we believe anyone interested in the topic of primary care behavioral health will benefit from the points that follow.

SUMMARY

1. Most PC medical appointments stem from psychosocial concerns. Primary care is the de facto MH system, as it is the setting where most patients with behavioral conditions seek care.
2. PCPs lack time and training to address the large volume of patients who seek help for psychiatric conditions, psychosocial problems, unhealthy lifestyles, and difficulties making needed changes to cope with chronic diseases.
3. While PCPs may refer to MH, specialty resources are increasingly scarce, and patients have difficulties accessing them. PCPs often respond by offering prescriptions, which seem like an adequate treatment but often are not and may actually create new problems for some patients.
4. The introduction of SSRIs resulted in an increase in the use of antidepressant medications for patients with behavioral problems, and the increased cost of such may have resulted in further financial insults to the collapsing MH system.
5. PCPs report job dissatisfaction, and recruitment is difficult, particularly to community health centers and to rural areas.
6. To address these problems, models have been developed for moving behavioral health services into primary care. The models vary with respect to the qualities of co-location, collaboration, and integration.
7. This book is about the Primary Care Behavioral Health (PCBH) model, which involves delivery of services by a new member on the PC team, the Behavioral Health Consultant (BHC). The PCBH model differs in many respects from traditional MH care and, by design, changes the delivery of PC services.

2

A PRIMER ON PRIMARY CARE

"Planning is as natural to the process of success as its absence is to the process of failure."

—Robin Sieger

Both of us trained and worked in traditional MH settings prior to entering primary care, and we felt comfortable there. We knew the lay of the land. Our offices were typically arranged in a long hallway, which was quiet most of the time, and sometimes doors even closed automatically. Rarely did unplanned visitors come into the immediate work area. When looking to socialize, we phoned or e-mailed a colleague, or went to the staff room to read, or have a beverage. If we didn't explicitly make this type of effort, the day could easily be spent in relative isolation in our office (which seemed quite nice because of the soft lighting and personal touches we had made to it!). Staff meetings were usually weekly and often involved case presentations. Therapy sessions were often intense, though they involved many of the same problems each day because we specialized in our areas of expertise. Patients with problems outside of those areas were usually referred to a trusted colleague. Workdays were enjoyable and at times challenging, but always much like the day before. When prompted by reception, we plucked patients one by one (or by groups of six or seven for a therapy group) from a waiting room, which usually was quiet and not very full. When patients didn't show, the time was used to catch-up on paperwork or read journals. The mission was clear: Diagnose accurately; write thoughtful and comprehensive reports; and treat, effectively, one client at a time.

Upon entering primary care, almost everything changed. The waiting rooms were huge and filled with people, and most of the little people were crying. Everyone called them patients, rather than clients. Staff consisted of nurses and nursing assistants, ward clerks, and other workers whose jobs we understood poorly. The workflow was quite confusing, with patients being whisked here and there by these staff persons, and we felt frankly uncertain about how to enter into it. The mission seemed quite different, and we strove to understand it while developing our own unique service. It was enough to make one's head spin, and as we tried to make sense of this novel work setting the noise level seemed to always undermine the creative process. However, with perseverance we discovered that we could become desensitized to children screaming and staff knocking on our door, and could even work effectively within the environment. We learned to work as part of a team, who welcomed us wholeheartedly, and began to enjoy the incredible variety of problems encountered. It was a rocky transition at times, but we actually began to enjoy this new environment as much as we had enjoyed our previous one. This experience is not unique to us but rather summarizes the experience most people have when they transition from specialty MH to the new world of PC. In this chapter, we hope to help the new BHC understand this new world a bit before entering it, by introducing the players involved and the unique PC mission.

THE PRIMARY CARE MISSION

The mission of primary care is to provide high-quality medical care to the ill and to prevent illness among the well. The Institute of Medicine (1996) proposed the following definition of primary care:

"Primary Care is the provision of integrated, accessible health care services by clinicians who are accountable for addressing a large majority of personal health care needs, developing a sustained partnership with patients and practicing in the context of family and community."

This comprehensive definition suggests that primary care is the foundation for health care delivery and emphasizes the critical role of a strong

PCP–patient relationship. In many communities throughout the USA, primary care is the patient's first point of entry into the health care system and the continuing focal point for all needed health care services. The vast majority of patient concerns and needs are addressed in primary care practices. Primary care is philosophically dedicated to the biopsychosocial model, meaning patient needs may be physical, mental, emotional, or social. Patients also may receive a gamut of services, including health promotion, disease prevention, health maintenance, counseling, patient education, and diagnosis and treatment of acute and chronic illnesses. Practice settings vary and can consist of a solo practice office, clinic, inpatient, critical care, long-term care, home care, day care, or school-based setting.

PROVIDERS AND MANAGEMENT IN PRIMARY CARE

Primary care physicians provide care to the undifferentiated patient from the time of the initial request. They form a strong personal relationship with the patient, and aim to continue responsibility for patient care as long as the patient continues to live in the community. They do not do so in isolation, however. A host of primary and auxiliary staff services exist to support them. After first providing an explanation of the different types of PCPs, we explain the roles of the most commonly encountered staff persons. Bear in mind, however, that all clinics are a bit different and might not have all of the staff positions described in this chapter.

Physician Providers

Primary care physicians are generalists, who share a commitment to improving the health of all members of a community. They have training in one or more primary care specialties, including family medicine, general internal medicine, and general pediatrics. Physician, as a term, applies to doctors of medicine (M.D.) and osteopathy (D.O.). *The Institute of Medicine 1996 Report on Primary Care* (Institute of Medicine of the National Academies, 1996) suggests specific competencies for PCPs, including periodic assessment of asymptomatic patients, screening and early detection of disease, evaluation and management of acute illness, evaluation and management or referral of patients with more complex problems, ongoing management of patients with chronic disease, coordination of care among specialists, and provision of acute hospital and long-term care services.

PCPs vary in practice styles, interests, and specialization areas. Older primary care physicians tend to have older patients, while younger doctors may tend to attract younger patients (Robinson et al., 1995). Provider panels vary in composition and size, and often reflect provider interest and skill areas. Some providers deliver babies and provide care for numerous young families, while others provide care to mostly older patients with multiple medical problems. Some providers enjoy treating patients with psychiatric disorders, while others have little interest in this area. Primary care clinics also vary significantly in accordance with their organizational structure, with most emphasizing team-based management (Taplin, Galvin, Payne, Coole, & Wagner, 1998) and others leaning toward a solo practitioner model. At this point, BHCs are most likely to work in clinics that employ multiple providers, and it is important that they learn about each provider's unique skills and interests as well as areas the PCPs are less comfortable with.

Nonphysician Providers

Nonphysician PCPs are generally either nurse practitioners or physician assistants. Their training is typically eighteen to twenty-four months of graduate work (i.e., after a bachelor's degree), and most nurse practitioners have a master's degree in advanced practice nursing. Their mission is often to support the work of physician providers by acting as an extension of them (hence the title "physician extender"). Their work, for example, might be to respond to the urgent care needs of patients in a specific physician panel or to see patients with common and less serious problems. However, in many clinic settings these providers have their own patient panels. Nurse practitioners and physician assistants do prescribe medicine, but are limited in the medicines and procedures they can utilize. Some clinics also have naturopathic physicians (ND), who function autonomously and have their own patient panels. Schooling for a ND consists of four years of graduate work, the first two of which are very similar to the first two years of medical school in terms of content. Naturopaths have a more narrow scope of practice than MDs and do not prescribe synthetic medicine.

In this book, the term "PCP" includes physicians as well as nurse practitioners, physician assistants, naturopathic physicians, and providers with similar credentials but slightly different professional titles. In other words, it includes those who independently make decisions about all aspects of patient care. In this definition, nutritionists, BHCs, acupuncturists, and some others may be "providers" but not "PCPs," because they do not govern all aspects of care.

Registered Nurses and Nursing Staff

Registered nurses (RN) provide invaluable team-building services in primary care. Possessing a bachelor's or an associate's degree, they often organize delivery of services from licensed practical nurses (LPN), medical assistants (MA), and certified nursing assistants (CNA). These other three members of the nursing staff have a high school degree plus specialized coursework (LPNs have the most and CNAs the least training). Together, this team of nursing staff members moves patients along from the beginning of a visit to the end. They often have a finger on the pulse of the clinic and will know where to find a PCP or a patient at any given time. A ward clerk is also a position in some clinics. These individuals answer the phone, triage calls, create schedules, and make appointments.

In many clinics, a RN is also responsible for triaging patients who desire same-day appointments, which might be done over the phone or in person. Diabetes education, some aspects of preventive education during well-child exams, and smoking cessation are all areas that might also be handled by a RN. Because the BHC can do some of this as well, talking with the RN to coordinate delivery of these services is important.

Clinic Administrators

Responsibility for all aspects of clinic operations rests with the clinic manager/director. These responsibilities include overseeing the budget, purchasing supplies, managing the property, and a great deal of personnel work. The manager usually supervises reception staff, billing staff, and maintenance personnel at a minimum. The manager also works closely with the clinic medical director (usually a MD) and the director of nursing (usually a RN). In some clinics, this tripartite meets with a "building committee" that considers all issues related to delivery of services.

Members of the building committee are usually elected by the department or area they represent (e.g., laboratory, imaging, billing, etc.).

The clinic medical director supervises the providers in the clinic and thus will usually supervise the BHC. He or she has a variety of responsibilities, ranging from provider recruitment, staffing and scheduling, to changing the clinic's model of care delivery. Efforts at introducing electronic medical records, transitioning to a different appointment scheduling design, or starting a new BHC service will all see heavy involvement from the medical director. The importance of having a medical director committed to innovation and quality cannot be overstated.

Small clinics may only have one nurse, but larger clinics or those that are part of a larger organization often have more, including a director of nursing. The director supervises charge nurses (i.e., those RNs in charge of a particular department, such as internal medicine) throughout the clinic, and each charge nurse supervises the nursing assistants (LPN, MA, CNA) in his or her area.

The Organization and Hierarchy of Primary Care

PCPs have "panels" of patients under their care. The panel is a basic element of clinic organization, as the goal is always to establish an ongoing patient–PCP relationship. Usually panels number from 1,500 to 3,000, and they are often adjusted to account for the types of problems seen by the provider. A provider who sees mostly older patients with complex problems will have fewer actual patients under his or her care than one with a less complex panel. Panels will sometimes be closed to new patients if a provider reaches maximum capacity. Providers cover for each other when on vacation, sick leave, etc., meaning they see patients from the absent provider's panel.

Another basic, if less formal, organizational characteristic of primary care clinics is the hierarchy. Medicine is steeped in hierarchy, sometimes in obvious ways as in the length of one's white lab coat. At other times, though, the hierarchy is felt but not expressed. As a newcomer to primary care, the BHC will likely feel a bit out of place and might not be sure where he or she fits in the hierarchy. Staff can be confused as well. If the BHC has a PhD, and is thus referred to as "Dr.," the matter gets even more confusing. Most BHCs will simply have to live with the reality that in the hierarchy of primary care they will not be on the same level as physician providers. This does not mean, however, that they will not be accepted or cannot be leaders in the clinic. Hopefully, as one uses the concepts presented in this book to achieve true integration, the hierarchy and barriers will become less and less important.

SUPPORT STAFF IN PRIMARY CARE

Some support staff positions (e.g., front desk staff) are similar in both primary care and specialty mental health, while others (e.g., ward clerks) are unique to primary care. Becoming familiar with these positions, and the people in them, is crucial to the success of a BHC service. We strongly recommend that a new BHC spend some time talking with key support staff about their role(s) in the clinic and how they can support, or be supported by, a BHC service.

Front Desk Staff Members

These are the first and last people to see most patients. When a patient enters the clinic for any provider, the front desk clerk obtains all necessary information and generates documentation for the visit. If electronic medical records are in use, he or she enters information on a computer showing that the patient has arrived. Whether communicated electronically or in some other way, the front desk clerk makes sure the nursing assistant knows when the patient is ready to be called back. When the front desk is short on staff, patients wait in lines and nursing assistants may not know in a timely manner that their provider's patients are in the clinic. At the end of a visit, patients are usually directed again to the front desk staff to turn in a billing slip and pay.

In many clinics, the front desk will be the ones to enter a BHC's same-day patients into the schedule. These are patients who were not scheduled with the BHC but who were referred for a same-day appointment during their PCP visit. Either the BHC or his or her assistant will need to notify the front desk of the same-day appointment, so that the appropriate documentation gets produced. Front desk staff members have a difficult job and may benefit from the assistance of the BHC. They are often the ones who check the insurance status of patients, tell the late-arriving patient that he or she cannot be seen, and keep a multitude of patient charts organized. Patients often express frustration to them and might view them as an annoying obstacle to care. At the end of a visit, when patients are eager to get home, they often must return to the front desk to pay. The BHC can cultivate relationships with front desk staff by suggesting strategies for handling angry patients, offering stress reduction workshops at lunch, and perhaps bringing them snacks during holiday times. Simply acknowledging the challenges of their job can go a long way.

Ward Clerks

Ward clerks are expert multitaskers who also have difficult jobs. They usually sit in the nursing station area wearing a headset and working at a computer while on the phone with patients. At the same time, they usually have a patient at the window with a request or concern and a nursing assistant at their side trying to tell them something. Be mindful of this when interacting with them. In some clinics, ward clerks create provider schedules and make changes to them, meaning they may be the ones to go to when scheduling same-day patients.

Nursing Assistants and Medical Assistants

Nursing assistants and medical assistants bring patients into exam rooms and complete various pre-visit activities with them. They take vitals, clarify the reason for the visit, get a list of current medications, and may ask screening questions about smoking or other problems. These team members are often the ones who will administer self-report measures, such as a depression measure, prior to the PCP visit. As such, they may need training from the BHC on how to administer and score measures the BHC introduces to the clinic. They also, by virtue of being the first clinical contact with the patient, might learn of patient concerns that could lead to a BHC referral. If empowered to bring such issues to the attention of the PCP or the BHC, they may generate referrals that otherwise would not materialize.

At the end of the patient–PCP encounter, the CNA may escort the patient to the next stop, such as the laboratory or the front desk. They also give patients information about resources, patient education pamphlets, etc., as directed by the PCP. For this reason, the BHC should ensure they have access to handouts on behavioral topics and keep them informed about relevant community resources. In this book, we use the term "certified nursing assistant" (CNA) consistently, but recognize that medical assistants may perform similar or even more responsibilities, consistent with their more extensive training.

Interpreters

Clinics vary in the way they address the issues related to interpreting. A private practice might have a less frequent need for interpreters and so might not have a strong system in place for this. Federally qualified health centers, which see a disproportionately high amount of non-English speakers, are required as a condition of their funding to provide interpreter services. In Hawaii, where patients speak any of ten or fifteen different languages, clinics tend to have multiple interpreters on staff. Clinics where many patients speak the same non-English language (usually Spanish in the USA) often try to hire staff who are fluent in that language. Interpreters from outside agencies are usually scheduled by the clinic to come to visits for patients speaking a less common language. In Chapter 4, we provide detailed guidance for working effectively with interpreters in BHC visits.

SUMMARY

1. The mission of primary care is to provide the majority of health care services to a group of citizens. These services include both intervention and prevention services and are by definition holistic.
2. Sustained and collaborative patient–PCP relationships form the basis for pursuing the primary care mission. Services are accessible, continuous, and team based.
3. There are various types of PCPs and a host of staff members to support their practice. As the PCBH model is new to primary care, BHCs will need to educate them about the service. Talking with each PCP and staff person about how to best promote collaboration and integration is a crucial part of starting a BHC service.

PART II

YOUR MISSION, SHOULD YOU CHOOSE TO ACCEPT IT

Soon after arriving in primary care one realizes how radically different the BHC job is going to be. Most will feel a bit overwhelmed in the beginning and wonder what they've gotten themselves into! However, by developing a solid sense of the PCBH mission, the requisite skills to learn or use, and some basic organizational concepts, the job will gradually seem less daunting. This part of the book aims to provide that information. We encourage you to use this section to create an operational manual for the new BHC service; one that defines basic policies and procedures. Creation of a manual can provide the sense of foundation so important to a new service, and helps one to gain a much clearer picture of the work that lies ahead.

3

A MISSION AND A JOB DESCRIPTION

"Make your work to be in keeping with your purpose."
—Leonardo Da Vinci

The mission of PCBH, in the broadest sense, is to improve the overall health of the population. This lofty goal is pursued in two ways: (1) by augmenting the usual preventive and direct care for behaviorally based problems; (2) through educational and systemic change efforts that improve the PC system's ability to provide such care. To the extent this mission is accomplished, PCPs and the system will be freed to attend better to the needs of the entire population.

Consider the example of a child referred for acting-out problems with his parents. The most immediate concern will be to help him or her (and his or her parents) with the presenting problem. At another level, however, one should also be thinking of ways the PC system might better discover or assist other children and their families with similar needs. Perhaps a new routine screening procedure could be implemented to detect child behavior problems better or different parenting information could be offered during well-child checks. Also important is to consider what about the individual visit could be used to enhance future care delivered by the PCP for similar problems. Could the PCP be taught how to deliver the relaxation procedure that was taught to the patient? Or, perhaps the PCP could benefit from learning the finer points of teaching Time-Out to parents. To achieve the PCBH mission, one needs to become adept at influencing not only patients, but also PCP colleagues and the system in general.

Fulfilling the mission of the PCBH model often requires a radical change in one's overall perspective and practice habits. To help guide this transition, this chapter provides a description of the core competencies involved in meeting the PCBH mission. These cover the domains of clinical practice, practice management, consultation, documentation, team performance, and administrative skills. These competencies can also be used to write a job description, which will often not be in place for a new BHC but can provide an important sense of grounding. In the hopes that the BHC service will expand over time, the chapter also provides suggestions for recruiting and interviewing BHCs. Lastly, given the concerns many new BHCs have about supervision and mentoring, we provide ideas for obtaining this as well as training and peer support.

THE CORE COMPETENCIES

Working in the PCBH model involves learning some new skills while applying some old skills in new ways. Each of the six domains described in this section contains distinct skills to master, which are summarized in the below table titled the "Behavioral Health Consultant Core Competencies Tool" (Strosahl & Robinson, unpublished) (Figure 3.1). These skills can also be reviewed in more detail in other sources (e.g., Strosahl, 2005).

Domain 1: Clinical Practice

The Clinical Practice domain is the largest of all six domains and requires a thoughtful review. The differences between clinical skills practiced in specialty MH versus in the PCBH model are obvious in some cases and subtle in others.

Apply principles of Population-Based Care. Learning the principles of population-based care is an important initial task for a new BHC. These principles underlie much of the rationale for the PCBH model but are often a new concept for providers trained in specialty MH. Traditional MH training is based on a case model that has different goals than a population

Behavioral Health Consultant Core Competencies Tool[*]

Use a rating scale of 1 = low skills and 5 = high skills to assess the BHC's (your) current level of skill development for all attributes within each of the following six domains. Place a checkmark in the column corresponding to the skill rating that best describes the BHC's (your) current skill level.

Domain	Attributes	Skill rating (1 = Low; 5 = High)				
		1	2	3	4	5
I. Clinical practice skills	1 Applies principles of population-based care					
	2 Defines role accurately					
	3 Identifies problem rapidly					
	4 Uses appropriate assessments					
	5 Limits problem definition					
	6 Focuses on functional outcomes					
	7 Uses self-management/home-based practice					

Figure 3.1. The Behavioral Health Consultant Core Competencies Tool.

Domain	Attributes	Skill rating (1 = Low; 5 = High)				
		1	2	3	4	5
	8 Interventions are simple, concrete and supportable by primary care team members					
	9 Shows understanding of relationship of medical and psychological systems					
	10 Shows basic knowledge of medicines					
	11 Shows knowledge of best practice guidelines					
	12 Provides primary care lifestyle groups or classes					
II. Practice management skills	1 Uses brief sessions efficiently					
	2 Stays on time when conducting consecutive appointments					

Figure 3.1.—*Cont'd*

Domain	Skill area	Skill rating (1 = Low; 5 = High)				
		1	2	3	4	5
	3 Completes treatment episode in 4 sessions or less					
	4 Uses inter-mittent visit strategy					
	5 Uses flexible patient contact strategies					
	6 Appropriately triages to mental health and chemical dependency					
	7 Uses primary care behavioral health case management strategies					
	8 Uses community resources appropriately					
III. Consultation skills	1 Focuses on and responds to referral question					

Figure 3.1.—*Cont'd*

Domain	Skill area	Skill rating (1 = Low; 5 = High)				
		1	2	3	4	5
	2 Tailors recommendations to work pace of medical units					
	3 Conducts effective curbside consultations					
	4 Assertively follows up with physicians, when indicated					
	5 Focuses on recommendations that reduce physician visits and workload					
	6 Presents brief lunch hour presentations in primary care					
IV. Documentation skills	1 Writes clear, concise chart notes					

Figure 3.1.—*Cont'd*

Domain	Skill area	Skill rating (1 = Low; 5 = High)				
		1	2	3	4	5
	2 Gets chart notes and feedback to physicians on same day basis					
	3 Chart notes are consistent with curbside consultation results					
V. Team performance skills	1 Understands and operates comfortably within primary care culture					
	2 Shows awareness of team roles					
	3 Readily provides unscheduled services when needed					
	4 Is available for on-demand consultations by beeper or cell phone					

Figure 3.1.—*Cont'd*

Domain	Skill area	Skill rating (1 = Low; 5 = High)				
		1	2	3	4	5
VI. Administrative skills	1 Understands relevant policies and procedures					
	2 Understands and applies risk management protocols					
	3 Routinely completes all billing activities					

*Note: This tool can be used by a clinical supervisor as part of a training and evaluation process and/or by the BHC for self-evaluation.

Figure 3.1.—*Cont'd*

health model. The basic definition of population-based care is "various approaches to medical care for specific groups identified by common demographic characteristics, risk factors, or diseases" (Lipkin & Lybrand, 1982). The population-based care model helps the health care system achieve basic preventive care, accessibility to acute care, and effective chronic disease management. Interventions based on this model might, for example, deploy new screening procedures to better identify members of a population with a certain problem (so treatment can be provided); or might attempt to better disseminate educational information (e.g., the risks of smoking) to a population, in hopes of lowering the incidence of a related chronic medical condition (e.g., lung cancer). Chronic disease management programs for high-impact problems such as diabetes or chronic pain or depression might also be population-based interventions.

An important goal of population-based care is to make a limited number of services available to many members of the population rather than providing intensive services to a selected few members. Intensive specialty interventions offer significant help to certain individuals, but the downside is that the majority of individuals needing help in the population go unidentified and/or underserved. These individuals, in turn, increase the health burden on the population and use up valuable healthcare resources. Population-based approaches thus attempt to reach more members of the population, if in a more limited manner, in hopes that small improvements in many may lift the overall health of the population. In a very fundamental way the approach is about resource utilization; i.e., finding ways for limited healthcare resources to reach as much of the population as possible.

The BHC should always be looking for opportunities to improve population health in the primary care setting. Following the seven steps below may help guide the process of developing new programs to achieve this:

1. Identify a condition that has a high impact on primary care practice
2. Form a committee of motivated PCPs and staff members to address the condition
3. Design a method for identifying members of the population that have the targeted condition
4. Select one or more measurable outcomes of evidence-based medical and/or BH practices for that condition
5. Assess outcomes of current practices
6. Design a new intervention that is feasible and represents a better value
7. Monitor outcomes and make changes as needed

Population-based care methods may improve health outcomes for numerous primary care patient groups, and prevention is often an objective. For example, Rabin (1998) developed a primary care-based intervention to help prevent sexual transmission of the Human Immunodeficiency Virus (HIV). (Sexual activity is the major source of HIV infections in the United States.) The intervention was manual based and included a train-the-trainers dissemination plan aimed at getting PCPs to conduct better risk assessment and risk reduction counseling regarding sexual transmission of HIV. The program did improve rates of PCP assessment and counseling, which in turn has been shown to make a difference for the large group of patients at risk.

Many other examples of population-based programs are available and, in most cases, the goal is improved risk-identification and behavioral counseling. Programs of this sort can often be incorporated into a "clinical pathway," which provides specific instructions to providers concerning a specific target population. We discuss clinical pathways and provide additional examples in Chapter 12. For now, readers should simply consider that BHCs need to trade-in the case model hat for a population-based care hat, and this requires on going attention during the first few years of practice. Clearly, the BHC will spend a good deal of time seeing individual patients in consultation, but much time should also be spent creating and implementing meaningful population-based initiatives. Robinson (2005a,b) offers a template to use in designing population-based care programs for common problems in primary care. A recent book, *Integrative Behavioral Health Care: Tools for Success in Primary Care* (Hayes, Fischer, & O'Donohue, 2002), and a concise summary of population care at the American Medical Association's website (www.ama-assn.org/ama/pub/category/6972.html) will also help the new BHC with this endeavor.

Define Your Role Accurately. Writing out and practicing a brief description of the BHC role helps one be ready to state it clearly to patients at the beginning of initial consultations. This description can also be conveyed to providers when talking with them about the BHC service. Chapter 7 provides specific wording that can be used, but for now simply keep in mind the importance of the introduction. Patients who have sought traditional counseling services in the past might need some extra explanation of the differences between a BHC visit and a counseling visit.

Identify Problems Rapidly. Initial consultations include about five to ten minutes for obtaining a social history and identifying health risk behaviors, followed by a focus on the identified problem. This means one needs to learn to hone in on the problem of concern quickly. Often the specific reason for referral will be clear, which helps immensely with problem identification (though sometimes the focus changes as the visit progresses). Other times patients are brought for a same-day referral by the nursing assistant at the request of the PCP, in which case the referral issue might not be known. The patient may know what the referral is about, but sometimes a quick trip down the hall to check with the referring provider is useful. In order to stay on time, the BHC needs to identify one or at the most two problems quickly and stay with them throughout the visit. If other problems come up that are significant, they can be noted in the Plan section of the chart note (e.g., "I recommend that Dr. Jones talk with patient about the risks and benefits of continuing to smoke, as patient is considering a change in this behavior in the next six months.")

Use Appropriate Assessments. Lengthy diagnostic or personality assessments are not appropriate for the primary care setting and are not a part of the PCBH model. However, brief self-report measures are often used, and the BHC should have some knowledge of those most appropriate for primary care. As a rule, measures should be directly pertinent to a referral issue or to the mission of the service and should require five minutes or less for administration, scoring, and feedback to the patient. If possible, the BHC or BHC assistant should ask assessment questions rather than passing out questionnaires, as this often improves accuracy and administration time. In Chapter 6, we review assessment tools appropriate for BHC visits, including quality of life and problem-specific measures. The number of measures used is best kept to a select few, so that PCPs might also learn to use them.

Limit Problem Definition. One of the more difficult transitions for MH providers coming from specialty MH settings is that of limiting exploration of problems. Many, if not most, of the patients seen in primary care have multiple complex, often chronic problems. The BHC's job, however, is to focus on the problem mentioned in the referral and to develop a strong intervention concerning it. Sometimes a complaint comes up that cannot be ignored (such as a statement of high suicide risk), but most of the information that will tempt diversion should simply be noted and left for a future visit.

Focus on Functional Outcomes. In PCBH work, the emphasis is on improving patient functioning, rather than eliminating symptoms. Rather than producing a diagnosis and administering a diagnosis-specific treatment protocol, BHC interventions are geared toward targeted interventions for improving behavior. If, for example, a patient complains that anxiety interferes with her or his ability to find work, a BHC may suggest any one of several generic anxiety management techniques to help with this problem, depending on the results of the functional analysis. The functional analysis process is discussed in more detail in Chapter 7, and is a powerful methodology for producing focused and effective interventions. Using a health-related quality of life scale that provides function scores for patient assessment (rather than diagnosis-based symptom checklists) can also help the BHC, the patient, and the referring provider maintain a focus on functioning.

Recommend Self-Management and Home-Based Practice. The PCBH model is a patient-empowerment model in which patients are taught skills briefly in consultations and asked to practice them at home. Thus, the BHC needs to be able to explain these skills and recommendations well enough in chart notes for the referring PCP to understand them. The hope is that he or she will reinforce the plan in subsequent visits. Helping the patient identify people who may support home practice, such as family members or friends, can also improve compliance with the plan.

Use Interventions that are Simple, Concrete, and Supportable. Primary care is not an appropriate place for subtle, complex interventions. Instead, one's work should be transparent, so that PCPs can learn what a BHC does and try it with their patients. Examples of interventions include collaborative goal setting for lifestyle change, teaching relaxation techniques, teaching and role-playing assertive communication, and developing reward plans for children, among others. Knowing how to do a functional analysis is fundamental to a BHC intervention, and we explain and demonstrate this in subsequent chapters. Though conducting this is not simple and requires training, the result should be an intervention that is clear and straight-forward. Over time, through written and oral communications and educational presentations, a number of PCPs will learn to use common behavioral interventions.

Explain the Relationship Between Medical and Psychological Systems. Helping patients understand how stress can influence health is often an important part of a BHC intervention. The stress-diathesis model is helpful for this, and should be something the BHC understands well. Most simply, this model states that stress is a normal and even helpful part of life, as long as the level of stress is in line with a person's skills for coping with it. When there is an imbalance and stress exceeds one's coping abilities, the person experiences physical and psychological problems and diminished quality of life.

Stress often plays a major role in illness and disease, and becoming informed about specific connections is an important core competency for a BHC. For example, understanding how stress might affect pain intensity for patients with chronic pain is a basic prerequisite for working with such patients.

Show Basic Knowledge of Medicines. Medication is perhaps the most common treatment in the primary care setting, and one of the most common areas for which BHCs need to seek additional training. Basic knowledge of the medications used in treating emotional and psychological disorders, as well as common side effects, is crucial. Additionally, at least a cursory knowledge of the most commonly used medications for other problems, and their potential psychological side effects, is helpful. Familiarity with prescription drugs with abuse potential is also important, and this is covered in depth in Chapter 13 of this book. Lastly, one should have some awareness of the herbs and nutritional supplements that are currently advocated for relief of mental and emotional problems. A highly useful resource for all medications is the *PDR Drug Guide for Mental Health Professionals, First Edition* (Siften, 2002).

Show Knowledge of Best Practice Guidelines. In recent years, more and more information is available to guide best practice in the area of PCBH, and keeping abreast of these developments is important. A good summary of them is in *Behavioral Integrative Care: Treatments that Work in the Primary Care Setting* (O'Donohoe, 2005). Springer Publishing may also soon start a journal for publication of articles related to PCBH practice. While awaiting a journal that is specific to PCBH, other helpful sources of information include the following journals: *Journal of Health Psychology, Annals of Behavioral Medicine, Journal of Consulting and Clinical Psychology, Cognitive and Behavioral Practice, Professional Psychology: Research and Practice,* and *The Behavior Therapist.* Though content in these journals is not always directly relevant to BHC work, much of it can be applied.

Keeping an eye on the journals that PCP colleagues read, and having some awareness of best practice guidelines they follow, is also important. There is a surprising amount of behavioral health research and practice information in primary care journals. Some of the best journals to monitor include *The Journal of Family Practice, The New England Journal of Medicine, JAMA,* the *Annals of Internal Medicine, Pediatrics,* and the *British Medical Journal.* One frustrating reality is that PCPs and BHCs tend to read on similar topics but from different sources. Being able to talk with PCP colleagues about an article in one of "their" journals helps the BHC overcome problems with language and conceptual differences and enhances understanding of the PCP perspective on problems.

Provide Primary Care Groups. Group services in primary care allow the BHC to offer more extensive contact to a larger group of patients, and often assume a different form than groups in specialty MH. Experience with running groups in specialty MH may be useful, but it is not a sufficient preparation for running them in primary care. There are several strategies for achieving consistently strong patient participation in primary care groups, and these are discussed at length in Chapter 12. For purposes of this section, suffice it to say the ability to deliver groups in a primary care setting is an important BHC core competency.

Domain 2: Practice Management Skills

This area of competence concerns time and resource management skills. Staying on time with brief visits and maintaining access for same-day visits is a crucial part of the PCBH model. The goal in the model is to meet with all referred patients immediately, even if it is just for five or ten minutes (but usually 20 to 40). Clearly, in some cases patients will be unable to stay or the BHC will be unavailable, but strong practice management skills should keep such problems to a minimum.

Use Brief Sessions Efficiently. Some BHC's use twenty-minute initial visits, others use forty minutes, and others fall somewhere in between. To complete work with a new patient in such limited time, the visit must be well spent. Whatever the allotted time, it should include charting and, if possible, in-person contact with the referring provider (so the allowed actual time with the patient will be less than the allotted visit time). We often write the time we start with a patient on our note sheet, so that we are able to track time and move along to various tasks as the consultation progresses. Detailed instructions for conducting both the initial and follow-up visits are provided in Chapters 4 and 7.

Stay on Time When Conducting Consecutive Appointments. This skill is complex, as some patients simply take longer than others. The trick is to speed up when possible, knowing that at times you may need to slow down. When follow-up patients are doing well, a visit might be concluded in ten or fifteen minutes. A straight-forward initial consultation may be possible in twenty minutes. Aiming to complete the most pertinent work rather than to fill the allotted time may help one to stay on time throughout the day. This is sometimes difficult for new BHCs who have been trained to use every minute in the fifty-minute hour, but in primary care if the goal of the visit has been accomplished, the visit can end. Observing how PCP colleagues manage a busy schedule can be quite instructive in this regard, as they are masters of using only the amount of time needed for a given problem!

Complete Treatment Episode in Four Sessions or Less. For most BHCs the modal number of patient contacts for any one referral will be one. However, a significant group of patients will probably return for two to four contacts. These patients might be working on a specific skill or simply desiring/needing more support. It is often helpful to tell patients that contacts are limited to four visits (though realistically a BHC may see a patient many times over the lifespan, as new problems develop or old ones recur).

Patients are usually accepting of a four-visit limit, particularly if told they may come for follow-up in three to six months to assess their success in maintaining skills learned. There is a very small group of patients with whom a BHC may have more than four contacts. These patients usually have severe and/or complex medical and psychological problems, and although they may see the BHC more often, the time allotted for visits may be decreased. We discuss details related to providing care beyond the usual one to four visits in more detail in Chapter 15.

Use an Intermittent Visit Strategy. With high-utilizing patients or those with significant needs, an intermittent visit strategy can help lessen the load on the PCP while maintaining or strengthening the patient's relationship with the clinic. In this scenario, the BHC "plays ping-pong" with the PCP, such that visits alternate between them. Very often the needs of these patients are more psychosocial than medical, which makes this a feasible strategy. If medical needs do arise during a BHC visit they often can be addressed in a quick collaboration with the PCP, thus helping the PCP avoid an unnecessary visit with the patient.

Use Flexible Contact Strategies. Direct patient care is but one of several strategies a BHC will use for teaching and supporting patients. Also important is to learn to deliver care via telephone calls, e-mails (with appropriate confidentiality safeguards in place), and letters. The BHC assistant (see Chapter 4) may help with delivery of some of these services. For example, BHC assistants may call depressed patients to assess success in implementing relapse prevention plans, or call patients implementing a behavior change goal set during a group visit. Alternative visit strategies are a good option for patients who have a poor track record of keeping follow-up appointments with PCPs or who have known challenges to transportation. They are also often used for patients working on less complicated issues such as quitting smoking or starting an exercise plan.

Triage to Mental Health and Chemical Dependency Programs. Many new BHCs feel confused about when to refer patients to specialty MH care. They often want to refer patients who seem to be more than the primary care setting can handle, and often the focus of the consult is on making that happen. Unfortunately, in today's resource-poor environment, triage of patients to specialty MH and chemical dependency programs can be difficult. Recent restrictions on the use of public funds may limit access even more to MH and substance abuse treatment, and some patients currently in treatment may be forced to drop out. For patients who are not eligible for specialty care, the only recourse is the primary care venue. Primary care clinics serving a more affluent, insured patient population may have more options than, say, community health centers, but even in such a scenario simply referring a patient to MH does not mean he or she will go (or continue to go beyond an initial appointment). For these reasons, referral to a specialty MH service is best regarded as an "add-on" to the BHC intervention. In other words, the BHC should plan on providing an intervention to all referred patients, even if part of the treatment plan involves referring the patient to specialty care.

Despite problems with patients accessing specialty care, a BHC should also strive to develop relationships with local MH and chemical dependency program leaders and learn about their services. Clearly some patients will benefit from referrals. Maintaining a basic awareness of the care limitations of common third-party payers, such as Medicaid and Medicare, is also important.

Use Primary Care Behavioral Health Case Management Strategies. In the PCBH model, traditional case management is not conducted. That is, the BHC does not assume ownership of patients and follow them on an ongoing basis for help with social needs. However, case management in the sense of connecting patients with social services when needed is frequently done. Quite often (especially in community health centers) a BHC will refer patients to agencies who can assist with various needs, including food, housing, child care, domestic violence support services, etc. A BHC assistant can also provide case management services. Case management can be an important task, particularly for the growing number of seriously mentally ill patients who can no longer access care in the community MH system.

Use Community Resources. Related to case management, keeping up to date on community resources is an important activity. Every BHC should maintain a list that is checked regularly, given that offerings change frequently. If available, a BHC assistant can do much of the updating. The BHC is also responsible for letting PCPs know about community resources that they might refer patients to. A brief list can be placed at the workstations of PCPs or possibly in exam rooms. Sometimes the leaders of community services will provide routine notification of offerings via mail, email, or phone if asked.

Domain 3: Consultation Skills

Consultation comprises skills in relating to PCP colleagues and conveying assessments and recommendations to them. It is a new set of skills for most BHCs, so competency in this area may be low initially. Monthly self-ratings on these skills can help promote and gauge growth.

Focus on and Respond to the Referral Question. Just as keeping a narrow and clear focus is important during patient visits, it also is important when giving feedback to PCPs. Feedback that wanders too far from the problem of concern will often fail to keep the attention of the PCP and is less likely to provide them with useful information. Limiting feedback to the referral question shows respect for the referring provider's concerns and makes the BHC job feasible.

Tailor Recommendations to the Work Pace of the Medical Unit. Most PCPs need to see over twenty patients daily to have an economically viable practice. As such, they appreciate recommendations that are clear and brief. Most PCPs will be interested in same-day verbal recommendations, while they still have a clear memory of the patient. However, PCPs will still need to rely on the chart note at the next contact, so the note should be consistent with the verbal recommendation and, whenever possible, use the same language that was used with the patient. A PCP can support a BHC's plan for behavior change or skill practice, but they should not be asked to review a patient's journal or other similarly lengthy material.

Conduct Effective Curbside Consultations. A curbside consultation is a brief discussion with a provider conducted spontaneously in a hall way, exam room, or provider's office. Such consultations may be initiated by the BHC or the PCP, and they usually last for less than five minutes. The content of the consultation may reference a specific patient or a specific care issue. For example, a PCP might ask how best to handle a specific patient who is refusing to take diabetes medications. Alternatively, the BHC might talk with a PCP who has a question about how, in general, to treat adult patients with ADHD.

Generally, PCPs will be easily pleased during consults because they are obviously feeling thwarted by the patient issue that led to their referral. However, there are numerous factors that can influence the effectiveness of a curbside consultation. These include the amount of time available, the possession of information needed to communicate well (e.g., hard copies of evidence-based guidelines), the clarity of the question being asked, and the relative value to patient care of the information being provided.

Be Willing to Assertively Follow-up with Physicians. Most of the time, consult recommendations can be provided to the referring PCP on a nonurgent basis, possibly even via a written chart note. However, there are times when interrupting a PCP who is in with a patient or contacting the on-call PCP will be necessary. An example is that of a child with a new diagnosis of ADHD who comes to the BHC after missing two follow-up appointments with the PCP. The child has not yet started a planned medication trial and is failing in school and getting into trouble for excessive talking and disturbing others. A case such as this would warrant interrupting the provider on-call to start the treatment while the patient is in the clinic. Other situations that may warrant interrupting a PCP are those involving urgent patient safety needs (e.g., an agitated patient who needs to restart medications) or important and urgent patient questions for the PCP (e.g., the patient can't remember if the PCP gave permission to increase the dosage of diabetes medicine). In some clinics the protocol for handling urgent patient needs is to contact the on-call PCP, but many PCPs prefer to be contacted personally if a question arises about one of their patients. In the early stages of a BH service the BHC should check his or her clinic's protocol for handling these situations.

Focus on Recommendations That Reduce Physician Visits and Workload.
A very important aspect of BHC work is to make the job of the PCP more
satisfying and feasible. Most PCPs have large patient panels and they struggle with patient access, so to the extent a BHC can reduce physician burden, the PCP's attention to population health issues can improve. There
are many ways to save physician visits and reduce their workload. For
example, facilitating a prescription for an antidepressant during a BHC
visit may save the patient a return trip to the clinic and save the PCP that
subsequent visit as well. Similarly, a BHC (instead of the PCP) might
follow-up with patients started on antidepressant medications to assess
treatment response and to further develop a behavioral intervention.
When a PCP desires to have personal follow-up in the near future with the
patient, the BHC may suggest that she or he see the patient on the same
day and just prior to the visit with the PCP. This allows the BHC to gather
information about treatment response and make the subsequent patient-
PCP visit shorter.

Taking/returning telephone calls from/to patients in distress, seeing
walk-in patients in emotional distress instead of or immediately preceding
the PCP, calling schools or MH providers to coordinate care plans, and
writing letters for patients are all additional ways the BHC might save PCP
time, though this is not an exhaustive list. One of us (PR) has begun classes
for chronic pain patients, during which a nurse provides patients with
monthly prescriptions that the PCP has written ahead of time. Patients
benefit from the class, while PCPs avoid having to see the patients monthly.

Prepare and Present Brief Presentations. Public speaking skills are helpful for a BHC to develop. This is an area that some prefer to avoid, especially in the new environment of primary care that may seem more
intimidating than the familiar environment of MH. However, occasional
presentations to PCPs during meeting times are an excellent way to adver-
tise the BHC service and increase understanding of what the BHC can
offer. Talks can initially be brief, and then gradually lengthen as one feels
more comfortable. The best topics are ones that PCPs have expressed
interest in, perhaps as a result of an informal survey. The lunch hour can
be a good time to schedule one of these, though more PCPs are likely to be
present at provider and staff meetings. Presentations should be kept short,
leaving time for discussion and application to a real-world case. If discussing clinical interventions, role-playing can be useful and fun, and is

best done with written scripts. The BHC can place handouts in the mailboxes of providers who did not attend, along with an offer to give them a brief overview of the presentation on an individual basis.

Domain 4: Documentation Skills

Chart notes from the BHC are part of the primary care medical record and should not be placed into separate MH or substance abuse sections. Remember one goal of a BHC service is to erase the line between physical and mental health and improve attention to the latter. Separating out sections of psychosocial information as somehow distinct from other types of healthcare information runs contrary to this goal. Plenty of sensitive psychosocial information exists in medical charts regardless of a BHC's input, so adding high quality information from a BH expert can only improve patient care.

Because charting is covered in detail in Chapter 7, this explanation of the Documentation competency domain is brief. The main points to consider are as follows. First, the format used by a BHC should be the same as the one used by PCPs in the clinic. (This will often be the SOAP format.) If charting by hand, chart legibly, but typing or dictating is the norm in many clinics. Notes should be brief and clear. We recommend that charting occur immediately after each patient visit, as delaying it usually results in a less concise and precise note. Curbside consultations, telephone calls, forms completed and letters written for patients should all be charted. Use of Electronic Medical Records (EMRs) is growing and improving the availability of charted information. This may be something a BHC has to learn to use upon starting in primary care.

Domain Five: Team Performance Skills

In traditional MH settings, providers often work in teams, such as the Brief Services team or the Child Services team, but teams in primary care may be organized differently. Review the description of the team players in primary care detailed in Chapter 2. In a small clinic, the team may be the entire staff, whereas in a larger clinic, the BHC may become a member of a department, such as the family practice department. If unclear, ask questions about your clinic's organization. Most important is to be a team player, not a "team of one," but for those coming from specialty MH this can entail learning some new skills.

Provide Unscheduled Services When Needed. In the primary care culture, providers tend to be available to each other and to offer help when needed. Perhaps this is because they are on the front line with limited access to specialists for back up. They often will see a patient for a colleague who is backed up, or make phone calls, or check labs for each other. The BHC will certainly at some point be asked to assist with a difficult situation or a crisis just as lunch hour begins or when preparing to head home at the end of the day. Part of being seen as a team member in primary care is saying "yes" when these situations come up (or, better yet, looking for situations where one can offer to help). The lunch "hour" is usually more of a lunch "ten minutes" or a lunch "as able" in primary care, and the clinic's closing time simply means it's time to work on charting or making phone calls. Demonstrating a willingness to work a bit harder or a bit longer or in ways not expected will go a long way toward helping a BHC be accepted onto the PC team.

Be Available for On-Demand Consultations by Beeper or Cell Phone. PCPs may see the BHC as more accessible and may refer more same-day patients if the BHC is available by beeper or cell phone (or possibly walkie-talkie). In large clinics, providers often do not have the time to walk down the hallway or to send a nursing assistant to find the BHC. The goal of a BHC service is to see as many on-demand consultations as possible, so the BHC needs to keep the phone or beeper on at all times and encourage PCPs to use it. If with a patient when a PCP calls or knocks at the door, the BHC can leave with a brief apology and step out of the room and into a private area to take the call. When talking with the PCP, obtain the identifying information for the patient being referred, listen for the referral question, and (if possible) go to the exam room so that the PCP can introduce the patient. If going to the exam room is not an option, the BHC can tell the PCP an approximate time that the patient will be seen, and formulate a plan as to where the patient will wait. When meeting with patients for the first time, the BHC may consider explaining that interruptions often occur during BHC visits. Most patients are accustomed to interrupted visits in primary care, but warning them and subsequently apologizing for interruptions are helpful nonetheless.

Domain Six: Administrative Skills

Understand Relevant Policies and Procedures. In this final domain of administrative skills the first area of import is familiarity with policies and procedures relevant to one's work as a BHC. Hopefully, readers will use the information in this chapter to develop a procedural manual that defines the BHC service well and provides a reference point when questions arise. Once developed, the manual can be revised as new opportunities arise and new services evolve. Including a statement about how revisions to the program manual will be made (e.g., by consensus of the BH team) may also come in handy. The manual should be given a thorough review annually.

Understand and Apply Risk Management Protocols. All primary care clinics have a risk management office or staff person who issues guidelines regarding management of risks. The BHC needs to be aware of these policies, especially as they pertain to his or her position. Policies involving management of aggressive patients or responding to psychiatric emergencies might even benefit from some tweaking by a BHC. We discuss these challenging circumstances in Chapter 13.

Routinely Complete all Billing Activities. While tedious at times, completing all activities related to billing on a daily basis is critical to the success of a service (for those services that bill). Diagnostic codes and procedures billed must match those in the chart notation and any billing problems (e.g., missing encounters) should be promptly addressed. Information on billing is presented in Chapter 4.

JOB DESCRIPTION

Creating a job description that includes the core competencies, as well as a policy for evaluating job performance, is an important part of launching a new BHC service. The title "Behavioral Health Consultant (BHC)" fits the position best, as it distinguishes this work from that of a therapist. However, some behavioral providers working in primary care use other titles, such as "Primary Care Psychologist" or "Primary Care Behaviorist." A basic job description is as follows:

"The Behavioral Health Consultant position requires an independent license to practice in a healthcare setting, such as a PhD in psychology, a MSW, or a Masters in counseling. The person in this position works as a primary care team member and delivers brief, consultation-based services to patients and PCPs using an integrated care model. This person adheres to the core competencies outlined in the PCBH program manual."

Doctoral-level providers typically have training in program development and evaluation, as well as in research, so they often lead the BHC service if the service includes more than one professional. The job description should include these responsibilities if this situation exists.

SUGGESTIONS FOR RECRUITING AND INTERVIEWING

For recruiting purposes the following description is recommended. It provides more detail to help the recruiting group attract the most viable candidates:

"*Behavioral Health Consultant*: Exciting new position as a primary care team member providing brief consultative visits to eight to fourteen patients per day and their primary care providers. Training and experience in evidence-based interventions and health psychology required. Must have a PhD in clinical or counseling psychology, a MSW, or a Masters in counseling, and be licensed or license-eligible in X state."

Hiring a BHC for the first time can be very challenging. Primary care administrators typically do not have a clear understanding of the mental health world or a clear idea of what to look for in a candidate. At the same time, most applicants probably will have little or no training or experience working in the PCBH model. There will likely be a deluge of applicants with a wide variety of backgrounds, which can all be very confusing to wade through. To complicate matters more, many applicants will have worked in medical settings in some fashion, yet lack the right background to fill a BHC position. The questions in Table 3.1 may help interview committees identify strong candidates, but we also recommend consulting with an experienced BHC—in another clinic or health care system if need be—regarding ideas for sorting the wheat from the chaff.

These are difficult questions and rare will be the candidate who provides impressive answers to all. The vast majority of candidates will have difficulty conceptualizing how to do abbreviated visits, will lack a clear

Table 3.1. Interview questions (and desired answers) for BHC position applicants

What are your thoughts about mental health care in general at the present time?
In the answer to this question, look for someone who sees problems with the
specialty model of care and wants to do something different (though might
have only a vague idea of what that would be). Candidates who say they want
to see more patients or extend services to a greater percentage of the population are on the right track. On the other hand, candidates who complain
about not getting reimbursed well or about restrictions from managed care
might not possess the vision that helps one succeed as a BHC.

Describe your ideal work situation, including the room and area of a building
where you would like to work and the types of patients you would ideally see.
MH providers are typically taught to maintain private, quiet offices, so don't
expect a candidate to suggest otherwise. However, the ideal candidate will say
he or she likes to be in the middle of the action and that variety is the spice of
life. Be skeptical of candidates who yearn for a narrow specialty practice or for
non-clinical activities (e.g., research or administration) or for a predictable
practice schedule. Also avoid candidates who would refuse to treat certain
problems. All providers have a comfort zone clinically, but those with the
widest zone and a willingness to expand it will work best.

If you only had 15 minutes to spend with a patient with marital problems who
is referred to you for insomnia, what would you do?
Most interviewees will express surprise and perhaps uncertainty when asked to
describe a 15-minute intervention, but nonetheless some answers are better
than others. Look for answers that stick to the problems at hand and that end
up with a reasonably clear self-management plan. A sound answer might suggest screening for common causes of insomnia, such as depression, but
should also include some sort of intervention that addresses the insomnia.
Suggesting a referral for counseling is an insufficient answer.

If you were asked to consult with a PCP about an 8 year-old child with attention
problems and behavior problems at school, what would you do?
Many mental health professionals have led a fairly specialized existence so those
who have worked primarily with adults might express unease when asked
about working with children. However, strong candidates will be open to
working with new populations and problems and will have at least a basic
idea of how to help. For example, the applicant might identify ways he or she
can help the PCP (e.g., contacting the child's teachers, recommending brief
standardized assessment tools, and meeting with parents), demonstrate an
awareness of diagnostic criteria for child behavior problems, and/or show
some familiarity with behavior modification techniques. A good follow-up
question could be to ask the applicant what he or she would say to a PCP who
believed the child had Attention Deficit Hyperactivity Disorder, Combined

Continued

Table 3.1.—*Cont'd*

Type. Again, look for answers that display an eagerness to help, a familiarity with basic behavior change techniques, and that ideally also recognize the time limitations in primary care. Simply suggesting a referral for counseling is again an insufficient answer.

If you were asked to consult with a PCP about an obese, adult patient with diabetes who is non-compliant with treatment, what would you do?

As with previous questions, many candidates will issue a disclaimer that obesity and diabetes have not been mainstays of their past work, yet they should show some basic familiarity with both and a willingness to engage with the patient. Ideal answers will mention approaches such as motivational interviewing or psychological acceptance of chronic disease, or may reference collaborative goal-setting approaches. Exploration of the patient's mood (e.g., to assess for depression) would also be a reasonable part of the plan. Detailed understanding of the medical aspects of obesity and diabetes should not be expected.

If the clinic manager came to you and asked you to be the lead for the clinic in developing a clinical pathway for chronic pain, what would you do?

Few candidates will be familiar with the term "clinical pathway," which means that one who is may be a strong candidate. If unfamiliar with the concept, a candidate should at least express an interest in learning about it. An impressive answer would include the importance of focusing on quality of life and functioning (in addition to pain intensity), and/or an awareness of the potential pitfalls of narcotic analgesics. Applicants who express an interest in or knowledge of novel interventions such as group visits will also likely be keepers. At a minimum, candidates should recognize chronic pain as something they can help with and be willing to work on issues at the systems level. Candidates who say they would not feel able to take on such a task should lose favor.

If the clinic manager came to you and asked you to be the lead for the clinic in developing a clinical pathway for substance abuse, what would you do?

Again, many applicants will be unfamiliar with the concept of a clinical pathway, but should at least be open to the idea once it has been explained to them. Listen for an awareness of the prevalence of substance abuse problems, a willingness to engage with them (even if lacking a strong experience base in the area), and some knowledge of empirically supported procedures for substance abuse. A promising applicant may suggest conducting motivational interviewing procedures, or at least show a familiarity with them in follow-up questioning. Very impressive would be ideas about how to get other staff involved in care, such as a mention of potential screening strategies or an interest in teaching providers and staff ways to intervene. Applicants who primarily focus on ways to refer patients out for specialized care may lack the creativity or flexibility desired in a BHC.

understanding of the primary care environment, and will have limited familiarity with some conditions commonly encountered in primary care. However, asking these questions can help interviewers gain a clear feel for which candidates are the best qualified and the best fit, and sometimes the questions prompt candidates who lack the basic preparation and interest to withdraw their application. These questions are best used as an addition to any standard interview questions.

JOB PERFORMANCE EVALUATION

Policies concerning job performance evaluation depend to some extent on an organization's hierarchy. In most circumstances, BHCs will report to the Clinic Administrator and the Clinic Medical Director. Annual evaluations ideally include written input from all PCPs in the clinic, the Director of Nursing, the Clinic Medical Director, other BHCs in the system (if applicable), a few staff members, and the Behavioral Health Assistant (if applicable). Chart reviews should also play a role in the evaluation, and Table 3.2 offers a form to use for this. Other evaluative measures such as patient and PCP satisfaction and BHC productivity and fidelity to the model are also important in the annual evaluation. Measurement approaches for these aspects of BHC job performance are discussed in detail in Chapter 15.

TRAINING

The area of PCBH is a new one, and it is growing rapidly. The most utilized consulting firm for training in this area is probably Mountainview Consulting Group, Inc., of which one of us (PR) is a co-owner. Mountainview was the chief vendor for the Bureau of Primary Health Care for several years and has also provided training for the U.S. Air Force, Navy, and Veterans' Administration. Their website (www.behavioral-health-integration.com) is a good one for finding information on training opportunities. It also includes a list serve, where interested persons can participate in ongoing discussions about issues related to primary care behavioral health integration. Common sources of training workshops in this field include the Association for Behavioral and Cognitive Therapies (ABCT; www.aabt.org), the Society for Behavioral Medicine (SBM;

Table 3.2. The primary care behavioral health chart review tool

Confidential: The purpose of this tool is to assure quality in documentation by Behavioral Health Consultants working in the PCBH Model.				
BHC:	MR#:		Date of service:	
Date of review:			Reviewer:	
	Yes	No	N/A	Comments
Documentation in medical record				
Entries are less than one 8.5 × 11 page (when printed) Each encounter contains written or electronic signature of the BHC In electronic medical record, all entries are signed within three working days				
Behavioral health documentation content				
Subjective includes referral question, functional analysis of problem Follow-up consultation notes indicate patient progress on target behavior identified in initial contact Objective includes description of patient behavior and/or outcomes instrument measure (e.g., Duke, PSC, PHQ-9) Assessment includes medical diagnosis by referring provider Plan includes homework and follow-up plan (next contact details, including with whom and what needs to be done by the provider at that contact)				

Continued

Table 3.2.—*Cont'd*

Feedback to BHC from reviewer (including any corrective action needed):

BHC summary of corrective actions planned:

---

www.sbm.org), and the American Psychological Association (APA; www.apa.org). The International Society for Traumatic Stress Studies (ISTSS; www.istss.org) also has regular primary care offerings at its conference and has a Primary Care special interest group. The Collaborative Family Healthcare Association (www.cfha.net) is also offering training programs consistent with the PCBH model in its annual conventions.

The challenge to finding training lies in finding people who are actually practicing the PCBH model. An incredible variety of primary care behavioral health "integration" approaches are in use around the country. To be sure, one can always learn something from a colleague practicing in primary care, even if he or she is utilizing a very different model. To find training in this model, however, look for colleagues who describe themselves as consultants and who use brief, functionally-focused visits in a co-located, collaborative, and integrated service.

SUPERVISION

In addition to annual job performance evaluations and regular self-assessments using the BHC Core Competency Tool, new BHCs working alone should seek out someone willing to provide clinical supervision. This is an important arrangement to make, given the novelty of BHC work. Ideally, supervision would include use of the BHC Core Competencies Tool and Chart Review Tool and observations of the BHC on a regular basis. Unfortunately, though, finding someone familiar with the model who can act as supervisor can be a challenge. The most likely places to find help are in community health centers and Veterans' Administration clinics, many of which utilize a PCBH approach. Hopefully, there will soon be organizations that help newer BHCs connect with more experienced BHCs, as the Mountainview Consulting Group's website does.

In the meantime, if no one is available to provide on-site supervision, phone or email supervision with another BHC might be arranged. Some might require compensation for the supervision, but many will simply offer to help pro bono, recognizing the difficulty of finding supervision. Be careful about assuming that anyone working in primary care can provide supervision. Many who work in primary care use a model other than the PCBH model, and such individuals are not likely to have a good enough grasp of this approach to be able to supervise. If given the BHC Core Competencies Tool, the Chart Review Tool, and a basic understanding of the model, they might be able to help as a last resort. But the ideal scenario is to have a mentor who knows this model well. More ideas for obtaining adequate experience, mentoring, and supervision are detailed in the chapter on ethics, Chapter 14.

SUMMARY

1. The core competencies involved in BHC practice can be grouped into six domains: clinical practice, practice management, consultation, documentation, team performance, and administrative duties. Each consists of a number of skills that can be quite different from those of specialty MH.
2. The core competencies form the basis for a BHC job description and a BHC service policy manual that should be written in the first months of a new BHC service. The Core Competency Tool can be used for initial and ongoing self-assessments of strengths and weaknesses and can also be used by supervisors in performance evaluations.
3. If interviewing applicants for a BHC position, identify those who possess some of the core competencies or who demonstrate good potential for learning them. In addition to the organization's usual interview questions, several specific questions can help sort out top candidates.

4. To establish a strong start, those new to this model should find a BHC in the community or via phone or E-mail to act as a clinical supervisor. Several mental health and medical journals are helpful sources of information, and some professional associations offer continuing education training in the PCBH model.

4

YOUR SERVICES, LOCATION, AND SUPPORT

"We are not what we know but what we are willing to learn."
—Mary Catherine Bateson

Everyone knows the saying, "The Devil is in the details," and upon entering a new BHC position the meaning of this becomes immediately clear. Questions will abound on any number of topics, such as where to place the BHC office, how to bill, how to schedule patients, and other technical yet important issues. This is particularly true for those who are beginning a new BHC service. Earlier chapters have outlined the rationale for the PCBH model, oriented the reader to primary care, sketched out a BHC job description, and suggested a training/supervision plan, meaning the next step is to begin answering the technical questions.

With this in mind, the current chapter begins with suggestions for finding a location in the clinic and determining who will help with BHC workflow. In small clinics the BHC may be fairly self-sufficient, but in larger clinics an assistant might be needed for various aspects of care. Recruiting and training an assistant will probably be the BHC's responsibility, so we cover ideas for accomplishing these tasks. Because clinic staff will need to know how to set up a scheduling template and billing process, including diagnostic and procedural codes to use, we also cover these topics in detail. The chapter ends with a discussion of general issues regarding billing for BHC services.

LOCATION, LOCATION, LOCATION

It can be a big surprise to enter a new clinic on the first day of work and discover that you have no office. However, this is a fairly common experience for those starting up a new BHC service. Owing to the novelty of the service, clinic administrators are often not certain where to place a BHC office and may simply decide to wait for input from the new hire. Believe it or not, this can actually be the best-case scenario. Office locations established by an administrator who does not understand the PCBH model will often be far from ideal. Having the opportunity to select one's own office location offers the possibility of getting a new service off to an excellent start.

However, new BHCs who trained in specialty environments (where the prized office was large and private) also run the risk of selecting a poor location for a primary care office. The pace in primary care is fast, and providers often do not have time to walk down several hallways, or a flight of stairs, to talk with the BHC. As a result, the best locations for a BHC are those that are easy to access and highly visible. Given the frequent space constraints of primary care clinics, one will not always have control over placement of the BHC office. However, to the extent control is offered, following the recommendations below will lead to optimal outcomes.

Get to the Heart of the Clinic

One of the first activities for a new BHC will surely be a tour of the clinic. During this tour, try to locate the heart of the clinic. What area do providers pass by most often? Where do they congregate? Is there a specific department (e.g., pediatrics or internal medicine or family practice) that seems especially busy? These questions help find the nucleus, and it is as close to this nucleus as possible that the new BHC should try to make a home. Setting up shop in the nucleus signals PCPs that the BHC is not a typical MH provider, but rather more like a primary care provider who wants to be in the middle of the action. Sacrifice space for accessibility, as space is often at a premium in primary care and being seen is more important than having leg room. Above all, avoid locating oneself in an administrative wing, as that will erect numerous barriers to referrals and runs contrary to the mission of the PCBH model.

Working Out of Exam Rooms

If a clinic has little to offer in the way of a designated space in the nucleus, consider working in an exam room. The advantages of this may outweigh the burdens. Working in an exam room may help develop a truly integrated service, from the perspective of both patients and staff. Instead of being the specialty provider in the quiet wing of the clinic that the "psych" patients are sent to, the BHC in the exam room is more likely to be viewed as a part of the primary care team. Using exam rooms also means the BHC will be in the middle of the action more often, where many opportunities to talk with providers exist. Daily changes in the availability of exam rooms also means the BHC will work in different parts of the clinic and can become acquainted quickly with many PCPs.

The challenge of working out of an exam room is getting access to office equipment. Often a BHC in this situation has a desk with a phone, computer, etc., in a separate location (one that cannot be used for patient visits, such as a shared space) and simply sees patients out of exam rooms. However, at other times the BHC might have no permanent space at all. If the latter is the case, a small rolling cart provides a place for charts and practice support materials such as books and handouts. A laptop computer can be carried for word processing, spreadsheets, and (if the clinic has a wireless network) the Internet. BHCs who work out of exam rooms usually get a permanent space when one becomes available, as they tend to make strong relationships with their new colleagues quickly and their colleagues become effective advocates for them. Clinics of the future will hopefully include planned space for the BHC in the heart of the clinic.

The Door is Open

If not talking with a provider or a patient, the door to the BHC office should always be open. When providers drop by, be sure to give them immediate attention. In provider meetings and in e-mails and newsletters, tell providers that the door is always at least figuratively open for them. Make it clear that interruptions are okay, even if they occur during a patient visit. This message will need to be repeated, as PCPs have often been trained in residency by specialty MH therapists who advised them to avoid interrupting therapy visits.

In primary care, patients almost expect interruptions, and sometimes interruptions even help the BHC develop a fresh focus upon returning to the patient. Providers will be brief when interrupting a visit; indeed, they interrupt because they do not have time to wait. The worst-case scenario is for a PCP to walk away frustrated because the BHC is unavailable. Accepting interruptions takes some getting used to, but most new BHCs come to prefer it over time because of the positive feedback from PCPs who marvel at their accessibility.

A final suggestion about the door (or cart, if using the floating exam room option) is to decorate it with information about the BHC service. For example, one might post brief summaries of important recent studies on primary care treatment of behavioral health issues, copies of recent BHC newsletters, handouts advertising parenting classes and other resources in the community, and, of course, the BHC schedule.

Make Your Office Look Like Primary Care

PCPs do not have fancy offices with couches and comfortable armchairs, and the BHC should not, either. Remember that one goal of integrating behavioral health into primary care is to break down the stigma of the former, and this task is made more difficult when the two look different. The more behavioral health care looks like primary health care, the more likely patients and providers will be to accept the former as part of the latter. Keep this philosophy in mind when deciding how to decorate and equip the BHC office.

As is typical for primary care, most spaces available for BHC visits will be small. If an office has been allocated for the BHC service, it will need two or three small office chairs. Often, a folding chair can be hung on a coat rack on the back of the door for use when seeing a family. A toy chest or basket is a good idea, as there are many children to see in primary care (a collection of stickers for handing out can be helpful, too). Bulletin boards are common in primary care, and can be quickly filled with information about community resources or BHC services. A computer or notebook will be important for accessing practice support materials, and ideally a printer will be close by. The BHC should also have access to a phone, and though it is best placed in the BHC office (for use with telephone visits with patients), this might not be possible. The phones used by

PCPs for patient calls are often located in a common area where staff and PCPs do their administrative work.

COMMON EXPENSES TO INCLUDE IN THE BUDGET

The most expensive items in the BHC budget will be technology related, unless hiring a Behavioral Health Assistant (see next section). Many health care centers are adopting electronic medical record systems, meaning the BHC will need materials necessary to interface with the clinic's technology. Usually the clinic will have an information technology office to assist with this. The materials in the previous section are also standard for an office. Otherwise, supplies such as printer cartridges, paper, behavioral health prescription pads, pens equipped with highlighters (for use in reviewing patient education materials with patients), a pager, and several reference books should be included. The following books are good resources for the BHC office: *PDR Drug Guide for Mental Health Professionals* (Siften, 2002), *Treatments That Work, Second Edition* (Nathan & Gorman, 2002), *Treatments That Work for Children* (Christophersen & Mortweet, 2003), *The Good Kid Book* (Sloane, 1976), *What Works for Whom* (Roth & Fonagy, 2005), *Clinical Health Psychology and Primary Care: Practical Advice and Clinical Guidance for Successful Collaboration* (Gatchel & Oordt, 2003), and *Behavioral Integrative Care: Treatments that Work in the Primary Care Setting* (O'Donohue, Byrd, Cummings, & Henderson, 2005). Most BHCs also keep favorite self-help books that they can show to patients when recommending them.

PRIMARY CARE BEHAVIORAL HEALTH ASSISTANT SERVICES

Once one has done the important work of establishing an office, the next issue to address may be obtaining practice support. In specialty MH settings, providers often go to the waiting area to retrieve patients after being notified of their arrival by a receptionist. In primary care, however, the pace is much faster and the BHC may need additional support. Most PCPs receive assistance from a variety of staff members. A PCP will usually have 0.33 to 0.5 Full Time Equivalent (FTE) support from a registered nurse, 0.33 to 0.5 FTE support from a ward clerk, and 1.0 FTE support from a nursing or medical assistant. A BHC may (depending on the ratio of PCP FTE to BHC FTE) need support from a Behavioral Health Assistant (BHA). The BHA's job parallels the work that a nursing or medical assistant performs for a PCP, and can be critical in clinics where the PCP to BHC ratio is large. In smaller clinics, the BHC may be able to meet the needs of the clinic with less or no BHA support. One of us (PR) works in a clinic that has 0.6 FTE BHC hours to support twenty-two medical providers; the other (JR) works in a clinic that has 1.0 FTE BHC hours to support five medical providers. Many clinics are staffed somewhere between these two scenarios. If in a clinic with a large PCP to BHC ratio, be sure to read the following section, as recruiting, interviewing, selecting, and training a BHA can be crucial to success.

Recruiting and Training a BHA

The minimal requirements for a BHA are a high school diploma and an interest in working in a medical setting providing service to patients with behavioral health issues. If in a setting where a significant number of patients speak a language other than English, try to recruit a BHA fluent in the non-English language most commonly encountered. Table 4.1 provides a list of questions for interviewing BHA candidates.

Answers to these questions may help gauge the ease with which a person can learn to perform the many tasks associated with BHC work. Often, nursing assistants who have interests in patients with behavioral health issues or who simply want to learn something new will apply.

Explaining BHA tasks to candidates during the interview can be a good way of defining this new position in the clinic. Table 4.2 provides a list of common BHA tasks.

Table 4.1. Questions for interviews with behavioral health assistant candidates

1. What is your experience working in medical settings?
2. What patients are most interesting to you?
3. How would you feel if hearing patients discuss personal issues?
4. How would you feel about asking patients survey questions?
5. How do you feel about calling patients on the phone?
6. What are your skills for working on computers?
7. How do you handle interruptions when you are working?

Table 4.2. Behavioral health assistant: Common tasks

1. Open the office door for the BHC in the morning
2. Get charts for the day's scheduled patients and locate any missing charts (if the clinic still has paper charts)
3. Call scheduled patients to remind them of appointment times (may be done in the morning of the appointment or the day before)
4. Schedule patients when they call for same-day or next-day follow-up BHC visits
5. Schedule patients for same-day visits referred by a PCP
6. Maintain copies of all outcome instruments and handouts used by the BHC
7. Complete pre-appointment assessments with patients.
8. Organize the BHC's patient visits; this includes obtaining the billing slip and chart, and taking these, the patient, and the results of the pre-appointment assessment to the BHC
9. Inform other departments/areas of the clinic when same-day appointments are available with the BHC (e.g., if there is a no-show or an open appointment time)
10. Assist with completion of forms for medical records, such as the permission form for release or exchange of information
11. Assist with completing referrals for services outside of the clinic
12. Maintain supplies for the BHC
13. Document patient no-shows and cancellations in patient charts
14. If asked by the BHC, contact patients who no-show or cancel to arrange follow-up
15. Send letters to patients who no-show for appointments
16. Assist with scheduling patients for return appointments (if patients want to schedule rather than calling later for a same-day appointment)
17. Assist with organizing BHC classes and group care clinics
18. Initiate calls to schools and other community organizations as requested
19. Update community resource lists on a quarterly basis
20. Organize patient education materials
21. At the end of the day, clean the room used for triage/pre-appointment activities

Once selected, the BHA will need at least eight hours of training specific to the tasks listed in Table 4.2. Often, the outgoing BHA (if applicable) will be able to do the majority of the training and the BHC can do fine-tuning over time. The BHC will often be the official supervisor for the BHA, and this requires that a BHC be familiar with the clinic's policies concerning supervision.

A Word about Interpreter Services

Particularly in community health centers, which tend to have a diverse patient population, the BHC will require assistance from interpreters. (Note that a "translator" transcribes written words into one language from another, while an "interpreter" works with spoken communication.) Whether the interpreter is the BHA or an interpreter that works with all of the providers in the clinic, some preparation for working together is important, given the unique nature of BHC interactions with patients. We recommend that the BHC schedule time with the interpreter at the outset of his or her service to discuss topics and techniques common to BHC visits. The two can plan where the interpreter is to sit and where the patient will sit during visits (recommended is to have the interpreter sit next to the patient so the patient and BHC must talk directly to each other). Also discuss during this time the importance of complete interpretation as opposed to summaries.

During visits, issues of etiquette are important. Ask the interpreter to ask the patient for permission to interpret prior to beginning the visit and to ask for patient evaluation of the interpreter services at the end of the visit (e.g., "Did I do a good job of interpreting for you today?"). Most interpreters will do this without prompting, but not all will. Especially during BHC visits, when patients are often distressed and talking rapidly and at length, one might also need to have interpreters interrupt patients so a word-for-word interpretation occurs. If this happens, take a few moments to explain to the patient the importance of accurate interpretation.

Some general points regarding the use of interpreters are also important to mention, not the least of which concerns BHC comfort with the presence of an interpreter. Although in specialty MH a provider may occasionally interface with interpreters, for most it is a rarity. Thus, the new BHC will likely need to learn to feel comfortable with this arrangement. This can seem like quite a challenge, given the brevity of BHC visits, because using an interpreter to repeat everything said by the BHC and the patient cuts deeply into an already brief visit. The presence of a third party in the room also takes some getting used to. Many BHCs feel self-conscious when an interpreter is present, and some interpreters are more professional than others. Completing the aforementioned preparatory work with the interpreter may help considerably, but be sure to address

concerns with interpreters immediately as they arise. Most BHCs habitu-
ate to the presence of an interpreter over time and learn to feel quite comfortable with them in the room.

There are other points to consider about using an interpreter effectively.
For starters, a BHC should always use an interpreter unless she or he is
completely fluent in the patient's language. Otherwise the tendency is to
say what one knows how to say rather than what one truly wants to say.
Also avoid using a family member or friend of the patient for interpreting,
unless absolutely necessary. Patients might not feel able to discuss certain
important issues with the family member or friend in the room, not to
mention the pressure unfairly placed on the family member or friend.
Typically such persons don't make very effective interpreters anyway, as
interpreting is actually a difficult skill that requires training and practice.
Some patients will refuse an interpreter, perhaps out of a desire to practice
English and perhaps out of pride, but be assertive about the need. Do recognize, however, that some patients and interpreters will not get along
because of class or cultural differences. The simple fact that the two speak
the same language does not imply other cultural or socioeconomic simi-
larities. Some interpreters may even subtly discourage certain topics of discussion that embarrass them (e.g., certain superstitious beliefs of a patient
from a similar background as the interpreter). Or, similarly, a patient
might avoid acknowledging certain beliefs or practices because of what the
interpreter might think of them.

Good interpreters are aware of these dynamics, as well as of their own
biases, and may discuss them with the provider as needed. They should
also explain cultural references to the provider as needed. For example, if
a patient refers to a national holiday in his or her home country, the interpreter should explain the holiday and perhaps the significance of it to the
provider. Even if interpreters are readily available in the clinic, all providers
should learn at least a few phrases of the most commonly encountered
language(s) as a show of respect for the patient's background (e.g., be able
to introduce oneself and handle basic greetings).

BHC SERVICES

A BHC service consists of three basic services: assessments, interventions,
and classes/groups. Initial visits often include both an assessment and an

intervention and, therefore, require more time than follow-up visits which may be limited to one or the other. Classes may occur in many formats, including as part of a clinical pathway or group care clinic. To create a scheduling template, the BHC may need to name these services and provide instructions concerning how much time to assign to each. Names are typically associated with abbreviations, e.g., BHFU for behavioral health follow-up. Visit length should be in the same increments used by PCPs in the clinic in order to simplify scheduling. In some clinics PCP visits are fifteen minutes and in others they are twenty minutes (occasionally clinics use other visit lengths, but these are the two most common). Thus, in clinics using fifteen-minute visit increments, an initial BHC visit might comprise two fifteen-minute slots, for a total of thirty minutes. Follow-up BHC visits in that same clinic might be fifteen minutes long. Work closely with the clinic scheduler/ward clerk and the clinic manager on establishing a schedule. Every clinic varies in how patients are scheduled, so the first step might be simply to ask for a brief tutorial on how this is done for the other providers.

Initial Contacts

As noted earlier in this section, initial contacts typically require two 15-(or two 20-) minute units. These may be labeled in the scheduling program as BHI or Behavioral Health Initial. Occasionally, when very busy, an initial contact may be completed in one 15- or 20-minute unit. Adjusting the time downward makes it possible for a BHC to see a walk-in patient when fifteen minutes are available and thirty are not (remember the importance of same-day access, even if for a very brief visit). When this is the best option, indicate that the BHI was fifteen minutes in length, rather than thirty, on the billing form. Chapter 7 also contains details on this practice.

Follow-up Contacts

Follow-up contacts, particularly with adults, are usually scheduled for one 15- or 20-minute visit. These may be referred to as BHFU or Behavioral Health Follow-Up on the scheduling program. When completing a reassessment and teaching a skill, such as progressive muscle relaxation, thirty (forty) minutes might be necessary for a follow-up visit. More often than not, thirty (forty) minutes will be required for follow-up visits involving tabulation and interpretation of questionnaire data, such as when diagnosing and planning treatment for Attention Deficit Hyperactivity Disorder. When planning a more intensive follow-up visit, ask the patient to schedule such. For regular follow-ups, patients may either be scheduled immediately after the initial visit or simply asked to call for a next-day or same-day follow-up visit when they are ready to return. Many clinics use Advanced Access principles (Murray & Berwick, 2003) for scheduling, in which patients are asked to call for an appointment on the same day one is desired. This model can be applied to BHC visits as well, and is discussed in detail in Chapter 7.

Allowing for Warm Handoffs

In order to see patients on demand, when a PCP identifies the need (sometimes called a "warm handoff"), the BHC schedule needs to be able to accommodate them. There are different strategies for accomplishing this. One strategy is to limit scheduled patients to two per hour. This allows room for one or possibly even two warm handoffs every hour of the day, because the show rate for scheduled BHC appointments ranges from 25 percent to 75 percent (it hovers around 70 percent in both of our clinics). In other words, there is a reasonable likelihood that a scheduled patient will not show, thereby creating time to see a warm-handoff patient. Another strategy is to create a schedule that attempts to match the supply of appointments with the demand for them. For example, warm-handoffs typically come in later in the day, so arranging a schedule that anticipates this need can be helpful. One of us (PR) leaves 10:30 to 12:00 and 4:00 to 5:00 open, to accommodate the warm-handoffs that proliferate at the end of the morning and again at the end of the afternoon. (This is one of the core strategies of an Advanced Access approach.) On the scheduling template, warm handoffs may be designated with the codes BHSDI (same-day initial contact patients) and BHSDFU (same-day follow-up patients).

Class Visits

There are a variety of behavioral health classes and group clinics that may be offered by a BHC. We devote Chapter 12 to a discussion of these. Note classes or groups on the schedule as BHCLASS or Behavioral Health Class. These usually vary from one to two hours, and they may be co-led with a teammate, such as a diabetes educator, dietician or PCP. The BHC may ask the staff member who creates his or her schedule to book group/class appointments for patients planning to attend, so that each receives a reminder call or appointment card (if the clinic's scheduling system generates these).

BILLING

Billing issues present some of the biggest challenges facing those starting a PCBH service. A clinic starting up a new service might not have a clear idea of how to bill for BHC services, and might expect the BHC to help with this. Alternatively, they might have an inappropriate plan, such as using Psychotherapy codes, which don't actually capture what a BHC does. Many PCBH services are started with grant money, but might have no clear future beyond the life of the grant. Determining the clinic's plan for billing and financial support of a PCBH program is an important task for the new BHC. Being prepared to offer guidance to the clinic on this issue is equally important.

To Bill or Not to Bill?

Truly progressive clinics may hire a BHC with no plan to use him or her as a direct revenue producer. Such clinics may view a BHC as a key member of the primary care team whose value comes in the form of saved PCP time, improved clinic functioning, increased patient and provider satisfaction, and quite possibly significant cost-offsets (see Robinson, 2002 for a discussion of cost-offset opportunities). Indeed, clinics attempting to initiate Advanced Access procedures have a great need for the types of services a BHC can provide, such as group medical visits, assumption of tasks typically done by PCPs, and substituting for PCPs during some follow-up visits (Murray & Berwick, 2003). There are many individuals in primary care who are paid not to produce revenue but to enhance team and system functioning, and including a BHC in this group is not a stretch. One of the greatest barriers to this happening may simply be psychological. MH providers have a long history of billing for services (in specialty settings), and thus both a BHC and his or her primary care administrators might have a difficult time envisioning any other arrangement.

Developing a Plan

Obviously clinics can figure out how to accommodate a BHC service, because many clinics currently have one. However, the funding strategies currently used vary widely. Because BHC services are still new in today's health care world, there is a great deal of variation in billing policies and strategies from state to state and from county to county within a state, making billing a challenge. Grant funding may be available for starting behavioral health services in primary care settings, particularly in federally qualified community health centers. Over the past decade, the Bureau of Primary Health Care has granted dozens of service expansion grants to community health centers. The grants have been for standard amounts, usually in the range of $100,000 to $150,000, and they are permanent increases in the clinic's funding.

Since clinics with four or five providers receive funding equal to clinics with twenty-five providers, financial pressure for billing and expanding services varies among clinics. One of us (PR) provides services to twenty-two providers with a 0.6 FTE BHC position and bills for services, while the other (JR) provides services to five providers with a 1.0 FTE BHC and does not bill. Of course, a lack of resources and services within a system creates more pressure for billing, yet even in clinics with a relative wealth of funds for initiating BHC services, billing is often an issue. Some seed grants require the clinics receiving grants to bill.

Whatever the situation in one's clinic—lucky or less so—developing a billing strategy is important. Patients will ask about the cost of BHC visits, and PCPs and BHCs need to provide a clear answer for them. A good billing strategy can minimize the financial obstacles to patients using BHC services, but a poorly designed one can be a significant barrier to care. To the extent patients are deterred from BHC visits due to cost, the effectiveness of the BHC in realizing cost-savings and other value to the clinic will be diminished. To develop a billing plan, one must first learn about billing slips and coding.

Billing Slips

Billing slips are printed forms that track the details of a patient's encounter in the clinic on the day of service. The person who first greets the patient (i.e., the receptionist) typically generates the billing slip. The slip goes to the provider who delivers the service, and this provider indicates procedure codes and diagnostic codes on the billing slip, accompanied in some clinics with information about planned follow-up. The patient or provider then takes the form to a billing staff member after the visit. Billing specialists submit the bill for payment, and a third-party payer responds by providing or denying payment. When payment is not made, the clinic billing specialist receives an Explanation of Benefit (EOB), which explains why payment was denied. There are almost 1,000 EOBs, so billing specialists deserve the title of specialists! We recommend that BHCs meet the group of people who do billing and maintain regular contact, as they will be the source of the most up-to-date information on how to get paid.

Codes

Third-party payers most commonly recognize the Physician's Current Procedural Terminology (CPT) system as the method for describing medical services in numerical codes for subsequent reimbursement. The CPT codes describe procedures, and delivery of a procedure requires that the provider of that procedure make a diagnosis. Therefore, BHCs, like PCPs, need to prepare to use a CPT or procedure code with an appropriate diagnostic code. At present, there are two series of CPT procedural codes that describe services provided by behavioral health providers. The newest series, codes 96.150 through 96.155 are Health and Behavior Codes. They are listed in the medical section of the CPT and were first included in the 2002 CPT. The older series, codes 90.801 through 90.899, are Psychotherapy Codes, and they are listed in the psychiatric section of the CPT manual. The Health and Behavior Codes best describe the procedures that BHCs provide. BHCs cannot bill for a Psychotherapy code and a Health and Behavior assessment and intervention code on the same day. In clinics where both psychiatric and BHC services are available, the BHC needs to use the code that describes the principle service provided. In a PCBH practice, the BHC focuses on quality of life and improvement of health even when patients have a psychiatric disorder. Thus, we both use the Health and Behavior Codes exclusively in our services.

The Practice Directorate and other key American Psychological Association representatives promoted inclusion of the Health and Behavior codes in the CPT manual (American Psychological Association Government Relations Staff, 2004). Practicing psychologists, nurses, licensed social workers, and other nonphysician providers, including licensed counselors in some states, are eligible to bill for applicable services and to receive reimbursement from Health and Behavior Codes. These codes apply to psychological services that address behavioral, social, and psychophysiological conditions in the treatment or management of patients diagnosed with physical health problems. Examples include patient adherence to medical treatment, symptom management, health-promoting behaviors, health-related risk-taking behaviors, and overall adjustment to physical illness (see the Health Care Financing Administration website, www.hcfa.gov). Most often, a physician will have diagnosed a physical health problem prior to referring to the BHC, and physical health diagnoses are represented by ICD-9 CM codes (*International Classification of Diseases, 9th Revision, Clinical Modification;* World Health Organization, 1996).

Table 4.3 lists the code numbers and names for the Health and Behavior Assessment and Intervention codes and reimbursement rates suggested by Medicare. The BHC uses the first code in the series, 96.150, for the initial assessment of a patient. In this assessment, the BHC evaluates biological, psychological, and social factors affecting the patient's physical health and any treatment problems. The second code, 96.151, applies to BHC re-assessment to determine a patient's condition and need for further treatment. Code 96.152 applies to BHC intervention services delivered to modify psychological, behavioral, cognitive, and social factors affecting a patient's physical health and well being. Examples include increasing patient awareness about his or her health condition and using behavioral strategies to support physician prescribed diet, exercise, or stress management regimens. For intervention services provided in a group format, BHCs use code 96.153. Examples include smoking cessation classes, group visits for adults with chronic pain and behavior change classes for patients with diabetes. Code 96.154 applies to intervention services that a BHC provides to a family with a patient present and 96.155 to intervention services provided to a family without the patient present. For example, 96.155 is the code that a BHC would use if providing service to family members of a medically ill patient if the patient is not present for the visit.

As mentioned earlier in this section, the BHC needs to record a diagnostic code(s) along with the procedural code on the billing form. The

Table 4.3. The health and behavior codes and reimbursement guidelines

CPT code	Service	1 Unit	2 Units
96.150	Assessment: initial	$26	$52
96.151	Reassessment	$26	$52
96.152	Intervention: individual	$25	$50
96.153	Intervention: group (per person)	$5	$10
96.154	Intervention: family w/patient	$24	$48
96.155	Intervention: family w/o patient	$23	$46

ICD-9 codes 290 through 31(which parallel DSM-IV-TR codes and apply to services provided to outpatients with a mental, psychoneurotic, or personality disorder) are not used with Health and Behavior procedure codes. BHCs use ICD-9 CM codes that do not specify a mental disorder when using the Health and Behavioral procedure codes. Because health and behavior assessment and intervention services focus on patients whose primary diagnosis is a physical health problem, BHCs use one or more codes that describe a physical diagnosis (e.g., diabetes, hypertension, sleep disturbance).

A physician—not a behavioral health provider—establishes a physical health problem. Therefore, the BHC should code physical health problems that have been identified by a physician prior to the delivery of BHC services. Consider the following example. Dr. Jones, a PCP, refers Nell (a patient) to Dr. Henderson, a BHC, because she has diabetes and is having difficulty making recommended changes to her diet. Dr. Jones notes that Nell has symptoms of depression as well. During the consultation visit, Dr. Henderson assists Nell with making changes to her diet. In the functional analysis, he determines that Nell overeats when she is sad, and they develop an intervention to improve her mood, as well as to limit portion sizes of her food choices. On the billing slip, Dr. Henderson would use the Health and Behavior Codes of 96.150 (initial assessment) and 96.152 (intervention) to describe procedures done. He would also use the ICD-9 code for diabetes, a physical diagnosis established by the PCP. The American Psychological Association website (www.apa.org) offers a crosswalk tool to help behavioral health providers locate appropriate ICD-9 CM codes for use with Health and Behavioral procedure codes.

Each of the Health and Behavior Codes is based on fifteen minutes of face-to-face contact with the patient. Consequently, BHCs code one unit per fifteen minutes of service. For example, a BHC would code two units of 96.150 or one unit of 96.150 and one for 96.152, as in the example given earlier, for a thirty-minute initial visit. When the time spent with a patient is between units, round up or down to the nearest unit. For example, if twenty minutes are spent with a patient, round down and indicate one unit, but if twenty-five minutes are spent, round up and bill for two units.

Documentation

Whatever is coded on the billing slip must be supported by documentation in the chart note, as inadequate documentation can lead to denial of payment or even charges of fraud. Historically, payers expect documentation to include at least the following areas when Psychotherapy Codes (as opposed to Health and Behavior Codes) are used:

- Date of service
- Length of encounter
- Description of the patient's mental state
- Description of the service provided
- Treatments implemented
- Response to treatment
- Provider signature

While not yet established, we will venture a guess at the documentation requirements that payers may specify for payment on Health and Behavior code services. These will likely include the following.

- Date of service
- Length of encounter
- Description of the patient's health-related quality of life
- Description of the service provided
- Interventions delivered or planned
- Treatment response (for follow-up visits)
- Provider signature

In Chapters 9 and 10, we provide examples of PCBH chart notes that support the use of Health and Behavior procedure codes.

Current Reimbursement Controversies and Problems

As noted above, clinics take different approaches to funding a BHC service. Some rely on grants, others on billing, and some do not charge for BHC services at all. For those looking to bill, the advent of the Health and Behavior Codes brings both opportunity and controversy. It will take time for the dust to settle and for payment issues regarding the codes to become more routine. Currently, though some practitioners are using the codes with success, many are finding it difficult to obtain reimbursement with them. We recommend that BHCs work with administrators and billing specialists to develop an initial billing strategy and then review it annually. To stimulate discussion of key issues with key players, such as the Chief Executive Officer, Chief Financial Officer, Clinic Administrator, and Clinic Medical Director, consider the following questions.

1. What is the clinic's mission for delivery of behavioral health services?

If utilizing the PCBH model, the goals of the service are to help patients improve their health-related quality of life and to improve the overall ability of the system to address the population's health needs. The BHC will see many patients, in brief visits, and help strengthen the delivery of care in general in the clinic. The BHC will also provide consultation services rather than psychotherapy services. If billing in this scenario, use of the Health and Behavior Codes is most appropriate. However, a clinic should also consider the barriers to BHC care that billing can erect. Some clinics will decide that the BHC will be of more value as a team player with completely open access and minimal barriers to care, and so will decide not to bill for BHC services. If the mission is to provide a traditional specialty model of MH care, with intensive individual care that is diagnosis based, the Psychotherapy Codes will be a better choice than the Health and Behavior Codes.

2. Who pays for what codes in my state?

Medicare reimburses for five of the six Health and Behavior Codes at present. The exception is 96.155 (family intervention without the patient present). Some private health insurance plans have begun to pay for these codes as well. Private insurance plans may have payment policies that are more or less restrictive than Medicare. Check with private insurers about their payment policies regarding these codes.

3. How much will I be paid for codes that I use?

The Medicare "Outpatient Mental Health Treatment Limitation" reduces Medicare's co-payment for MH services from 80 percent to 50 percent. This limitation applies specifically to services provided to outpatients with a mental, psychoneurotic, or personality disorder identified by an ICD-9 CM diagnosis code between 290 and 319. The Medicare "Outpatient Mental Health Treatment Limitation" does not apply to services provided under the Health and Behavior Codes; therefore, health and behavior assessment and intervention services are reimbursed at 80 percent. Table 4.3 lists nationwide Medicare reimbursement rates for one and two units. Typically, initial appointments with the BHC require two units, while follow-ups require one. In regards to 96.153, the total group fee equals the reimbursement amount ($5.00 per unit) multiplied by the number of persons in the group, such that a one-hour group (four units) with ten patients would be billed at $200 or $20.00 per patient.

According to the APA Practice Directorate, Medicare reimbursements to psychologists for the Health and Behavior codes recently topped $6 million and seventeen private insurance carriers now accept the codes for reimbursement (3-1-05 mailing from APA Practice Directorate). New BHCs should contact the local Medicare carrier to get specific reimbursement amounts for the State in which they practice, because the national rates are subject to geographic adjustments.

4. What are the options for reimbursement for uninsured patients who receive BHC services if I submit Health and Behavior Codes?

To answer this question, the BHC needs to learn about his or her clinic's sliding scale payment plan and what happens when patients fail to pay for other services. If you work in a community health care setting, there may be opportunities for increasing the capitation rate the clinic has with State funding sources. The clinic could ask for an increase in their base rate of funding based upon offering a significant number of new services. (The services coded with Health and Behavior codes will be new services.) Whatever the plan, one needs to be certain that it is the same for patients with and without insurance.

Getting Paid

If billing for BHC services is the plan, the new Health and Behavior Codes provide an opportunity for that to happen. Our advice in two phrases is: be proactive and be persistent. Prior to submitting a bill, contact the payer and explain the PCBH model. Work closely with the billing department on an ongoing basis, to stay current on developments in the dynamic reimbursement environment. Obtain information as soon as possible from the Center for Medicare and Medicaid Services (CMS) regional office about billing Medicare codes.

If there are problems with reimbursement from private third-party payers, bill and then appeal the Evidence of Beneficiary or EOB. For denials from Medicare, contact the local Medicare carrier to explore the problem. Medicare offers health professionals an appeals process at the local level. Most Medicare carriers have websites that provide information on appeals. Beyond the local Medicare level, the BHC and/or billing specialist may contact the office of the CMS in the local area for help. So, in a word, persist!

Professional organizations may also be able to support efforts to find stable financial ground for a PCBH service. The American Psychological Association, a leader in development of the Health and Behavior Codes, is actively seeking information from psychologists who use these codes. Psychologists may contact the Practice Directorate's Government Relations Office at (202) 336-5889 to discuss issues or problems.

SUMMARY

1. Before starting clinical work, the new BHC and the system's or clinic's leadership group need to set the best foundation. Policies regarding the location of the BHC in the clinic, administrative support of the practice, and the budget are important to establish early. These should be documented in the BHC program manual.

2. The location and look of a BHC office is important. It should blend well with the primary care environment and be in the heart of the clinic. Some BHCs see patients in exam rooms.

3. A new BHC needs to work closely with the clinic manager and schedulers to create a schedule template and a list of services. The process for scheduling same-day patients (also called "warm hand-

offs") and group visits may need ongoing attention as the service develops.

4. Some clinics bill for services, others rely on grants, and still others do not bill at all for BHC services. There are many issues related to billing that will probably be worked out over the next decade. The Health and Behavior Codes are a positive development and are appropriate for BHC use, but many have had problems obtaining reimbursement with them. Chart documentation must match billing slips.

PART III

A HORIZON AND A COMPASS

As described in earlier chapters, the mission of the PCBH model is not merely to provide direct patient care but also to improve the delivery of healthcare, for all problems and all people, within the primary care system. Pursuing this mission requires a rethinking of some old concepts and practices. Since 1946, the World Health Organization (WHO) has defined health as "... a state of complete physical, mental, and social well-being and not merely the absence of disease or infirmity." Yet, while tremendous efforts have been made toward eliminating disease, little effort has been made toward creating health. There have been many successes in disease elimination, yet one of three Americans now lives with one or more chronic diseases. Rather than focusing on ridding ourselves of suffering, the need exists to focus on creating health. Lifestyle issues form the core of such a change, meaning the BHC is uniquely positioned to help achieve it.

In this part of the book, Chapter 5 discusses first how the design of the fully integrated PCBH model reflects a different conceptualization of health, one that attempts to correct the stifling of behavior change issues that has occurred in healthcare. From a PCBH perspective, the process of achieving good health is a social activity that occurs within biopsychosocial constraints rather than a biomedical activity occurring within social constraints (Waltner-Toews, 2001). We then introduce theories and therapies that the BHC will rely on in patient visits, as he or she attempts to paint a new horizon for the primary care system. In Chapter 6, we present screening and assessment strategies, which provide the compass the BHC will need in order to pursue that new horizon.

5

THEORETICAL MODELS AND THERAPEUTIC APPROACHES FOR INTEGRATED CARE

"Medicine is not only a science; it is also an art. It does not consist of compounding pills and plasters; it deals with the very processes of life, which must be understood before they may be guided."
                                                    —Paracelsus (1493–1541)

Behavioral health services delivered in primary care may look in some respects like those in traditional mental health, but they deviate significantly in other respects. One important difference concerns the role of the DSM diagnostic system. While this system forms the cornerstone of the MH system, it is not a part of the PCBH model. The goal of PCBH is to avoid the problems inherent in the medical model approach, which has stigmatized behavior problems and pushed behavior change technologies off of the healthcare stage. Through true integration into the frontline of the nation's healthcare system, a BHC is well-positioned to help move behavior change technology to the fore.

Another difference lies in the way clinical interventions are delivered. Clinical practice in the PCBH model relies on approaches that can be adapted to the unique demands of primary care. Newer evidence-based approaches including mindfulness, motivational interviewing, and acceptance, are commonly used or adapted, as are traditional behavioral techniques such as relaxation and communication skills training. Although these models and practices are applied in specialty mental health as well, by its very definition as a "specialty", mental health favors lengthier and broader applications with a more intensive change focus. Applications in the PCBH model are more restrained and geared toward smaller changes in a larger number of people.

Although up to now there has not been a consistently applied theoretical approach or practice among BHCs, in this book we hope to begin the process of standardization. As in specialty mental health, PCBH practitioners cannot currently stipulate that "X" problem requires "Y" intervention. After all, medicine is both a science and an art, and this is certainly true for BHC work as well. The clinical work of the BHC combines a solid theoretical grounding with a dash of creativity to adapt empirically-supported interventions to the primary care setting. In the pages that follow, we aim to introduce the philosophies of health that guide PCBH work and the clinical approaches that comprise it.

CURRENT DILEMMAS IN HEALTH

Before launching into the clinical theories and techniques that underlie the PCBH approach, some background on the need for a different conceptualization of health should prove helpful. Though space prohibits a detailed discussion, this introduction will hopefully give the reader a basic idea of the model's roots.

The Advent of Miracle Medicine

Until the advent of "miracle medicine", the relationship between patient and provider was at the heart of health care. For millennia, healers in various cultures offered psychological interventions to community members. But the discovery of antibiotics, anesthesia, and surgery in the 20th century changed much of that. It introduced new possibilities and, while offering physicians the opportunities to save more lives, it also created new problems (Bolls, 2004). Many once fatal illnesses became curable, but living longer has not always meant living better.

As a result of miracle medicine adding years to lives, behavioral technology has become a highly relevant tool for adding quality to lives. The one-third of Americans that are now living with chronic illness must make numerous behavior changes to improve or even maintain their diminished state of health (yet only about half do). While patients and their doctors struggle to manage chronic conditions, educators and researchers look upstream to see what behavioral technologies might prevent them. Diseases of lifestyle and behavior are the major threats to health today (Matarazzo, 1982; McGinnis & Foege, 1993). Behavioral choices around diet, exercise, smoking, substance abuse, and sexual behavior factor prominently in heart disease, cancers, obesity, respiratory problems, and HIV infection. The authors of Healthy People 2010 (U.S. Department of Health & Human Services, 2000) emphasize the central role of behavior change technology in promoting health and in reducing disease morbidity and mortality rates.

Yet, many of those living with chronic conditions secretly hope for, or openly demand, a magic bullet—a pill or procedure—that will allow them to achieve good health and avoid pain, suffering, and behavior change. Rather than developing and disseminating behavioral technology, society has responded to this demand by looking to the pharmaceutical industry for help. They have, in turn, seized on this opportunity, creating ever more products to feed the demand.

As people live longer with more diseases, the quality of the patient–provider relationship has deteriorated. It has changed to a less intimate and busier one, and while people long for a medical cure for almost all discomforts, providers are often unable to deliver one. The ability of the doctor–patient relationship to produce change has become limited while the concept of patient-driven lifestyle change seems sometimes to have been lost. Though one focus group of patients after another would declare that the idea of the physician as the sole person responsible for one's health is ridiculous, this notion pervades our distribution of health care resources, training programs, and the day to day delivery of services (Bolls, 2004).

The Diminishment of Behavioral Health Approaches

Why have behavioral scientists been unable to capitalize on the opportunities presented by the fallout from miracle medicine? The importance of self-driven behavior change in preventing and managing chronic conditions has been spelled out again and again, so why has the field failed to find a role in society equal to that of the pharmaceutical industry? The reasons for this are many and complicated, and remedies will require changes in multiple aspects of society and healthcare. However, some of the obvious barriers can be overcome by the type of integrated care that the PCBH approach involves. These barriers include a culture of specialization and separation, the prominence of avoidance strategies in our society, the inadequacy of models for evaluating health care costs, and the "biomedicalization" of mental health care.

The origins of most health problems usually include a variety of behavioral, social, environmental, and biological factors. However, health professionals tend to work in camps organized by specialization. To choose targets and agree on future priorities, such as more attention to behavioral technologies, better teamwork will be needed. Behavioral health providers must have more of a presence in the health care system, instead of living in the separate world of the MH care system. Theories are also needed that promote an understanding of how to create "self-protective action"—that is, strong, sustained behavioral repertoires that enhance health and reduce risk of illness (Ewart, 2004). Rather than applying a theory that singles out the mind or a specific body system for change, an integrative theory is needed that (1) places the individual in a broader environmental context, (2) organizes important social and individual mechanisms of behavior change, (3) indicates how these components interact with one another, and (4) suggests how they might be activated and coordinated to support health-protective activity (Ewart, 2004). Work has begun in this area, as evidenced by new contextually sensitive behavioral research (see the discussion of "third-wave" behavior therapies later in this chapter), but much more work will be needed.

Promotion of the idea that suffering is part of life and part of pursuing health is also pivotal to a view of health that supports behavior change. People living longer with chronic diseases such as arthritis, diabetes, hypertension, and others will need to learn how to experience the suffering inherent in losing functional abilities if they are to enjoy the days added to their lives by today's medicine. Forgoing the chocolate cheesecake for a cup of herbal tea is a mild form of suffering that can help the octogenarian to walk on arthritic knees. Unfortunately most current approaches in healthcare are geared more toward avoidance of suffering, be it physical or psychological, rather than learning to live well with it. Medicines aimed at eliminating anxiety or alleviating chronic back pain often produce more problems than they help with (see Chapter 13), and promote the notion that life cannot be lived until suffering is gone. One of the most important missions for a BHC is to dignify suffering and teach providers and nurses to teach patients to suffer well and escape the avoidance trap.

In the meantime, as people live longer and without much availability of behavioral technologies, health care costs will certainly continue to escalate. Research is needed for calculating health care costs that include the cost-offset effects of providing behavioral services. Nicholas Cummings anticipated the unfortunate "side effects" of miracle medicine in his work with the Kaiser Foundation in the 1960s (Cummings & Follette, 1968; Follette & Cummings, 1967). In this work, he predicted the need for a more prominent role for health–behavior change efforts in the future. He also demonstrated the effectiveness of behavioral interventions in reducing the cost of providing medical care to large and diverse populations of medical patients. Unfortunately, providers, patients, and insurance carriers have been slow to integrate this information into practice.

Part of the reason this has failed to catch on surely has to do with the "biomedicalization" of behavioral health. For a variety of political, economic, and scientific reasons, the (bio)medical model continues to exert a great deal of influence on the medical community, including primary care and mental health (Strosahl, 2005). From a biomedical perspective, health is a state of freedom from disease. The medical provider attempts to diagnose a specific disease based on a cluster of signs and symptoms and to provide a disease-specific treatment that eliminates those signs and symptoms. However, labeling clusters of symptoms as syndromes is meaningful only to the extent that it links with etiology, prevention, course of illness, and treatment response. In physical medicine, when this model hasn't worked, researchers have sometimes been able to go beyond it. Medical researchers demonstrated this ability in the case of cancer and the basic work on oncogenes. In this work, when attempts to suppress cancer symptoms kept running into roadblocks, researchers turned instead to understanding how cancers emerge and proliferate.

Behavioral research may need a similar change in focus. Quite simply, the syndrome strategy has not worked well because there are multiple causes that lead to common outcomes and single causes that lead to multiple outcomes for most behavior disorders. Yet, we continue to rely on the idea of syndromes. The Diagnostic and Statistical Manual of Mental Disorders, 4th Edition (DSM-IV) (American Psychiatric Association, 1994) is hundreds of pages in length yet has questionable reliability. As early as 1949, we learned that three psychiatrists faced with a single patient and given identical information at the same moment were able to reach the same diagnostic conclusion only 20 percent of the time (Ash, 1949). Thirteen years later after multiple revisions resulting in more and more pages of syndromes, agreement had only inched up to between thirty-two and forty-two percent (Beck, 1962). Most recently, the American Psychiatric Association received funding from the MacArthur Foundation for a broad reliability study of the DSM-IV TR, and while the research phase of the project was completed, findings were not published (Spiegel, 2005).

With hopes of greater prediction and control, behavioral health and medical providers purchased over a million copies of each of the first three versions of the DSM. Proponents of the behavioral disease model worked with pharmaceutical companies to develop powerful medications to address the numerous specific disorders listed in the DSM. Unfortunately, though it was good for the pharmaceutical industry, the popularization of the syndrome idea probably delayed rather than furthered progress toward creation of a meaningful basic behavioral science. Like the early cancer researchers, a focus on symptom reduction has stood in the way of furthering a science capable of identifying meaningful functional processes in behavior. Applying the medical model to mental health has instead resulted in basic accounts of behavior that are too vague or global to be of scientific value, such as psychoanalytic and brain-behavior models.

A variety of other issues have also contributed to behavioral health's diminished role in health care and research. For example, the popular idea of health as a state of being free of disease has promoted the false notion of a "cure" for all problems. This notion of a cure has placed the burden for health on the healthcare provider rather than promoting individual behavior change. The well–sick distinction also has contributed to stigma, which can have an insidious effect on all levels of healthcare and deter individuals from seeking help with behavior change (Corrigan, 2004). The reality is that health and loss of it are best described as dynamic. Even a dental cavity is in a state of flux and can recover somewhat with care.

A good definition of health might be the one proposed by Last (1988), namely, "a state characterized by anatomical, physiological, and psychological integrity; ability to perform personally valued family, work, and community roles; ability to deal with physical, biological, psychological, and social stress; a feeling of well-being; and freedom from the risk of disease and untimely death." Such a definition emphasizes the individual's capacity to respond and adapt, and encourages a focus on the interconnectivity of human health with the health of other entities. Fortunately, the fully integrated BHC is in a unique position to retrain health care providers in their conceptualizations of health and behavior.

The Role of PCBH in Promoting a New Model

An increased focus on creating health using behavior change technologies is clearly warranted but it faces significant barriers. The PCBH model, with its blend of co-location, collaboration, and true integration, is uniquely suited to help break down these barriers. For starters, the very presence of a BHC in a primary care clinic signals a shift from a specialization and separation model to an integrated care model. In striving for true integration, the goal of PCBH is to not only influence any one individual's care but the care delivered by the providers and system in general. Once integrated, the BHC can address system barriers, such as those discussed above, to the application of behavior change technologies. Providers can be made more aware of the prominence of avoidance strategies (and their unintended negative consequences), and the problems of conceptualizing mental health problems from a medical model perspective. The BHC can also develop a strong plan for evaluating the financial impact of adding integrated behavioral services to the clinic. (Strategies for program evaluation are in Chapter 15.)

Consider the clinical approach used in BHC visits, which attempts to avoid the problems inherent in using a medical model for behavioral issues. The PCBH approach focuses on improving functioning rather than on eliminating a presumed "disorder" or "disease". Practitioners of this model speak, for example, of teaching a patient with concentration problems techniques for improving the concentration; the focus is not on finding a supposed "cause" of the concentration problem, such as depression, ADHD, obsessive-compulsive disorder, etc. This approach often resonates with PCPs, who (despite being trained in the disease model) often make medication decisions based on functioning. Many have an inherent skepticism about the DSM diagnostic system. They develop questions about the diagnostic system when they realize, for example, that one medication (e.g., Zoloft) can be used to treat several supposedly distinct disorders (e.g., depression, chronic pain, posttraumatic stress disorder, panic disorder). This is a phenomenon that often does not compute for those trained to link specific syndromes to specific treatments. Though they might not readily perceive this in themselves, PCPs often naturally de-emphasize diagnosis when prescribing and instead focus simply on what "works" (i.e., what improves functioning). This pragmatism and skepticism can easily be capitalized on by the BHC to help PCPs move away from a stigmatizing diagnostic approach that holds empty promises of cures and move toward more functionally-based conceptualizations of behavior problems.

Note that the PCBH approach we are describing is not antipharmaceutical. Rather, it is about changing how behavioral problems are conceptualized in the primary care arena. There clearly are numerous pharmacological approaches with demonstrated effectiveness for the treatment of behaviorally based problems, and in many cases the role of a BHC is even to help patients comply with a medication plan. Improving a PCP's understanding of how to work with patients using behavioral techniques will hopefully help decrease the *inappropriate* use of medications, but in a biopsychosocial model there will always be a place for medication treatments.

THEORIES AND THERAPIES RECOMMENDED FOR THE BHC

The remainder of this chapter is divided into brief reviews of the concepts and approaches most commonly used by a BHC in clinical practice. The Stress-Coping-Vulnerability model and research on styles of coping are discussed, as they reinforce the notion that people suffer in similar ways, regardless of the context for the suffering. This model also helps PCPs understand coping in ways they can readily assess and address. Motivational interviewing and problem-solving techniques, for example, provide for a pragmatic approach to functional improvement, regardless of the presenting problem. The "third-wave" behavior therapies represent a new advance that aims to help people suffer better (or function better while suffering). By combining competence in traditional and newer behavior therapies, the BHC will be well-equipped to handle the myriad of problems seen in primary care.

We assume that our readers have working knowledge of well-established behavioral and cognitive-behavioral therapies, so have omitted details of them (though they are mentioned). For most of the selected theories and approaches only a very basic description is provided. A lengthier description is, unfortunately, beyond the scope of this book. However, considerably more detail is provided on acceptance and commitment therapy (a third-wave approach) because its concepts are likely to be new to many readers and they are referenced frequently throughout this text. Readers are encouraged to seek out more training in all of these areas, especially new and emerging approaches. Appendix A provides a list of recommended readings for each of the models and techniques discussed.

When selecting an intervention during a patient visit, remember that primary care is ultimately a place for pragmatists. This is true whether one is a BHC or a PCP, and whether using medicines or behavioral interventions. Whether one chooses to use a motivational intervention, a traditional behavioral intervention or a third-wave approach depends on multiple factors, such as functional analysis findings, provider knowledge, receptivity of the patient, time available, and what has been tried by the patient before (among others). The goal of the following sections is simply to highlight theories and approaches that will be useful for the BHC's armamentaria. The more familiar one is with these, the more able he or she will be to rather quickly create interventions that work and that can be taught to primary care colleagues.

Stress-Coping-Vulnerability Model

Stress-coping-vulnerability models see humans as existing in a dynamic environment that involves responding to both internal and external stress with stress-buffering or coping responses. Problems with functioning arise in the interplay of three major social and psychological realms: (1) recently occurring stresses that can vary in magnitude from daily hassles to major life events, (2) personal dispositions that influence the individual's reactivity to the stresses (including genetic vulnerabilities, resources, and liabilities resulting from remote learning histories), and (3) the individual's repertoire of coping skills (e.g., stress management, assertiveness, problem-solving, mindfulness, values clarification focus, etc.). Behavior problems occur when the individual encounters stressful events and experiences that heighten vulnerability and overshadow the individual's skills for coping (Scodol, Dohrenwend, Link, & Shrout, 1990). Through the lens of the medical model, a person's presentation may suggest psychopathology that requires medications. From a stress and coping framework, the same person may be seen as experiencing a shift in stress-coping equilibrium and in need of a behavior change plan to correct that.

A central assumption of this model is that most psychologically healthy or normal people have symptoms of dysfunction, just as physically healthy people at times have aches and pains. The preponderance of difference between a person who receives a label from the dozens available in DSM-IV TR and the person who doesn't, centers on the person's skills for coping with problems. These skills presumably are learned over a lifetime of interacting with one's environment, through such processes as modeling, operant conditioning and classical conditioning. In some cases skills learned are adaptive and health-protective, as in the case of someone who learns to go for a walk when stressed. In other cases skills learned may be maladaptive, as in the case of someone who learns to drink alcohol when overwhelmed by stress. But in all cases, the behaviors are presumed learned in a completely natural fashion, with no prejudgment on the inherent value of the behavior. Value judgments regarding behaviors are made only with respect to whether the behavior functions to promote or to detract from health. An individual who exhibits insufficient or maladaptive skills for coping is not presumed to be pathological or diseased, but rather in need of skills training.

Teaching PCPs. Unlike most medical providers who are trained in a medical/disease model, most behavioral health providers have training in brief and strategic therapies and/or cognitive behavioral therapy, both of which originate from the Stress-Coping-Vulnerability model. In fact, most empirically-validated cognitive behavioral treatments have coping and stress-reduction skill development at their core (Strosahl, 2005). In contrast, most PCPs have been trained in a disease model that suggests use of the DSM-IV (as a method for identifying specific mental diseases) and prescribing medications as a method for curing disease. Teaching them the stress-coping-vulnerability model can help PCPs adopt a better-rounded, and possibly more effective, approach to identifying, conceptualizing, and treating behavioral problems.

Informal case discussions and more formal case presentations (e.g., during meetings) provide a good format for teaching PCPs to talk with patients about brief stress management techniques. Most PCP's already talk about stress with their patients, but may welcome the Stress-Coping-Vulnerability framework as one that is less pathologizing and stigmatizing than a traditional disease model. Many will also welcome instruction in standard Cognitive Behavioral Therapy (CBT) interventions that stem from a Stress-Coping-Vulnerability model. Teaching stress management interventions (e.g., relaxation training, problem-solving, scheduling of pleasurable activities, personal assertion skills) will often be appreciated. Not all providers will be interested, but many will try talking about these techniques with patients rather than focusing immediately and solely on finding a medication.

Several years ago, in response to the overwhelming need for more behavioral health care, the Australian government gave PCPs support for learning a group of "Focused Psychological Strategies". The PCPs were trained in these strategies and then delivered them in the course of their work (Jackson-Bowers & McCabe, 2002). The 2002 Medicare Benefits Schedule (MBS) for Australia included codes for PCPs who participated in the "Better Outcomes in Mental Health Care (BOiMHC)" initiative (Commonwealth Department of Health and Ageing, 2002). In the Australian model, focused psychological strategies included psychoeducation, motivational interviewing, behavioral therapy (including behavior modification, exposure techniques, and behavioral activation), cognitive interventions (including cognitive analysis, challenging, and restructuring), relaxation strategies (including progressive muscle relaxation and controlled breathing), skills training (including problem-solving, anger management, social skills training, communication training, and parent management training), and interpersonal therapy. In Australia, PCPs who complete training and practice with some supervision are credentialed to provide these interventions in thirty-minute visits for up to six sessions in any twelve-month period (Hickie & Groom, 2002). We mention this initiative because it provides an excellent list of skills a BHC might wish to work on with interested PCPs. In this country, PCPs will not usually be able to utilize these approaches in thirty-minute visits, but the more of these approaches they understand the more agile they become during visits with patients.

Most of the standard cognitive-behavioral techniques mentioned above will be familiar to readers. However, two that might not be, motivational interviewing and problem-solving therapy, deserve some elaboration. Both are approaches that can be widely applied in the PCBH model and are important to teach to PCPs as well.

Motivational Interviewing. Motivational Interviewing (MI) (Miller & Rollnick, 2002) is perhaps best described as a "way of being" with patients that has the goal of helping them identify problem areas and improve motivation to change those areas. It can be a powerful intervention for patients ambivalent about making a behavior change. Various techniques comprise MI, including reflective listening, open-ended questioning, and summarizing of the positives and negatives of a proposed behavior change, all with the goal of eliciting self-change statements *from the patient.* The goal in MI, in other words, is for the patient to start talking about why he or she would benefit from change instead of the provider doing so. This is quite different from the approach often seen in medical settings, which typically involves dictums from a provider and expressions of disappointment or (worse yet) lecturing when patients resist change. In MI, the provider asks questions in a nonjudgmental, curious manner so as to help the patient examine the effect(s) of a problem behavior on his or her health or life goals. If resistance to change is encountered from the patient, this is considered a provider problem rather than a patient problem. Resistance simply indicates the need for the provider to shift tactics with the patient.

Though first used to treat addictions, MI is also proving useful for facilitating lifestyle change for health promotion and chronic disease prevention. It is not intended to replace traditional educational or other provider-directed interventions, but instead is best used as a preparation for them with patients who are ambivalent. Some patients will make changes based solely on an educational intervention by a provider, but for the many who express ambivalence, MI will be much more effective than attempts to lecture or shame the patient to change.

Teaching PCPs. For PCPs accustomed to a hierarchical doctor–patient relationship in which they direct patients to make changes, the transition to MI interventions can be challenging. The task is made doubly difficult by the time constraints in primary care, which leave many PCPs feeling the best they can do is to simply tell patients what changes to make. One way to address these concerns is to remind PCPs of the time spent on repeated unsuccessful efforts to provoke patient change. Repeated efforts to convince an ambivalent patient to quit smoking, for example, could go on for years, adding up to a significant chunk of time spent. That time would likely be better spent using a MI approach in each visit, which is more likely to produce change and to produce it faster. Remind PCPs that MI is not an intervention that needs to be conducted in addition to the usual education, but rather in place of it for patients who are ambivalent.

Another important point to teach PCPs relates to the stages of change model, which underlies much of MI. In this model, readiness for change is not construed as fixed but rather as a fluid state that ranges from precontemplation to maintenance of a change. Thus, if an intervention helps move a patient closer to change it is considered a success, even if the patient continues to lack complete readiness for change. Many times PCPs become frustrated when patients fail to actually complete a behavior change, not realizing that the patient might actually be moving closer to making that change. In these cases the PCP misses the opportunity to reinforce important approximations to change.

Handouts that simplify MI for time-strapped PCPs can be helpful. For example, a handout might suggest specific questions to use to ascertain a patient's level of readiness for change, along with one or two interventions for each level of readiness. Of course, in some cases, PCPs will prefer to simply have the patient see the BHC to discuss readiness to change. This is certainly better than a busy PCP resorting to telling a patient what to do and moving on.

Problem-Solving Therapy. A behavior therapy approach that grew out of the work on coping, named Problem Solving Therapy (PST), is invaluable for work in the PCBH model. Originally applied to depression, PST has been effective in reducing distress in a variety of populations, including cancer patients (Nezu, Nezu, Felgoise, McClure, & Houts, 2003). Early research that contributed to development of PST showed the following: (1) negative life events often result in an increase in problems, (2) the degree to which one effectively copes with these problems is a function of his or her problem-solving ability, and (3) effectively resolving problems decreases the likelihood of experiencing depression symptoms (Nezu, 1986). The basic purpose of PST, then, is to teach patients how to effectively solve problems.

There are five components to the PST approach. The first, problem orientation, is a bit different from the other four. Problem orientation is geared toward providing patients with a rational, positive, and constructive set to problems in living and to problem-solving as a means of coping with them. The goal is to change attitudes or beliefs that can preclude work on the other four components. Patients are also taught to use emotions as cues for identifying the existence of a problem and to inhibit the tendency to respond automatically to problems (engaging instead in the problem-solving process). The remaining four components teach patients (1) problem definition and formulation (breaking a problem down into specific parts and identifying specific goals), (2) generation of alternatives (brainstorming a list of possible solutions), (3) decision-making (evaluating possible consequences of the alternatives and selecting the most optimal ones), and (4) solution implementation and verification (evaluating the solution outcome after its implementation).

Many patients seen in PC can benefit from a problem-solving approach, particularly if they already identify a problem and utilize problem-focused coping. Many of these patients simply need some help brainstorming possible solutions or help sorting through the alternatives. The PST approach also works nicely in the context of group visits for chronic conditions. In some group visit models (see Chapter 12), a PCP and BHC can work together to problem-solve with patients who, by nature of their attendance at the group, likely recognize the existence of a problem and are seeking ways to manage it.

Teaching PCPs. Many PCPs are excellent problem-solvers themselves, a quality that perhaps led them into medicine or perhaps results from their medical school training. As such, they tend to understand the PST approach rapidly and may be more likely to use it than some other interventions. A twenty-minute presentation during lunchtime or at a provider meeting that focuses on the four problem-solving components (excluding problem orientation) may be all that is needed to prompt some PCPs to try PST. We recommend excluding the problem orientation component for a brief talk because it is a bit more complicated, and less straight-forward than the other four components.

The Role of Coping Styles in Selecting an Intervention

The coping interventions described above, meaning the standard cognitive-behavioral approaches, will often rapidly help patients achieve improvements in functioning. Patients who employ a problem-focused approach to problems tend to respond readily. They are typically open to reviewing and applying problem-solving strategies, using relaxation techniques, or practicing self-guided exposure. These patients often need minimal assistance from the PCP or BHC beyond initial instruction and support. Even patients needing a motivational intervention may be problem-focused and may utilize a cognitive-behavioral intervention once ready. The problem with such patients is simply that at the time of the BHC encounter they are not yet motivated to approach the problem.

However, patients with strong behavioral patterns of avoidance may benefit less from the interventions that originate from the stress-coping-vulnerability model. Rather than addressing a problem, the patient utilizing avoidance-focused coping will prefer instead to avoid all aspects of it (including even thinking about it). He or she may go to extraordinary lengths to avoid facing a problem and the unwanted emotions that accompany it, and may be singularly focused on eliminating the unwanted emotions (without a clear idea of how). For patients such as these, a different approach (described in the upcoming section on "Third-Wave Behavior Therapies") might prove more helpful. Table 5.1 displays basic differences in the presentation of problem-focused versus avoidance-focused patients.

Teaching PCPs. Providers may inadvertently support entrenchment in emotional and behavioral avoidance patterns, rather than making a closer evaluation of the patient's stance toward distress and suffering in general. When a PCP says, for example, "You certainly have a lot of anxiety about dealing with your boss at work. Perhaps you should take some time off," the message to the patient is that stress is something to be avoided and that avoidance of problems is helpful. Patients with strong avoidant patterns of coping typically do not benefit from such advice. They are often unclear in their goals and may have not focused on valued directions in life for quite

Table 5.1. Differences between problem-focused and avoidance-focused patients

	Problem-focused	Avoidance-focused
Problem identification	Clear definition of problems, ownership of problems	Blame shifted to others
Generation of solutions	Capable of brainstorming, evaluating options	Feels victimized, prefers the provider offer a solution
Implementing plan	Capable of forming, implementing and evaluating a step-by-step plan	May agree to a plan, such as taking medicines, but often struggles with implementation
Resolution	Attends follow-up	May avoid follow-up until condition worsens

some time. These patients often persevere in ineffective problem-solving behaviors and rely on strategies to avoid thinking or feeling. Helping PCPs to recognize these problems in patients can lead to significant changes in patient–provider interactions.

In teaching PCPs about problem- versus avoidance-focused coping, a handout of Table 5.1 can be helpful. Emphasize to PCPs that patients utilizing problem-focused coping are good candidates for standard cognitive-behavioral interventions, including problem-solving therapy, whereas those using avoidance-focused coping may need an alternative, acceptance-based approaches, such as those explained next.

Third-Wave Behavior Therapies

To be optimally effective in primary care, knowledge of all facets of behavior therapy is crucial. In addition to traditional behavior therapy approaches, several new directions for behavior therapy have emerged over the last two decades, and these so-called third wave behavior therapies are the focus of this section. In the third wave, behavior therapists are exploring nontraditional areas, such as acceptance, mindfulness, cognitive diffusion, and values. Third-wave approaches question basic assumptions about mental illness and suggest that suffering and struggle are characteristic of people whether they have mental problems or not (Hayes, 2004). The direction of intervention is toward helping individuals live value-driven lives, rather than to be symptom-free. These approaches include Acceptance and Commitment Therapy (ACT) (Biglan, 1995; Hayes, Strosahl, & Wilson, 1999), Functional Analytic Psychotherapy (FAP) (Kohlenberg, Kanter, Bolling, Wexner, & Parker, 2004), Mindfulness Based Cognitive Therapy (MBCT) (Segal, Williams, & Teasdale, 2002) and Dialectical Behavior Therapy (DBT) (Linehan, 1993).

To understand what these approaches might offer that is unique from earlier behavior therapies, we need to consider the first and second wave approaches briefly. The first wave addressed the scientific weaknesses of the then current nonempirical clinical traditions, such as psychoanalysis. These first wave approaches focused directly on decreasing harmful behaviors and increasing helpful behaviors and relied largely on principles of operant and classical conditioning. The second wave continued with direct change efforts guided by social learning theory and included cognitive as well as behavioral and emotive targets. Cognitive therapy emerged in the second wave, and the focus of technology development was on changing the individual's problem behaviors by changing the thoughts presumed to cause and maintain them. As a part of the third wave, both behavioral and cognitive camps are now evaluating techniques that emphasize context. The introduction of this concept has spurred the development of a host of experiential procedures that may actually enhance the effects of first and second wave behavior therapies.

One of us (PR) trained in Acceptance and Commitment Therapy (ACT) in the early 1990s and incorporated it into day-to-day BHC work. The other (JR) is learning and applying ACT strategies with success in primary care. Therefore, we often use ACT to illustrate the use of third wave technology in a PCBH practice in our clinical chapters (i.e., Chapters 9 to 12). We do want to say that many standard first and second wave behavioral interventions are also helpful, but we have weighted the clinical chapters toward third wave technologies to give readers ideas for applying them in primary care.

ACT is built upon a theory involving five core processes (see Figure 5.1), all of which have been demonstrated in ACT's companion science known as Relational Frame Theory (RFT) (Roche, Barnes-Holmes, Barnes-Holmes, Stewart, & O'Hora, 2002). RFT involves an experimental analysis

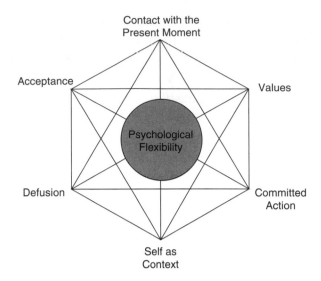

Figure 5.1. Acceptance and commitment therapy: Core processes (Reprinted with permission from Hayes & Strosahl, 2004).

of human language and cognition, and RFT findings suggest that "cognitive fusion" and "experiential avoidance" are both ubiquitous and harmful (Hayes, 2004). ACT strategies target (1) cognitive fusion (i.e., being unable to separate one's sense of self from one's emotions, thoughts, and feelings); (2) experiential avoidance (i.e., using any of a host of cognitive, emotional, and behavioral strategies to avoid direct experience of unpleasant feelings, thoughts, and sensations); and (3) psychological flexibility (i.e., the ability to choose a direction and behave in the world in ways that are consistent with that direction despite experiencing unwanted thoughts, feelings, and behaviors that are contrary to the direction).

With the use of ACT strategies and exercises, patients acknowledge and experience discomforting internal events while behaving in ways that are consistent with valued directions in life, including the fundamentally important value of good health. While not essential, good health may empower pursuit of other valued directions such as loving relationships, meaningful spiritual pursuits, satisfying work, and restorative leisure. All of these can add immeasurably to well-being, even when health deteriorates.

From an ACT perspective, patient deficits in psychological flexibility are by-products of the domination of verbal functions (such as rules like, "If you don't like it, get rid of it"), which are amplified by the culture. The culture, of course, may declare that no one should experience pain and that crying is a sign of weakness. In ACT terminology, patients may fuse (i.e., merge) with verbal phenomenon, and diffusion strategies (i.e., those that help a person have a sense of self that is larger than the self that suffers) are needed to help them recontextualize their experience of the verbal phenomenon. From an ACT perspective, all humans engage in experiential avoidance, as it is built-in to human language. Technically, experiential avoidance is the tendency to attempt to alter the form, frequency, or situation sensitivity of historically produced negative private experience. It occurs even when it causes psychological and behavioral harm. It is clinically important for the BHC to understand that negative private experience includes unwanted emotions (such as anxiety and depression), thoughts (such as, "I'm not good enough and I'm all alone and nobody is helping me"), and bodily sensations (such as rapid heart beat, sweating, bloating, dizziness, and shortness of breath).

Patients who lack psychological flexibility have difficulties acting in ways that are inconsistent with what their minds say and tend to ignore the lessons inherent in their experience. The same may be equally true of providers, who can persevere in offering treatments that are supposed to work, but are not working for a particular patient. A patient may not know that he or she can play with a grandchild and laugh while hearing the mind say, "I am a failure; a fake; my grand child is sick and tired of me." He or she might not realize it is possible to take a walk and perceive the beauty of the trees while hearing the mind insist, "I am in pain; this pain is dangerous; it will get worse; I can't take it any more." A PCP may similarly not know that he or she can refuse to make a referral for an unneeded procedure while hearing the mind warn, "You could be wrong; best not to take a chance; what would your colleagues think if... ?." It is often the patients who are lacking psychological flexibility that bring providers into contact with their own deficits in psychological flexibility.

When patients fail repeatedly in efforts to solve problems and reduce stress, they experience greater emotional distress and respond with greater emotional and behavioral avoidance; i.e., greater suffering. In their primary care visits, they receive more intensive treatment. Unfortunately, the treatment given may help them continue to avoid the experience of failing to solve problems of living as well as the accompanying physical and psychological discomfort. In conducting a functional analysis, one easily perceives this humiliating pattern of failure and avoidance among patients who struggle with substance abuse, chronic pain, recurrent depression, generalized anxiety, and other problems. Many others are demoralized by their lack of success in creating better mental and physical health. They do not know that they lack skills needed to solve overwhelming problems; they persevere in applying ineffective strategies; they blame themselves (and sometimes their health care providers); and they continue to live with little hope in dissatisfying life contexts. These patients often cannot stop what they are doing to address stressful circumstances, even though their strategies are not working. They struggle with learning from their experience and tend to be caught up in their minds, often rigidly adhering to rules that may be present in the culture but which in actuality are not supported by the experience of most members of the culture. For example, chronic pain patients often subscribe to the commonly held notion that with the discoveries of miracle medicine, no one should have to suffer pain.

The cost of cognitive fusion and experiential avoidance for health care is probably huge, as these problems may drive unnecessary primary and specialty care and contribute a great deal to provider burn out. ACT and other third wave approaches acknowledge and often integrate older behavioral traditions while focusing on second order and contextual change. The shift from form to function is an important advance, particularly for health care patients who lack flexible and effective repertoires for addressing stress. For these patients, use of ACT and other third wave strategies may energize the impact of first and second wave behavior therapies, and thus, improve patient outcomes and provider satisfaction. The patient with diabetes who makes gains in psychological flexibility can tolerate anxiety about disease and death, clearly identify personal values, and then show behavioral actions consistent with those values. The provider who trains in psychological acceptance may be more capable of experiencing his or her discomfort in response to the chronic pain patient's request for narcotic medications and to choose a response based on dearly held principles of medicine, even while feeling intensely uncomfortable with the patient's affect. Within the core processes of ACT, we may find keys to creating the psychological flexibility that will help patients and providers let go of the magic bullet notion that suffering can be eliminated.

While all patients want to be healthy, patients with deficits in psycho-logical flexibility are poorly equipped to create the health status they desire and they often live in contexts that fail to support health-promoting behaviors. Some are unaware of what they do to pursue health, so cannot build upon their repertoire of health-promoting behaviors. Perhaps even more are blind to the cost of their daily efforts to avoid confronting the anxiety-provoking topic of health. Lacking the prerequisite skills for rising to the level of awareness where intention and choice are possible, they con-tinue on. Meanwhile, providers of primary care may inadvertently rein-force their continuation of an unworkable struggle. To help the growing segment of the population who face these challenges, the BHC needs to employ powerful therapeutic strategies and to be able to teach these to PCPs trained in the old symptom-elimination mode.

Teaching PCPs. Many PCPs will be receptive to learning about behavior therapy strategies. They know the limitations of their standard interven-tions and seek more empowering approaches. The BHC will be able to make some behavioral interventions more transparent than others, and thirdwave behavior technologies may be somewhat of a challenge to teach, as some concepts directly contradict common medical training. For example, one of us (PR) had a PCP say to her after a series of lunch-hour ACT trainings, "Do you know how hard it is to do what you are asking us to do! We are trained to be problem solvers and to eliminate symptoms." The BHC needs to be prepared to ask, "And when that doesn't work, what do you do?" as this is the question that can help PCPs explore new options.

While most PCPs will not want to read a book on CBT or ACT, many might read a book chapter and later perhaps a self-help book (e.g., Hayes & Smith, 2005). The Hayes and Strosahl (2004) book has chapters on ACT in medical settings and using ACT with patients with chronic pain, and these and/or the new self-help book on ACT (*Get Out of Your Mind and into Your Life*) might be acceptable reading material for a lunch hour study group.

SUMMARY

1. In this chapter, we challenged our reader to reconsider the traditions of making diagnoses and working to eliminate symptoms. These traditions have combined with other factors to advance the pharmaceutical industry at the expense of behavior change research

and funding, while promoting the false notion of a "cure" and discouraging self-driven change. The PCBH model strives instead to help patients improve functioning by developing a repertoire of health-protective behaviors with ongoing support from their PCP.

2. To make progress in meeting the challenges facing healthcare today, several problems must be overcome. These include the culture of separation and specialization, the prominence of avoidance strategies in our society, the inadequacy of models for evaluating health care costs, and the biomedicalization of mental health. As a fully integrated participant in primary care, the BHC is well-positioned to chip away at these.

3. A variety of theories and therapies are used and/or adapted for patient care in the PCBH model. These include both traditional cognitive-behavioral and newer "third-wave" approaches. These help improve functioning regardless of diagnosis, and as such they fit well with the PCBH model. Most can be easily taught to PCPs.

4. Newer, "third-wave" behavior change technologies such as ACT, mindfulness, functional analytic psychotherapy, and dialectical behavior therapy promote living in a more immediate and present manner while acting in the world in ways that reflect deeply held values. These approaches have much to offer BHCs and PCPs alike.

6

MEASURES FOR A PRIMARY CARE BEHAVIORAL HEALTH PRACTICE

"The force that through the green fuse drives the flower Drives my green age."

—Dylan Thomas

Self-report tools are a mainstay of many specialty mental health practices and training for administering and interpreting them constitutes a significant chunk of a psychologist's training years. As a result, new BHCs are often dismayed to learn that psychological testing is not generally a part of the PCBH model. There is certainly a role for self-report tools to play in primary care, though, meaning one's training in assessment can still be put to good use. While the MMPI will not be a part of the BHC's toolkit, the ability to select and appropriately use brief self-report tools can come in quite handy.

In primary care, self-report measures can be important for a variety of reasons. Brief measures can be used to help detect behavioral problems, such as alcohol misuse, that might otherwise go unnoticed. They can also be useful for planning individualized interventions and evaluating the impact of interventions in follow-up. Further, the use of measures may provide another way of influencing PCPs. When a BHC uses tools such as quality of life measures that exemplify the "green fuse" of health, mental and physical, it helps PCPs reconceptualize their definition of "health" to be more inclusive of behavior. In some cases, PCPs will also follow suit and begin using measures to improve their own accuracy in planning and evaluating care. With these possibilities in mind, this chapter provides guidelines for the use of self-report measures in primary care. We introduce measures that are used commonly for various problems and suggest how BHCs can use them optimally and best "sell" them to their PC colleagues. Implementation of effective measurement tools, whether used routinely or when indicated, can enhance the delivery of services by both BHC and PCP.

PLANNING SCREENING AND ASSESSMENT ACTIVITIES

Though often confused, the terms "screening" and "assessment" actually refer to separate processes. Screening is conducted to identify individuals at risk of a health condition or having significant signs of one. Typically all members of a population are screened, though a population may be narrowly defined. For example, when screening for depression, one could screen all patients in a clinic annually or only those at higher risk, such as patients with diabetes. Assessment refers to the procedure applied to individuals who screen positive. The goal of assessment is to confirm the presence of the health condition and measure its severity. Screening and assessment efforts can both improve patient care in the primary care clinic, but their introduction may meet with resistance from some members of the team. Typically this resistance stems from fears of an added work burden. The good news is that with some creativity, flexibility, and persistence, any initial resistance can usually be overcome. To help ensure that new clinic-wide screening efforts succeed, consider the following guidelines before getting started.

Guideline 1: Get Buy-In to Pilot a Measure

Providing presentations on the evidence for screening and assessment, along with identifying staff or PCP opinion leaders with an interest in the area, will usually provide enough buy-in to pilot a measure. While pilot studies can be time-consuming, they may save time in the long run. They often identify glitches and build support, which helps with subsequent dissemination efforts. They can also provide a sense of what is feasible for the primary care setting, including what is feasible for the BHC. For example, if half of the clinic's patients screen positive for depression in the pilot study, what adjustments will the BHC need to make if the screener is routinely used?

Guideline 2: Make it User Friendly

Successful screening and assessment activities involving PCPs rely on clear answers to who, what, when, where, how, and how much time. The following list of questions can be used as a checklist to help plan for PCP-based screening. Both here and throughout the rest of the chapter ideas are provided for how to answer these questions.

1. *Who will ask the screening or assessment questions?* The BHC or BHA can complete all assessments associated with BHC visits, but who will be responsible for them during PCP visits? Support staff selected for this task (often medical/nursing assistants) should be responsible for maintaining the supply of measures and keeping them organized, as well.

2. *What are the conditions of concern at a clinic?* While screening for dementia may be a priority for providers at a clinic that serves a large group of older patients, another clinic may have more concerns about substance abuse. Also, most clinics already screen routinely for some problems, so the questions to answer may be whether the extant system could be better and/or whether screening for additional problems might be warranted.

3. *When will the screening or assessment occur?* Should it be done as needed, when a problem is suspected or identified? Or could it be done routinely, at a designated interval? If given routinely, what is the most workable interval for the clinic? Keep in mind that some patients visit the clinic frequently while others rarely do, so a screening system should try to capture all patients without becoming burdensome to patients and staff.

4. *Where will screening occur, and where will any paper measures be stored or located?* Consider placing measures in hanging files on the BHC office door or in exam rooms. Many providers will begin, with a minimum of encouragement, to use measures if they are available

in clearly labeled files (e.g., "Adult PHQ-9, English"; "Age four to fourteen Child Screener, Spanish"). Completion of measures usually occurs in the exam room, but could it be done in the waiting room or even at home before an appointment?

5. *How will screening and assessment results be scored, communicated to providers, and entered into the medical record?* Measures used during PCP visits may be scored by a medical/nursing assistant in the exam room before the PCP enters, or by the PCP during the visit. Clinics using electronic medical records may want to build room for screener scores in provider templates or even have patients complete the screener on the computer in the exam room.

6. *How much time will screening and assessment require?* If screening is lengthy and has a negative effect on PCP productivity, it will not be viewed favorably. Measurement activities for PCP visits, including administration, scoring and scoring documentation, need to require less than five minutes to meet the PC feasibility criteria.

When efforts to launch screening and assessment activities fail, it is often the result of a poorly organized plan or a failure to address feasibility issues. Think through the above issues carefully, with the help of the ideas in the rest of this chapter, and conduct a pilot effort to identify and address implementation problems.

Guideline 3: It's All About the Functioning

In politics the line might be, "It's the economy, stupid!" but in primary care that changes to, "It's the functioning, stupid!" The goal of screening and assessment is not generally to make a DSM-based diagnosis, as that often holds little value over and above a functional assessment for either the BHC or PCP. Instead, the goals are to (1) identify "problems" (rather than diagnoses) that often go undetected in primary care but that have a negative effect on health (e.g., family violence, alcohol misuse, etc.); (2) help the PCP to select the most appropriate medication to use, while minimizing the likelihood of adverse side effects (e.g., screening for a history of mania before starting a selective serotonin reuptake inhibitor); and (3) measure treatment response over time. Attempting to use traditional psychological assessment tools, such as personality inventories or exhaustive symptom-based diagnostic checklists will take up far too much BHC time, and is simply not appropriate for a BHC service. Rarely will the finer points of a diagnostic assessment change much in a PCP's treatment plan. Primary care is a world that revolves around pragmatism, and the best way to fit into that world and to be helpful is to think functionally.

Guideline 4: Select the Right Measure

A plethora of options exists when it comes to finding self-report tools for most problems. Finding ones that work in primary care, however, can be more challenging. In the sections that follow, we offer specific measures for the reader's consideration, but ultimately the choice of which to use will depend on a clinic's preferences and resources. When selecting a measure, the following characteristics are the most desirable:

- *Brevity.* Both BHC and PCP visits require brief measures. Questionnaires with more than twenty items are probably too lengthy.
- *Translated versions exist.* This is particularly important in federally qualified health centers, which tend to serve very diverse patient populations. At least make certain measures are available in the non-English language encountered most frequently in the clinic.
- *Available for free or at low cost.* Owing to the volume of patients seen, clinics will burn through copies of measures quickly. For this reason, measures available publicly for free, such as via download from the internet, often make the most sense. Given the wide selection of good quality measures available at no cost, one needs some compelling reasons to choose one that must be purchased.
- *High quality.* Psychologists are trained to be very selective in the assessment instruments they use, and for good reason. In the primary care clinic, measures chosen for use will be completed by thousands of patients, and they will often play a central role in treatment planning. Be sure to examine carefully the psychometrics of all measures being considered for use.
- *Appropriate reading level.* A widely-used measure should probably require a maximum of 8th grade reading skills. Patients who are unable to read may not convey this to the BHC, choosing instead to

answer random or only selected questions. Patients whose language is not English are actually less of a concern because they are more easily identified and can then be matched with an interpreter who can help with completion of the measure.

- *Easy to score.* This is related to the "brevity" concept, in that measures requiring a lot of time to score are not usually feasible in primary care. Bear in mind, however, that some measures have a small number of items but a complicated scoring procedure. These are often less desirable than measures that produce, for example, a single tallied score.

Although a measure chosen by a BHC might not possess all of the above qualities, the more of these that are present the greater the likelihood that the measure will work in the primary care setting.

SCREENING TO DETECT SPECIFIC PROBLEMS

For any PCP, detection of behavioral problems can be difficult. In Chapter 1, we discussed the various factors that contribute to this problem, such as brevity of visits and stigma associated with emotional issues, among others. Yet, most patients with behavioral problems are seen exclusively in primary care settings, meaning the only possibility for treatment may depend on detection by PCPs. Fortunately, identifying patients at risk for poor health outcomes may enable early effective treatment and improved outcomes. While primary care resources may be too limited to support comprehensive treatment for the huge group of patients who present with behavioral concerns, detection of problems and delivery of brief interventions may improve clinical outcomes for a large number of primary care patients, who might otherwise receive nothing (e.g., Katon et al., 1996).

With this in mind, there are several areas worthy of consideration for routine screening in primary care, including mood problems, alcohol misuse, cognitive impairment, exposure to violence, eating problems, and pediatric behavioral problems. Indeed, the most common, and most commonly missed, behavioral problems in primary care are depression, anxiety, alcohol abuse, and cognitive impairment (Halverson & Chan, 2004). Though all are certainly worthy causes, even raising the idea of screening routinely for all of the aforementioned problems in a primary care clinic would rather quickly win a BHC some enemies. Thus, in this section, we discuss the arguments and evidence for screening for these problems and others, in hopes that the reader will gain ideas for getting the most bang out of the screening buck.

A case can be made for focusing on any of the common problems. However, in arguably the most comprehensive series of reviews on this topic to date, the U.S. Preventive Services Task Force (USPSTF) found the most support for routine screenings for depression and alcohol misuse (Pignone et al., 2002; United States Preventive Services Task Force, 2004). They found insufficient evidence to recommend for or against routine screening for family violence, drug abuse, cognitive impairment, or pediatric behavior problems. Their review does not include recommendations regarding screening for some other common problems, such as anxiety. The USPSTF is a nongovernmental panel of topical experts assembled by the U.S. Public Health Service to review scientific data and provide recommendations to practitioners. The recommendations of the panel, for a host of problems, can be found online at www.preventiveservices.ahrq.gov or via the National Guideline Clearinghouse at www.guideline.gov. The recommendations of the American Academy of Family Physicians for clinical preventive services all derive directly from the work of this task force, so it is a good resource for BHCs. Their findings and recommendations differ in some cases from those of prominent associations, but nonetheless their review was an impressive one and many PCP's are aware of the recommendations.

Considering the USPSTF findings, if one is searching for an evidence-based strategy for screening, the choice might be to implement routine screenings for depression and/or alcohol misuse for starters, then consider building in routine screenings for other problems later if desired. However, given the importance of buy-in from staff and PCP's, a choice based on their preference may prove more productive than one based on the evidence.

One important distinction to make for this section is that of "routine" screening versus "indicator-based" screening. The former refers to inquiry that is done on a planned, regular basis from healthcare provider to patient about a particular problem. It might be done verbally or with paper-and-pencil methods, and the target is all members of a given population. The latter, in contrast, is conducted only when signs or indicators of a problem exist. Thus, for example, routine screening for domestic violence might mean that all patients are asked about it in paperwork that is completed prior to every physical exam. Indicator-based screening would mean that patients get asked about domestic violence if a PCP suspects it based on behavioral or physical or other signs. The USPSTF reviews were mainly conducted to determine the evidence for routine screening. For many problems the use of the measures for indicator-based screening will be helpful, even if the evidence for routine screening is less clear.

In the paragraphs that follow, we discuss possible measures to use as screeners, which are displayed in tables according to problem. Where necessary, we elaborate in the text on measures in the tables, but we have purposely tried to avoid dragging the reader through a narrative about each measure. Our selection of measures is not exhaustive, only suggestive, but we have tried to include the most "primary care-friendly" tools that have adequate psychometric properties. Those described as "free online" in the tables can be accessed from a variety of websites, so rather than direct the reader to a specific site we recommend an online search using the title of the measure. Various formats of most measures can be obtained, so the reader can choose which best fits his or her preferences. Of note, there are often no clear empirical indications for selecting one measure over another. Reviews concerning depression and alcohol misuse, for example, found no reasons to recommend one screener over another for universal use (Pignone, et al., 2002; USPSTF, 2004). Suggestions for selecting a measure are discussed in Guideline #4, discussed earlier in this chapter, and the tables include as much relevant information as possible to allow for an informed selection.

Depression

Depression is common in primary care, and evidence suggests that routine screening improves detection of depression by 10 to 47 percent (Pignone et al., 2002). Bear in mind, though, that detection of depression does not in and of itself improve patient outcomes. In fact, when screening is associated with only feedback to the provider, the benefits of screening often disappear. Only when detection by screening leads to an effective intervention, which includes some sort of improved follow-up relative to usual primary care, do clinical outcomes improve (U.S. Preventive Services Task Force, 2002). This sort of follow-up is, of course, exactly what a BHC can provide.

In Table 6.1, which lists common depression screeners, one item to elaborate on is the "2-question screen." Asking two simple questions about mood and anhedonia ("Over the past two weeks, have you felt down, depressed, or helpless?" and "Over the past two weeks, have you felt little interest or pleasure in doing things?") may be as effective as using longer paper-and-pencil instruments (Whooley, Avins, Miranda, & Browner, 1997). This obviously can be the simplest way to screen and the most likely to gain favor with PCPs. The questions could be asked during the patient interview, by a nursing assistant or the PCP, or could be embedded within larger questionnaires already used by the clinic (such as questionnaires completed prior to physical exams). The Patient Health Questionnaire–9 (PHQ-9; Spitzer, Kroenke, & Williams, 1999) uses a 2-question screener, with optional administration of seven follow-up questions when screening results are positive.

The USPSTF (2002) review found insufficient evidence to recommend for or against routine screening for depression among children or adolescents. However, depression is quite common in children, with up to 20 percent experiencing an episode of major depression prior to age eighteen (Lewinsohn, Hops, Robers, Seeley, & Andrews, 1993). Further, the American Academy of Pediatrics does recommend regularly asking about depression during adolescence (American Academy of Pediatrics, 2000). Unfortunately, of the screeners validated for use with this population in primary care, many must be purchased. The Center for Epidemiological Studies-Depression Scale for Children (CES-DC) might be the best value, as it is available free, has a Spanish version, and requires only five to ten minutes to complete. Another option is to administer the Pediatric Symptom Checklist (PSC), which is a global behavioral screen rather than a depression-specific one. Both of us use the PSC at every child and adolescent visit and find it helpful for both screening and treatment response-monitoring. The PSC comes in several forms, including the original thirty-five-item measure (Jellinek et al., 1999), a seventeen-item version (Gardner et al.,1999), and a self-report version for children age eleven and up (Pagano et al., 2000).

Table 6.1. Depression screeners

Screener name	Used for	Reference	Brief description
Beck Depression Inventory for Primary Care (BDI-PC)	Depression in medical patients	Steer et al. (1999), www. psychcorp.org	7 items; purchase online
Patient Health Questionnaire-9 (PHQ-9)	Depression in medical patients	Pinto-Meza, Serrano-Blanco, Penarrubia, Blanco, & Haro (2005) and Spitzer et al. (1999)	Validated for phone use; 9 items; free online
2-question screen	Depression	Whooley et al. (1997)	1 interview question about depressed mood and 1 about anhedonia
Geriatric Depression Scale (GDS-15)	Depression in older adults	Friedman, Heisel, & Delavan (2005)	15 items; for cognitively intact adults over age 65; free online
Center for Epidemiological Studies— Depression Scale for Children (CES–DC)	Depression in adolescents	Fendrich, Weissman, & Warner (1990) and Radlof (1991)	20 items; 6th-grade reading level; for 12–18 year-olds; free online
Pediatric Symptom Checklist (PSC)	Global behavior problems in kids	Gardner et al. (1999), Jellinek et al. (1999), and Pagano, Cassidy, Little, Murphy, & Jellinek (2000)	Three versions; free online

Alcohol and Drug Problems

Alcohol and other substance use disorders are often chronic conditions that progress slowly over time, meaning primary care clinicians are in an ideal position to screen for them through their regular, long-term contact with patients. However, many patients pass through primary care without attention paid to their substance use. In a nationwide study, 94 percent of primary care physicians missed or misdiagnosed alcohol-abusing patients (i.e., when presented with early symptoms of alcohol abuse in adult patients, the physicians failed to include substance abuse among the five diagnoses they offered; National Center on Addiction and Substance Abuse, 2000). This represents a serious missed opportunity, given that estimates of the prevalence of alcohol misuse problems in adult primary care patients range from 4 to 29 percent (U.S. Preventive Health Services, 2004). Though most who use alcohol do so in moderation and without resulting problems, the cost of alcohol misuse is numerous health and social problems and more than 100,000 deaths per year (U.S. Preventive Health Services, 2004).

As mentioned earlier, the USPSTF guidelines recommend routine screening to detect alcohol misuse, in general, in all adult primary care patients. They also recommend brief interventions in primary care for those with patterns of risky and/or harmful use. A "brief intervention" as classified in the guidelines is an initial contact of at least fifteen minutes followed by at least one follow-up. As in the case of depression, this is exactly the sort of service a BHC can provide if a patient screens positive for risky or harmful drinking. The definition of "risky/hazardous" drinking is more than seven drinks per week or 3 per occasion for women, and more than fourteen drinks per week or four per occasion for men. "Harmful" use describes those experiencing physical, social, or psychological harm from alcohol use but not meeting DSM criteria for abuse or dependence (Reid, Fiellin, & O'Connor, 1999).

For adolescents, the USPSTF concluded that insufficient evidence exists to recommend for or against routine screening for alcohol problems. However, some other groups such as the American Medical Association (1997) and the American Academy of Pediatrics (1997) do recommend it. Similarly, the last USPSTF review on the topic of routine screening for drug abuse (in both adults and youth) found insufficient evidence to recommend for or against the practice, but the AMA and AAP recommend it be done annually for adolescents. The USPSTF is currently updating their recommendations on the topic of routine drug abuse screening.

Many measures have been developed for substance misuse screening, but Table 6.2 focuses on the most frequently used and/or recommended ones for primary care. In the column labeled "Used For," measures are categorized according to whether they are designed to detect more problematic use ("disorders") versus any level of problem ("misuse") and whether they are geared toward alcohol or drug screening or both. The Substance Abuse and Mental Health Services Administration's Center for Substance Abuse Treatment (CSAT) also offers a number of primary

Table 6.2. Screeners for alcohol and drug problems

Screener name	Used for	Reference	Brief description
CAGE	Alcohol disorders	Ewing (1984)	4 items, can be asked in interview or with written questions
CAGE-Adapted to Include Drugs (CAGE-AID)	Drug and alcohol disorders	Brown & Rounds (1995)	Adaptation of the CAGE to screen for drugs
Alcohol Use Disorders Identification Test (AUDIT)	Alcohol misuse	Saunders, Aasland, Babor, De la Fuente, & Grant (1993)	10-item questionnaire; free online
1-question screener	Alcohol misuse	Williams & Vinson (2001)	1 question about date of last heavy drinking episode
TWEAK	Alcohol misuse for pregnant women	Chang (2001)	5 items; detects lower levels of use that may pose risks to fetus
Rapid Alcohol Problems Screen plus Quantity and Frequency items (RAPS4-QF)	Alcohol disorders	Cherpitel (2002)	Maybe better than CAGE for diverse patient populations
CRAFFT	Alcohol and drug misuse in adolescents	Knight et al. (1999)	Maybe better than CAGE for adolescents

care screening tools and recommendations as a part of its Treatment Improvement Protocol (TIP). Several measures can be viewed at their website: http:/www.ncbi.nlm.nih.gov/books/bv.fcgi?rid=hstat5.section.45979.

The CAGE is the most widely used and best known screener for alcohol problems and is helpful for patients with low literacy skills because it can be done via direct questioning. Less well known is the CAGE-AID, which is simply an adaptation of the original CAGE in which patients are also asked about drug use. The acronym "CAGE" invites yes–no responses for the following (the CAGE-AID includes the words in parentheses):

- Have you felt you ought to *Cut* down on your drinking (or drug use)?
- Have people *Annoyed* you by criticizing your drinking (or drug use)?
- Have you felt bad or *Guilty* about your drinking (or drug use)?
- *Eye*-opener: Have you ever had a drink (or used drugs) first thing in the morning to steady your nerves or to get rid of a hangover?

Acknowledging just one of these experiences is 90 percent sensitive for detecting an alcohol-related disorder, with specificities ranging from 50 percent to 90 percent. Using one positive item as the criterion, the CAGE-AID is somewhat more sensitive than the CAGE but less specific, but in general is a good measure (Brown & Rounds, 1995).

One limitation of the CAGE is that it often performs less well among women, minority, and adolescent populations. The RAPS4-QF, an alternative that is now being evaluated in an international screening project, outperformed the CAGE across all gender, ethnic, and service-utilization groups (except blacks and Hispanics) in detecting alcohol abuse (Cherpitel, 2002). The CRAFFT (Knight et al., 1999) is superior to the CAGE for use with adolescents in primary care, and has the added advantage of screening for both alcohol and drug misuse (Knight, Sherritt, Harris, Gates, & Chang, 2003). Its format is similar to the CAGE, as it is an acronym of the first letters of key words in the test's six questions:

Have you ever ridden in a *CAR* driven by someone (including yourself) who was "high" or had been using alcohol or drugs?

Do you ever use alcohol or drugs to *RELAX*, feel better about yourself, or fit in?

Do you ever use alcohol or drugs while you are by yourself, *ALONE*?

Do you ever *FORGET* things you did while using alcohol or drugs?

Do your family or *FRIENDS* ever tell you that you should cut down on your drinking or drug use?

Have you ever gotten into *TROUBLE* while you were using alcohol or drugs?

A positive screen for alcohol or drug disorders is considered to be endorsement of one of these items.

The TWEAK is also similar to the CAGE in design, but is recommended specifically for screening pregnant women for alcohol misuse in primary care. Its letters stand for:

Tolerance: "How many drinks does it take before the alcohol makes you fall asleep or pass out? If you never pass out, what is the largest number of drinks that you have?" (5 or more drinks = 2 points)

Worried: "Have your friends or relatives worried about your drinking in the past year?" (Yes = 1 point)

Eye-opener: "Do you sometimes take a drink in the morning when you first get up?" (Yes = 1 point)

Amnesia: "Are there times when you drink and afterwards can't remember what you said or did?" (Yes = 1 point)

K/C Cut down: "Do you sometimes feel the need to cut down on your drinking?" (Yes = 1 point)

A score of 2 or greater is considered a positive screen.

Similar to depression, there is some indication that a 1-question screen ("When was the last time that you had more than X drinks in one day," with X = 4 for women and X = 5 for men) may be an effective screener for problem alcohol use (Williams & Vinson, 2001). A positive screen is an affirmative in the past three months. From a practical standpoint this might be used as a brief screen, which if positive would trigger use of one of the more extensive screens, such as the AUDIT, which could be administered by a nursing assistant or the BHC.

Anxiety

Difficulties with anxiety may be even more common than depression among primary care patients, and providers probably detect only one in four patients who present with an anxiety disorder (Lang & Stein 2002; Sherbourne, Wells, Meridith, Jackson, & Camp, 1996). Providers are trained first and foremost to detect medical problems, and patients with anxiety problems are often more likely to make somatic complaints than to report psychosocial problems. For this reason, patients with anxiety problems may make detection even more of a challenge for the busy, medically oriented PCP, who is expected to be able to detect any one of 100 medical conditions on any given day. At the same time, anxious patients who have a medical diagnosis may use more care than nonanxious patients with the same diagnosis and may be more likely to be referred to specialists.

Unfortunately, there is a paucity of anxiety screeners appropriate for a primary care setting. No brief measure exists that covers all three components of anxiety (cognitive, somatic, and behavioral), meaning one would need to either combine various screeners or risk missing entire subgroups. The Beck Anxiety Inventory, for example, focuses on somatic symptoms, and the Penn State Worry Questionnaire focuses on cognitive symptoms. Both require about five minutes to complete. The Fear Questionnaire helps assess severity of common phobias and related anxiety and depression symptoms and takes ten minutes to complete. If combined in order to assess all components of anxiety, the total time for administration would be about twenty minutes, which is obviously too long for primary care. One alternative is to ask a few key questions representative of each anxiety domain (e.g., "Do you worry a great deal, even about things you don't think you need to worry about?"; "Do you have chest pain or dizziness and does this frighten you?"; "Do you avoid situations in order to avoid feeling afraid?"; "Have you ever experienced an event where you thought you or a loved one might die and do you avoid remembering this?"). Unlike the cases of depression and alcohol misuse, however, the use of single questions such as these has not been investigated for anxiety. We supply these questions only as suggestions derived from our anecdotal experience.

Cognitive Impairment

Dementia is a large and growing problem and it often goes undiagnosed in its earlier stages. Studies suggest that most patients with dementia go undiagnosed in primary care, and that from 1.8 to 12 percent of primary care patients over age sixty-five have undiagnosed dementia (Agency for Healthcare Research and Quality or AHRQ, June, 2003a,b). In fact, more than 50 percent of patients with dementia have never been diagnosed by a physician (AHRQ, 2003; Valcour, Masaki, Curb, & Blanchette, 2000). Yet, if detected early, six to twelve months of treatment with cholinesterase inhibitors can modestly slow the decline of cognitive and global clinical functioning in patients with mild to moderate Alzheimer's disease (Boustani, Peterson, Hanson, Harris, & Lohr, 2003). Relatedly, intensive multicomponent caregiver interventions may delay nursing home placement of patients who have the good fortune to have caregivers (Boustani et al., 2003). For these reasons, some have advocated for routine screening for cognitive impairment (especially dementia) in primary care. This might be particularly helpful in clinics seeing many older adult patients.

The USPSTF review (AHRQ, 2003) found insufficient evidence to recommend for or against routine screening, though. They cite concerns about the questionable feasibility of routine screenings and the potential harms, such as being incorrectly labeled as demented. They also cite concerns about known problems with the specificity of current screening instruments. Additionally, though the drug therapies referenced above may help slow cognitive decline, the USPSTF notes that their effects on actual functioning are unclear and, at best, small.

Regardless of whether one decides to screen routinely for cognitive decline, indicator-based screening may still be needed when a PCP suspects a problem. Table 6.3 provides a list of screeners for detecting problems with cognitive functioning. The Mini Mental Status Exam (MMSE) is the most widely recognized screening tool for cognitive impairment (Folstein, Folstein, & McHugh, 1975). The MMSE is not a diagnostic instrument for delirium or dementia, so positive screens need further assessment. It can also be useful for annual tracking of decline with Alzheimer's patients, who lose three points per year on average. The MMSE is difficult to deliver within the time constraints of primary care, but it is fairly commonly used there nonetheless. Other screeners that require less time have been devel-

Table 6.3. Screeners for cognitive functioning problems

Screener name	Used for	Reference	Brief description
Mini-Mental Status Exam (MMSE)	Dementia	Folstein et al. (1975)	30 items, takes 5–10 minutes; purchase at www.parinc.com
Clock-Drawing Test (CDT)	Dementia	Shulman (2000)	Free online; maybe better than MMSE for non-English speaking patients
Functional Activities Questionnaire (FAQ)	Dementia	Pfeffer et al. (1982)	Assesses functioning rather than cognition; completed by caregiver
Confusion Assessment Method (CAM)	Delirium	Inouye et al. (1990)	4 items; free online

oped to assess cognitive functioning, but most of these have not been evaluated for use in primary care. One of these is the Clock-Drawing Test (CDT; Shulman, 2000). Despite little study of its use in primary care, it is a well-known and simple instrument that might make a good substitute for the MMSE when the patient is non-English speaking and without an interpreter (Borson et al., 1999). In this test, the patient is given a pencil and paper and asked to draw a clock face with numbers, and to display the hands so they show a time of 11:10. Scoring is based on whether the clock face is a closed circle, if numbers are in their correct positions and are all present, and if the hands point to the correct time.

As an alternative to assessing cognitive functioning, the Functional Activities Questionnaire (FAQ; Pfeffer, Kurosaki, Harrah, Chance, & Filos, 1982) uses caregiver feedback to assess everyday life functioning to screen for dementia. Again, a limitation is that it has not been studied well in primary care, but it generally has sensitivity and specificity similar to the MMSE and is easy to use with patients of diverse backgrounds. Of course, another important limitation of the FAQ is that many patients do not have a caregiver.

If screening for delirium, rather than dementia, the Confusion Assessment Method (CAM; Inouye et al., 1990) is often viewed as the standard (Schuurmans, Deschamps, Markham, Shortridge-Baggett, & Duursma, 2003). It focuses on assessing four key signs of delirium including symptom acuteness/fluctuation, inattention, disorganized thinking, and altered consciousness level and can be used by trained nonphysicians. It has not been widely studied or employed in primary care.

Exposure to Violence

Family violence is ubiquitous, and consists of child, spousal, and elder abuse. Women are at a particularly high risk of violence, and are the largest single group of posttraumatic stress disorder (PTSD) sufferers in the U.S. (Brown, 1993). In surveys, 31 percent of U. S. women report a history of abuse at some point in their lives (The Commonwealth Fund, 1999), most often by a person known to them (Kilpatrick, Edmunds, & Seymour, 1992; Norris, 1992). Many female victims of violence show up in primary care at some point, and many seek care exclusively in a primary care clinic. Indeed, over 20 percent of female primary care patients report histories of completed rape (Koss, Woodruff, & Koss, 1990) and around 23 percent report histories of physical assault or battering (Hamberger, Saunders, & Hovcy, 1992). For a variety of reasons, female victims of violence are more likely to turn to their PCP for help than other professionals, including mental health counselors, police officers, or lawyers (Koss et al., 1990; Mehta & Dandrea, 1988). Unfortunately, they often go under-detected there (Elliott, Nerney, Jones, & Friedmann, 2002).

Men can also be victims of violence, and their detection may be even more challenging as they may be less likely to present to primary care and less likely to exhibit behaviors (such as crying) that invite PCP involvement. They may even engage in behaviors that discourage PCP and nursing staff from screening activities, such as acting angry, frustrated, or impatient. Women are seven to fourteen times more likely than men to sustain severe physical injury at the hands of an intimate partner (Muelleman, Lenaghan, & Pakieser, 1996); meaning men might not have obvious physical signs of abuse.

There is no doubt that child abuse is also a significant problem. The Adverse Childhood Experiences (ACE) study, a large and high-quality retrospective study of 18,000 adults, showed that 11 percent had experienced physical abuse, 11 percent emotional abuse, and 22 percent sexual abuse during childhood (Felitti et al., 1998). This study showed adverse childhood experiences to be much more common than recognized or acknowledged and even was able to link them to adult health a half-century later. At the same time, children who are experiencing abuse often show no clear signs of it, and they have a probability of about 50 percent of denying it if asked (Fergusson, Horwood, & Woodward, 2000). Indeed, in the ACE study, most participants had not revealed their adverse circumstances to PCPs during childhood. The obvious conclusion is that much child abuse is undetected.

Just as poorly recognized may be the problem of elder abuse. It can take many forms, including physical, sexual, and psychological abuse, financial exploitation, and neglect (AMA Council on Scientific Affairs, 1987), and could be perpetrated by a range of family members (spouse, adult children) or by nonfamily caretakers. It is possibly fairly common, with one study finding a prevalence of 3.2 percent for just the problems of physical violence, verbal aggression, and neglect (Nelson, Nygren, McInerney, & Klein, 2004). However, self-report by the elderly is sometimes compromised by cognitive impairment and/or overshadowed by other medical problems in the healthcare setting (Nelson et al., 2004).

Although improved detection of family violence is clearly important, especially in primary care, the best process for doing so is less clear. Screeners must be very sensitive and specific because of the implications of false positives. In the case of child abuse, extant paper-and-pencil screeners have been criticized for their lack of established validity across healthcare settings and non-English speaking populations and for their questionable feasibility for primary care (Nygren, Nelson, & Klein, 2004). These all focus on assessing the parent(s) rather than the child directly. Similarly, none of the screeners currently developed for detection of elder abuse have been extensively validated or validated for use in primary care, and no screener for intimate partner violence (IPV) has been validated using verified abuse outcomes (Nelson et al., 2004).

Probably the best bet for improving detection of most types of family violence is to help PCPs be more alert to signs of it and more comfortable asking about it when signs exist. This approach fits well with the recommendations of the American Medical Association (1992a, 1993) and the

American Academy of Pediatrics (1991) for child abuse, and of the American Medical Association (1992b) for elder abuse. These organizations encourage providers to be vigilant for signs of abuse and to ask about it when suspected. There are too many types of indicators (injuries, medical findings, emotional/behavioral characteristics of a victim, emotional/behavioral characteristics of a perpetrator, situational characteristics) and too many types of abuse (physical, emotional, sexual, neglect) for us to summarize here. Instead, a good source of information on these are the AMA Diagnostic and Treatment Guidelines (1992a,b, 1993), from which a training session for PCPs could easily be developed.

For IPV (Interpersonal Violence), however, the American Medical Association (1992c) recommends routine screening of all female patients. Thus, if routine screening is done for any type of family violence this might be the most empirically-supported area to do it for. Studies of women in general and women survivors of IPV suggest that most do favor healthcare providers asking about domestic violence (Gielen et al., 2000; Nicolaidis, 2002). The Family Violence Fund, a prominent national domestic violence advocacy organization, has an extensive collection of resources that can help train providers to ask about domestic violence. Much of the collection is available at www.endabuse.org. They also produced an excellent video that is available for training PCPs. The AMA's recommendations also include a straight-forward and useful guide to screening for and responding to IPV (Brown, 2002).

Tables 6.4 and 6.5 provide, respectively, examples of common barriers to identifying IPV and of helpful screening questions for PCPs to ask. This information can make for a productive training geared toward improving PCP screening for IPV. Content of the tables is derived from the Family Violence Fund's publications, the AMA's Guidelines (Brown, 2002; 1992c), and two peer-reviewed publications (Elliott et al., 2002; Sugg & Inui, 1992).

Attention-Deficit Hyperactivity Disorder (ADHD) in Children

As with other behavior problems, ADHD care is often delivered exclusively in the primary care setting by pediatricians and family practice providers. Although the former tend to feel more comfortable managing ADHD than

Table 6.4. Physician and patient barriers to identifying IPV

Physician qualities that reduce screening	Patient barriers to identification
Low estimated prevalence of IPV in one's practice	May be literally held captive in home
Lack of confidence for handling IPV issues	May lack money or means of transportation to go to physician visits
Fear of offending patients	Fear that revelation will jeopardize her safety
Belief that abused women will volunteer a history of violence	Thinking she is to blame for the abuse
PCP gender (males less likely to screen)	Shame and humiliation about the abuse
Forgetting to ask	Cultural, ethnic, or religious influences on her response to
Less likely to screen patients from higher socioeconomic class	abuse and her awareness of viable options for help
Perceived inability to "fix" IPV	Witnessed IPV as a child, doesn't recognize it as abuse or see a
Lack of time during visits	way out
Lack of recognition of the social and psychological costs of abuse	Belief that injuries are not severe enough to mention
Thinking it is not a physician's place to intervene	Financial reliance on the batterer
Believing the woman must have provoked the abuse	Abuse may be infrequent, tempered by sincere apologies and loving
Frustration with women who do not leave abusive relationships	moments
Disbelief because the alleged batterer is known by the PCP to be pleasant, concerned	Hope that the batterer will change
	Fear of being blamed
	Poor understanding of the relationship of stress (from the abuse) to her physical symptoms

the latter do, the assistance of a BHC can add much to the assessment and treatment process of either. As mentioned throughout this book, the BHC model de-emphasizes diagnosis-based assessment in general, but the case of ADHD is a bit different. Medication plans notwithstanding, schools often require a diagnosis of ADHD in order for a child to access special services, meaning a thorough assessment should be conducted. Even time-strapped PCP's often take more than one visit to assess for ADHD, so they are typically pleased to have the assistance of a BHC.

Table 6.5. Recommended questions for IPV screening

Framing questions

(These set the stage for direct questioning)

1. "Because violence is so common in many people's lives, I've begun to ask all my patients about it."
2. "I'm concerned that your symptoms may have been caused by someone hurting you."
3. "I don't know if this is a problem for you, but many of the women I see as patients are dealing with abusive relationships. Some are too afraid or uncomfortable to bring it up themselves, so I've started asking about it routinely."
5. "Some of the lesbian women and gay men we see here are hurt by their partners. Does your partner ever try to hurt you?"

Direct verbal questions

(Asked alone, face-to-face, in a direct and nonjudgmental manner)

1. "Are you in a relationship with a person who physically hurts or threatens you?"
2. "Did someone cause these injuries? Was it your partner/husband?"
3. "Has your partner or ex-partner ever hit you or physically hurt you? Has he ever threatened to hurt you or someone close to you?"
4. "Do you feel controlled or isolated by your partner?"
5. "Do you ever feel afraid of your partner? Do you feel you are in danger? Is it safe for you to go home?"
6. "Has your partner ever forced you to have sex when you didn't want to? Has your partner ever refused to practice safe sex?"

Screening for ADHD routinely is not typical practice. Rather, ADHD is a problem that might be detected during the course of a more global behavioral screen, followed by a more detailed assessment. Unfortunately, many of the instruments used to assess specifically for ADHD in specialty care are too time- and labor-intensive for primary care. However, an excellent set of materials for assessment and intervention, called the "ADHD Toolkit," is available at the website of the National Initiative for Children's Healthcare Quality (NICHQ), http://www.nichq.org/nichq. These tools were designed specifically for primary care and include instruments for initial and follow-up assessments by parents and teachers. The assessment instruments are widely known among PCPs as "Vanderbilts" because they are titled the NICHQ Vanderbilt Forms. Items help evaluate for conditions that are commonly comorbid with ADHD, including conduct disorder, oppositional defiant disorder, and depression/anxiety problems. Follow-up assessment forms include questions about possible medication side effects.

Working in concert with the PCP, a BHC can collect pertinent history on a child being assessed, distribute and subsequently collect and score the Vanderbilt assessment forms, talk with the school, and collect and review collateral school data such as report cards or standardized test scores. Thus, for many BHC services, this assessment process will look more like the type of assessment that would be conducted in a specialty setting. One of us (JR) even has a weekly hour-long visit in which he and the pediatrician together conduct ADHD evaluations.

ADHD in Adults

More and more adults are presenting to primary care complaining of ADHD symptoms though, like childhood ADHD, this is not a problem clinics typically screen for. Significant residual effects do linger in at least 30 to 50 percent of adults who had ADHD in childhood (Searight, Burke, & Rottnek, 2000), and maybe even in the majority (National Institute of Health Consensus Statement, 1998). Often adult parents will become suspicious that they have ADHD if their child is being evaluated for it (Ratey, Greenberg, Bemporad, & Lindem, 1992). Accurate diagnosis of ADHD in adults is often challenging because of symptom overlap with other conditions. Because of this, and because treatment may include long-term use of a drug with potential for abuse, many PCP's are reluctant to treat adults with ADHD. However, given the frequency with which this complaint surfaces, it is not a topic that can be dodged, and thus PCPs will probably be appreciative if a process to help with assessment is developed.

An assessment process that works well in many clinics is to first have the BHC gather history and then administer an adult ADHD brief self-report tool. Of the extant screening tools for adult ADHD, perhaps the best for primary care is the Adult Self-Report Scale (ASRS) which was developed by the World Health Organization (WHO) in 2003 and is widely available online. The ASRS reflects symptoms that adults with ADHD complain of, which may differ significantly from those in child-hood. The ASRS requires ratings on a 4-point scale for eighteen items so it takes little time to complete. It is scored with a simple tally and scores (one for Inattention and one for Hyperactivity/Impulsivity) are com-pared to a cutoff score. If the screen is positive, the BHC or PCP can ask additional questions about degree of impairment, presence of symp-toms during childhood, and the consistency of symptoms over time. The ASRS is also helpful in evaluating the effects of treatment. Three other popular self-report measures for adult ADHD include the Wender Utah Rating Scale, the Copeland Symptom Checklist and the Brown Attention Deficit Disorder Scale for Adults (Searight et al., 2000). However, with the briefest of these (the Brown scale) requiring ten to twenty minutes to complete, the length of these measures may be pro-hibitive for primary care.

If an initial history and results of the self-report tool are suggestive of ADHD, the BHC might ask the patient to return for a second visit with old school records and/or with a parent or someone who knew him/her during childhood (to establish an early onset and consistent course of symptoms). Records of previous treatment, if available, should also be brought or ordered, and the BHC might ask the PCP to order a urine drug screen to assist in ruling out substance abuse as a confounding problem. Quite often PCP's reluctant to treat ADHD in adults will be more recep-tive to the idea if the BHC can provide this level of assessment, and it can usually be accomplished during usual BHC visit times (though it might take more than one brief visit).

Eating Problems

Eating problems occur commonly among young adults and teenagers, particularly females. They occur in all ethnic groups but are most common among whites in industrialized nations. Eating problems are particularly common in young women with type one diabetes mellitus. As many as one third of these women may have diagnosable eating disor-ders, a problem that places them at high risk of resultant microvascular and metabolic complications (Walsh, Wheat, & Freund, 2000). The USP-STF did not review the literature on screening for eating problems and so has no recommendations regarding it. However, the American Medical Association's Guidelines for Adolescent Preventive Services (GAPS; 1997), among others, does recommend annual screening for eating disorders among eleven to twenty-one-year-olds. As a result, some PCPs will want to do this, and the BHC should be able to recommend a screening process.

The AMA recommends that patients be assessed for eating problems if any of the following are found: weight loss greater than 10 percent of previous weight; recurrent dieting when not overweight; use of self-induced emesis, laxatives, starvation, or diuretics to lose weight; distorted body image; or body mass index (BMI) below the fifth percentile. However, they do not recommend specific screeners to use in the event one of these problems is present. A good option may be the five-item "SCOFF" (Morgan, Reid, & Lacey, 1999). The SCOFF questions include:

"Do you make yourself *Sick* (induce vomiting) because you feel uncomfortably full?"
"Do you worry that you have lost *Control* over how much you eat?"
"Have you recently lost more than *One* stone (14 lbs.) in a three-month period?"
"Do you think you are too *Fat*, even though others say you are thin?";
"Would you say that *Food* dominates your life?"

A positive response to two or more questions is suggestive of anorexia nervosa or bulimia nervosa. The PCP could administer the SCOFF to patients who present with one of the initial warning signs, or could simply refer such patients to the BHC who might in turn administer the SCOFF along with his or her functional assessment.

METHODS FOR SCREENING

The method for deploying behavioral screeners for adults and youth will vary from clinic to clinic, depending on preferences, needs and resources. For the most studied problem of depression, no particular routine screening interval has emerged as superior to others (Pignone et al., 2002), so some clinics screen annually, while others screen only during physical exams. Physical exams generally occur frequently during childhood, less frequently during early adulthood and middle-age, and then more frequently again as one enters late adulthood. Thus, some might feel that behavioral screening during physicals will be too frequent early and late in life, and too infrequent at other times. Nonetheless, physical exams do provide an excellent platform for screening and addressing behavioral needs. If used during physicals, the screening tool can be included with the other paperwork patients are usually asked to complete. Some clinics have patients complete a questionnaire package prior to an appointment for a physical, in which case adding a behavioral screener might be less of a problem for patients (though this might still be resisted by providers, who will have to review the screener during the appointment).

Screening during physical exams can be made much easier if a group visit format is used. One of us works in a clinic that regularly holds health fairs for kids, the focus of which is to get kids in for needed physicals. The clinic now routinely mails the Pediatric Symptom Checklist (PSC), as well as other paperwork, to parents in advance of the health fair. During the fair, the BHC maintains an open schedule and briefly sees any child (with parents) who screens positive on the PSC. Typically the PSC is scored by the PCP during his or her visit with the patient, but it can also be scored by a medical assistant or other staff person, or by the BHC, before the patient meets with the PCP. These fairs always lead to referrals that would likely not have materialized otherwise.

As an alternative to routine (i.e., annually or during physicals) screenings of all patients, a clinic might focus mostly on at-risk populations. The USPSTF review found support for this practice, suggesting that routine screening for depression might be most productive for patients with a history of depression, unexplained somatic symptoms, comorbid psychological conditions, substance abuse, or chronic pain (U.S. Preventive Services Task Force, 2002). If a clinic is using electronic records or a registry to track care of some chronic conditions, routine screening and subsequent referrals of these patients is made easier.

A third option is "passive screening" for behavioral problems. Passive screening encourages patients to self-identify problems rather than relying on the provider to identify them. A common passive screening strategy is to place signs in a waiting room or exam rooms describing signs or symptoms of a particular problem. For example, a sign might ask, "Do You Have Symptoms of Depression?" and then proceed to describe the symptoms of depression and encourage the patient to inform his or her PCP if a number of these symptoms are present. Similarly, a brochure could be included as part of an informational packet given to patients just prior to a physical exam. The flyer might list symptoms of depression and encourage the patient to discuss them with the PCP during the physical. For domestic violence, providing pins for PCPs and nursing staff to wear that indicate availability of service to victims of violence is a simple and efficient approach, yet possibly powerful in helping victims to self-identify. Although passive screening provides a way of working around PCP's who might be reluctant to address behavioral issues, it might not help with patients who for one reason or another are reluctant to raise concerns themselves.

ASSESSMENT FOR TREATMENT PLANNING AND EVALUATION

Besides screening to improve detection of behavioral problems in primary care, self-report measures can also be used to aid treatment planning and evaluation of treatment response. This is true for interventions provided by both BHC's and PCP's, though in this section we primarily focus on the latter.

Medication Planning

Consider the case of depression. Depression is very common in primary care, and PCPs are most likely to prescribe medication as a treatment. However, several studies suggest that almost half of the patients PCPs diagnose as having major depression and in need of antidepressant medication do not meet research diagnostic criteria for major depression (Katon et al., 1995, 1996). Thus, using a depression self-report tool may help avoid overprescribing by the PCP. A PCP may be more likely to use watchful waiting strategies successfully, or to develop behavioral plans to improve functioning, if a self-report measure suggests subclinical levels of depression.

Various possibilities for brief assessment of depression were covered in the screening section on depression earlier in this chapter, and these will not be reviewed again here. Both of our clinics use the Patient Health Questionnaire-9 (PHQ-9; Spitzer et al., 1999) to obtain measures of symptom severity and impact on functioning, and have guidelines for interpreting this in exam rooms. Incorporating the PHQ-9 into clinical pathways can do a great deal to further PCP development of skills for treating depression, to improve patient outcomes, and to save health care dollars (for discussion, see Robinson, 2003).

Another way self-report tools may aid medication planning in primary care is to help avoid adverse treatment consequences. The case of mania provides an excellent example of this. Bipolar disorder is under-detected in primary care, and prescribing a SSRI for a person with manic episodes may lead to adverse outcomes (Das et al., 2005). In a recent study in an urban general medical clinic, 9.8 percent of primary care patients screened positive for lifetime bipolar disorder (Das et al., 2005), meaning this is a fairly common problem. The Mood Disorder Questionnaire (MDQ; Hirschfeld et al., 2000) is available free online from various sources and may be used to screen for a history of mania before starting a treatment course with a SSRI for depression.

Another use of the MDQ, as well as some other brief screening tools, is to aid the PCP in the proper selection of medicines. Patients presenting for help in primary care often have complicated histories and complain of chronic symptoms that can fit with several different diagnostic categories. Left alone, a PCP may have a very tricky job determining which medicine to try, but with the aid of self-report tools the better options often become clearer. For example, a patient who presents with rapid, pressured speech and complaints of chronic agitation and poor concentration might end up with vastly different prescriptions, depending on the treating PCP. One might prescribe an SSRI (for depression), another might try a mood stabilizer (for mania), a third would perhaps try a psychostimulant (for attention-deficit hyperactivity disorder), while a fourth might decide to use a benzodiazepine (for anxiety). Although self-report tools do not in and of themselves provide definitive diagnoses, they often help narrow the range of medications for a PCP to consider. For example, for this patient the MDQ and/or a depression measure and/or the ASRS might prove quite helpful. With just a few extra minutes added to the evaluation, the odds of the PCP selecting the most appropriate medication almost certainly improve. Ideally this patient would also see the BHC for more history-gathering before starting treatment, but this will not always occur.

Many in the specialty mental health sector would express dismay at such an assessment, proclaiming—with some legitimacy—that much more assessment needs to be done to plan treatment with confidence. However, the reality of today's healthcare system is that very few patients will receive such detailed assessment before being started on a treatment plan, and it is within that reality that one operates in primary care. In this scenario, the addition of a few brief screeners to the treatment planning process may make a great deal of difference relative to primary care as usual.

Measuring Treatment Response

A final reason for using self-report tools in primary care is for the assessment of treatment response. "Treatment" can refer to either services delivered by a PCP or by the PCP and BHC in conjunction. Using measures in this way helps PCPs and BHCs communicate with each other regarding treatment progress, provides patients with feedback regarding change, and offers a more objective assessment of that change for all involved. It also may lead to the creation of a database that can be used for program evaluation purposes, which are discussed in Chapter 15.

Assessing Response in Adults. For assessing treatment response in adult primary care patients, we recommend that a measure of health-related quality of life (HRQOL) be used at all BHC visits. The concept of HRQOL refers to a person's or group's perceived physical and mental health over time (Moriarty, Zack, & Kobau, 2003). Measuring it helps the BHC and anyone else who sees the scores to understand the impact of an illness and/or disability on a person's day-to-day quality of life, as well as how life might be changing in response to treatment. In our clinics, HRQOL is assessed in all BHC contacts with patients aged eighteen and over. Given the right tool, it could conceivably be assessed at all PCP visits as well. Although we advocate for HRQOL to consistently be the focus of treatment response monitoring, sometimes PCPs want to measure change in a specific problem instead, such as depression. In such cases, use of the condition-specific measures described earlier (e.g., the ASRS, PHQ-9, MDQ, etc.) can be helpful. These can be administered as needed by either the PCP or BHC during follow-ups.

For regular assessment of HRQOL, a number of widely used and well-studied tools exist (See Table 6.6). Both of us use the DUKE Health Profile (Parkerson, 1996), and examples of its clinical utility are provided in a later chapter on adult consultations. The DUKE requires less than five minutes to administer and score, and is available in over a dozen languages. While it has only seventeen items, it generates ten scale scores. One of us (PR) routinely reports eight scale scores in chart notes for initial and follow-up visits, while the other (JR) uses the DUKE clinically to guide discussion with patients, but does not record scores in charts. The decision of whether to score and document results will probably have a lot to do with how much administrative support (such as a BHA) the BHC has, but if possible it can be very helpful.

Useful scale scores to document include (1) Function Scale Scores for Physical Health, Mental Health, Social Health, and Perceived Health, and (2) Dysfunction Scale Scores for Anxiety, Depression, Pain, and Disability. Higher scores on the Function Scales indicate higher levels of function or better health, while higher scores on Dysfunction Scales indicate higher levels of dysfunction or more severe symptoms of psychological distress, pain, and disability. The DUKE manual discusses how to use other helpful features, such as an Anxiety/Depression scale and a measure of social

Table 6.6. Measures of health-related quality of life (HRQOL)

Measure	Reference	Brief description
DUKE Health Profile	(Parkerson, 1996)	17 items; free with author permission
Healthy Days Questions (HRQOL-4)	Moriarty et al. (2003)	4 items; free online; less studied with individuals
Brief Disability Questionnaire	Von Korff et al. (1998)	8 items; validated across cultures in primary care
Short Form-12 (SF-12)	Ware, Kosinski, & Keller (1996)	12 items; obtain license at www.iqola.org, probably for cost

support. Permission to use the DUKE clinically can usually be easily obtained by contacting the author at Duke University. Instructions for electronic scoring are in the manual, and if using electronic medical records a clinic could potentially integrate DUKE scoring into the system (Parkerson, 1996).

A briefer alternative to the DUKE is the HRQOL-4, also known as the Healthy Days questions (Moriarty et al., 2003). The Centers for Disease Control and Prevention introduced this four-question measure of HRQOL in the mid-1990s, and it has been used extensively since then. Though mostly used for large-scale population health research, it has also been found to be helpful for tracking individual change (Currey, Rao, Winfield, & Callahan, 2003). Figure 6.1 displays the HRQOL-4 or Healthy Days questions. The only scoring is a summary "unhealthy days" index, which is obtained by adding the respondent's physically and mentally unhealthy days (questions 2 and 3), with a maximum score of 30. Thus, if a patient reports four physically unhealthy days and two mentally unhealthy days, the unhealthy days score is six; and if a patient reports thirty physically unhealthy days and thirty mentally unhealthy days, the unhealthy days score is the maximum, 30. An alternative "healthy days" score is preferred by some, and is calculated by subtracting the number of unhealthy days

---

1. Would you say that in general your health is:
   Excellent   Very Good   Good   Fair   Poor
2. Now thinking about your physical health, which includes physical illness and injury, for how many days during the past 30 days was your physical health not good?
3. Now thinking about your mental health, which includes stress, depression, and problems with emotions, for how many days during the past 30 days was your mental health not good?
4. During the past 30 days, for about how many days did poor physical or mental health keep you from doing your usual activities, such as self-care, work, or recreation?

Figure 6.1. Healthy days questions (HRQOL-4).

from thirty. A meaningful change for a given individual over time is considered to be a change of 1 day, and a change of 2 days is considered twice as meaningful as 1. Its brevity makes the HRQOL-4 a tempting measure, but of course what one gains in time one sacrifices in the extent of information obtained.

Other alternatives for assessing HRQOL in primary care include the Brief Disability Questionnaire (Von Korff, Ustun, Ormel, Kaplan, & Simon, 1996) and the SF-12 (Ware et al., 1996). The former measures health-related disability while the latter is a measure of overall health status.

Assessing Response in Youths. Treatment response may also be tracked in children. As with adults, some may choose to use symptom or problem checklists while others will focus on HRQOL measures. The Pediatric Symptom Checklist (PSC, PSC-17, or PSC-Y) mentioned earlier is a good problem checklist that can be used at pediatric visits. All versions can easily be completed in the waiting room, with total time for administration and scoring less than five minutes using a simple tally procedure. The PSC can be downloaded in English or Spanish at http://psc.partners.org/. A Chinese version is also available (e-mail mmurphy6@partners.org). Both the self-report and longer parental report versions consist of thirty-five short statements of problem behaviors, including both internalizing and externalizing problems. The respondent rates how often these problems occur, and a score of zero, one or two is then assigned to ratings of never, sometimes, or often. Higher scores indicate higher psychosocial dysfunction, and age-based cut-off scores are provided.

The KINDL(R) questionnaire (Ravens-Sieberer & Bullinger, 1998) is an option for the BHC that wants to assess health-related quality of life in children and youth. It provides options for self-assessment and parent-assessment and is appropriate for children aged 8 to 16. It can require up to ten minutes for completion, though, which is a bit long for primary care. It may also be administered in the form of an interview (face-to-face or by telephone) but again this takes considerable time. The KINDL(R) questionnaire consists of twenty-four Likert-scaled items associated with six dimensions: physical well-being, emotional well-being, self-esteem, family, friends, and everyday functioning (preschool/school). It also produces a total score. For permission to use the KINDL(R) for free, contact Dr. Ulrike Ravens-Sieberer (e-mail: ravens-siebereru@rki.de or ravens@uke.uni-hamburg.de).

TIPS FOR TEACHING PCPS TO USE BEHAVIORAL MEASURES

As mentioned earlier, PCPs often show interest in screeners and assessment instruments when presented with evidence about their usefulness and when their completion is feasible. When introducing measures to PCPs and staff members, remind them of the World Health Organization (WHO, 1946) definition of health—"Health is a state of complete physical, mental, and social well-being, and not merely the absence of disease or infirmity." Explain that the choice of measures for the BHC service reflects a desire to contribute useful information to individual patient care and to introduce some objectivity to treatment planning. In other words, help PCPs to understand that the measures are relevant to them. Many PCPs will welcome the use of measures as a replacement to the "shooting from the hip" that they often have to do when dealing with behavioral issues. However, a lot of reinforcement and gentle prodding might be needed to get new assessment or screening processes started. Making repeated presentations on screening and/or assessment, routinely charting assessment results, and frequently referring to assessment results during consultations with PCPs can help.

Choosing measures that have broad applicability and normative data from primary care will also boost credibility and improve the odds of obtaining meaningful information. Also remember to ensure assessment instruments are readily available to PCPs, that nursing staff know how to administer and score them, and that PCPs have ready access to information from them.

SUMMARY

1. Assessment using self-report tools in the PCBH model does not involve lengthy diagnostic or personality tests.
2. The primary uses of self-report measures in the PCBH model are for screening and assessment. Screening might be routine or indicator-based, and might be done with the entire clinic population or with

subgroups. Passive screening can also be helpful. Assessment helps establish the presence of a health condition and its severity.

3. Keys to successfully implementing the use of self-report tools are to get buy-in from staff, develop workable processes, and find measures that are functionally-focused and appropriate to the primary care environment.

4. Although many problems may be routinely screened for, the evidence is most supportive of routine screening for depression and alcohol misuse.

5. The U.S. Preventive Services Task Force (USPSTF) is an independent, nongovernmental panel that issues recommendations regarding screening and brief interventions in primary care. Recommendations of the American Academy of Family Physicians (AAFP) come directly from their work and most PCPs are familiar with it.

6. Measures can also be used to help PCPs to select the right medication, decide when to prescribe, avoid adverse side effects (such as mania), and monitor treatment response.

7. When tracking treatment response, use of health-related quality of life measures is ideal, though sometimes more narrowly focused symptom checklists can be helpful.

8. Most PCPs will not expect the BHC to use objective outcome measures in intervention planning and evaluation and will not view such measures as relevant to their own work. Persistence and patience will be needed to help PCPs gradually learn to use behavioral measures in their own practice.

PART IV

THE ADVENTURE BEGINS

At long last, we are ready to discuss patient care! While previous parts of the book focused on defining the PCBH model and getting organized, this part begins the clinical focus. Owing to the newness of PCBH work, this part thoroughly details the content of patient visits, including how to introduce oneself, what types of questions to ask (and not to ask), and when to schedule follow-ups. Specific practice tools are also introduced to help guide individual care and practice management efforts. In Chapter 7, the functional analysis process is explained, as it is the focus of initial consults, and templates are provided for interviewing patients and dictating notes. Directions for charting are also included. Chapter 8 provides a Start-Up Checklist to structure first-year practice activities, and suggests a tool and process for overcoming barriers to patient referrals. Also provided are written materials to help PCPs and staff understand the full potential of a BHC service, with the goal of keeping their interest in the service strong. The intent of these chapters is to help the new BHC have a structured approach to growing a successful and busy service from Day 1. Let the adventure begin as we dig into the daily life of the Behavioral Health Consultant!

7

PRACTICE TOOLS FOR THE BHC

"Deliberation is the work of many men. Action, of one alone."
—Charles de Gaulle

Assuming a basic understanding of the territory of primary care, the operational structures necessary for supporting a BHC practice, and the theories, interventions, and measures for practicing in the PCBH model, this chapter gives structure to PCBH clinical work. This is where deliberation turns to action. Hopefully this "nuts and bolts" content will complement the theoretical material of previous chapters and begin to help the reader envision how PCBH practice actually is conducted.

INITIAL CONSULTS

The term "initial consult" probably seems simple enough to define, yet in reality it can be a bit fuzzy. Is the first visit with a patient for marital problems considered an "initial consult" if he has been seen before by the BHC for obesity? What about the patient seen one year earlier for headaches who is now seeing the BHC again for headaches? This is more than an issue of semantics, because the structure of an initial consult varies significantly from that of a follow-up. Details of the differences between the two will hopefully become clear as this chapter progresses, but the most significant difference is that the initial consult includes both a functional assessment and an intervention, while a follow-up includes only the latter. Thus, determining which category a visit falls into has ramifications for the focus of the visit and the amount of time required. We will come back to this issue in a few pages, after first providing a more complete picture of the content of initial consultations.

An initial consultation comes in one of two forms. It may involve a same-day patient, as in when a problem is identified during a PCP visit and the BHC sees the patient immediately afterward. It could also involve a scheduled patient, as in the case of a patient who could not stay to see the BHC after an earlier PCP visit or a patient referred on a day the BHC was absent. Ideally, at least half of the patients seen in a given day will be same-day referrals. To strive for this, PCPs need to learn to find the BHC immediately after identifying a referral issue and at least introduce him or her to the patient. Even if the patient cannot stay, this display of teamwork demonstrates to the patient the close working relationship between the two providers, boosts the credibility of the BHC, and increases the likelihood that the patient will actually schedule to see him or her. All too often, patients who are simply told to see the BHC, but are not introduced, fail to show for an initial consult. (Additionally, too many scheduled patients can create problems with access, a problem doubly frustrating if patients fail to show.)

Ideally, all referred patients will be seen immediately, but in reality this is not always possible. Patients often cannot stay, and sometimes the BHC's schedule is too full. However, like the saying, "A bird in the hand is better than two in the bush," seeing a patient for even a brief five- or ten-minute consult can be preferable to simply asking him or her to schedule a consult. As one's consultation skills improve, providing a very brief yet meaningful consult becomes easier to do. Whatever the length of the visit, an initial consultation should always include a brief explanation of the BHC's role, an assessment of the patient's functioning with respect to the referral issue, a brief social history, and recommendations tailored to the referral issue.

The Introduction

Each initial consult begins with an introduction to the BHC service to ensure the patient understands the BHC's role and what to expect from the visit. This is particularly important given the differences between a BHC visit and what patients might have experienced with more traditional MH visits. Introductions actually come first from the PCP, when he or she refers the patient, meaning that if the BHC has been effective in teaching PCPs how to refer, all involved may be spared from misunderstandings. (See Chapter 8 for suggestions on training PCPs to refer patients.) For purposes of the BHC's introduction of his or her services, Figure 7.1 offers a scripted introduction. Obviously the wording will be modified to fit one's usual way of speaking, but the key components of the script should be maintained. Key components include a summary of the BHC's credentials, an explanation of his or her role as a consultant, the length and structure of the visit, and the likelihood that this may involve a single visit only. A brief reference to the BHC's role as a mandated reporter is optional. We often include it, as it only takes seconds.

Some BHCs may delegate explanation of BHC services to the Behavioral Health Assistant (BHA), when one is available. In such cases,

---

"Hi, my name is _____. I am a (psychologist, social worker, counselor, etc.) and I work as a consultant to patients and providers in the clinic. I would like to explore the concern that you and your provider have and then make recommendations to both of you. This should take about thirty to forty[a] minutes. Many patients simply follow-up with their provider after meeting with me, but sometimes I ask a patient to return for a few visits if we plan to work on a new coping skill. I do not provide psychotherapy services. Instead, my job is to help your PCP help you to manage stress and make lifestyle changes. (*Optional*: Like the other providers, I will help you get help if you tell me you are in danger of harming yourself or someone else.) Do you have any questions?"

[a]As noted in Chapter 4, the number of minutes in BHC schedule templates may be fifteen or twenty minutes per unit, and an initial consult usually involves two units of service

---

Figure 7.1. A behavioral health consultant's introduction.

occasional checks should be done to assure that the BHA is staying close to the script. Some BHAs rush through and omit parts on busy days or gradually truncate the introduction as a service grows busier. Figure 7.2 displays a script that may be used by a BHA. Again, the wording may be changed to fit one's usual language, but the key components should be maintained.

If the introduction was delegated, the initial consult should begin with, "Do you have any questions about this service?" Patients often ask questions about the cost of the service at this point. They may also ask why they were referred. Sometimes patients do not understand a PCP's reasoning in referring, sometimes the PCP was unclear about the reason when discussing it with the patient, and sometimes patients are simply expressing their discomfort with being referred to a BH provider. Be ready to explain the referral reason, which hopefully was discussed with the PCP but

---

"Hello, my name is ____ and I am the assistant for (Dr., Ms., Mr.___). She or he is a (psychologist, social worker, counselor, etc.), and works as a consultant to patients and their providers in the clinic. She or he will explore the concern that you and (Dr., PA, ARNP___) have, and then make recommendations to you and your provider. This should take between thirty and forty[a] minutes. For many patients, follow up after meeting with (Dr., Ms., Mr.___) will be with their provider, but sometimes (Dr., Ms., Mr.___) asks a patient to return for a few visits to learn a new coping skill. This is not a psychotherapy service. Instead, (Dr.'s, Ms.'s, Mr.'s___) expertise is in helping patients manage stress and make lifestyle changes. (*Optional:* Like other providers, (Dr., Ms., Mr.___) will help you find help if you tell him/her you are in danger of harming yourself or someone else.) He/she will answer any questions you have.)"

[a]As in Figure 7.1, an initial consult usually involves two 15- or 20-minute units of service.

Figure 7.2. A behavioral health assistant's introduction of BHC services.

otherwise might be documented in the chart. If it is unknown, another option is to ask the patient, "Do you have any ideas about why (Dr., P.A., ARNP___) might have referred you?" This can open discussion about issues that the patient might view as important, even if they are not exactly sure of the reason(s) for the PCP's referral.

Less commonly, patients may express concern about information being relayed to the PCP or placed in the medical chart. To reassure patients without misleading them, explain that your goal is simply to tell the provider what he or she needs to know in order to best help the patient. Regarding charting concerns, try to reassure the patient that only information necessary for coordinating care will be documented and explain that much BHC notation is devoted to planning and recommendations. Sometimes important issues can be conveyed to the PCP without putting them in a chart note, but it is best not to promise this (if it is important enough to tell the PCP it probably should be in the chart).

Another option to help patients understand BHC services is the creation of a brochure that introduces services. The brochure might be placed in the waiting room or exam rooms and include a suggestion that patients talk with a PCP if interested in a referral. This can be especially helpful for new services trying to grow the number of referrals. Figure 7.3 provides an example of content appropriate for this type of brochure. We recommend putting this content onto colored paper to catch attention and perhaps, if one's computer skills are up to the task, adding eye-catching graphics.

Introducing and Completing Behavioral Health Measures. Prior to both initial and follow-up BHC visits, patients are usually asked to complete a routine self-report measure. One way to increase patient acceptance of this process is to explain that it is akin to the routine taking of vitals (e.g., blood pressure and weight) prior to medical visits. In larger clinics where the ratio of BHC hours to PCP hours is leaner, a BHA might complete the appropriate assessments prior to the visit. Whether done by the BHA or the BHC, the measures are best scored prior to the actual visit so that results may be shared with the patient. In the initial consult, health-related quality of life scores help inform the design of the intervention and, for patients who return for follow-up, they provide a way to assess change.

We are pleased to have a Behavioral Health Consultant (BHC) in our clinic!

Her or his name is _____ and she or he is a (psychologist, social worker, etc.).

Services from the BHC include:

- Problem-solving stressful life problems
- Stress reduction skills, such as relaxation techniques
- Parent training
- Help coping with the diagnosis of a chronic disease, such as diabetes or cancer
- Help with changing important behaviors, such as tobacco use or problematic alcohol or drug use
- Coaching in developing a healthy lifestyle
- Assistance with behavior changes to help manage chronic problems, such as hypertension, obesity, and ADHD
- Tips on preparing for difficult medical procedures
- Techniques for improving sleep
- Skill training to improve marital and parent–child relationships
- Strategies for coping with care of a sick or impaired loved one

Services from the BHC do not include:

- Court evaluations
- Custody evaluations
- Psychotherapy

BHC consultations:

- Require a referral from your provider
- Are usually fifteen to forty[a] minutes in length
- May be available on the same-day as the request

BHC consultations cost the same amount as your co-pay for a visit with your PCP[b].

Questions? Your provider will be happy to answer them.

[a,b]This information may vary from one clinic to the next

Figure 7.3. Content for a brochure introducing BHC services.

What to Ask

Because of the relatively short time allotted for conducting an assessment, making recommendations and charting, questions must be limited to what is most essential. Using an interview template can improve efforts to focus on key questions and avoid questions that are less relevant to the referral concern. Figures 7.4 (Life Context Questions) and 5 (Functional Analysis Questions) are templates that together form the backbone of an initial consultation. These templates are flexible and can be used with a child, adolescent, or adult patient by making suggested variations in the questions.

Our clinics both use a "SOAP" format for chart notes (discussed later in this chapter), and thus the final note should have sections labeled "Subjective," "Objective," "Assessment," and "Plan." Using the same format as that of the PCPs is crucial for communicating information easily. Additionally, using a template can help the PCP to read and comprehend consultations more quickly. They will learn to expect certain types of information in specific locations, and this can save them time and increase the likelihood of their reading more of a note. Both of these templates are illustrative, and can be applied in varying ways to fit the

---

SUBJECTIVE (S):
1. Life Context:

Referring Provider: PCP: Reason for Referral:

Patient Age: Marital Status/Grade: Job/School:

Quality of family relationships?

Quality of social relationships?

Job/School Satisfaction:

Lives with?   Where?   For how long?

Health Problems: Medication Compliance:

Health Risks: Tobacco products?   Alcohol?   Other drugs?

Recreation?   Relaxation?   Sleep?   Diet?   Exercise?

Worry/Stress?

Figure 7.4. Template for life context questions.

1. Describe the target behavior
   a. Onset
   b. Frequency
   c. Duration
   d. Intensity
2. Describe activities or times when the behavior is most likely to occur
   a. Where is the behavior most likely to occur?
   b. Are there times when the behavior rarely occurs?
   c. With whom is the behavior likely to occur?
   d. What is most likely to be occurring just before the behavior occurs?
   e. Is there one thing that triggers the behavior?
3. What skills or changes might make the behavior less likely to occur?
4. What happens after the behavior occurs, in terms of patient experience and the behavior of others?
5. Is there a predictable pattern of behaviors leading up to the target behavior?
6. What has the patient tried to do to help the problem? Has it worked?

Figure 7.5. Template for functional analysis questions.

visit's flow. Rarely does one progress through them in a rigid question-by-question fashion. Each template is described in the following sections.

Life Context Questions. The section of the template likely to be the most different from initial visits conducted in specialty MH is the "Subjective" section. This section consists mostly of life context questions, also referred to as the patient's "history." Many of the questions included here are similar to those asked in specialty MH, at least in terms of topics covered. But while the questions might appear similar, in the PCBH model only about five to ten minutes is spent on them in order to keep the focus on the referral problem. These same areas might be probed for the better part of an hour in a specialty MH session. Assessing life context in such a small amount of time requires the BHC to keep the questions flowing and avoid unnecessary follow-up questions.

New BHCs will probably feel as if a lot of material is being left out of this assessment, given the detail of most specialty MH assessments. Certainly, deviations from the template do occur, and often these do yield helpful information. At times, such as when the BHC knows there are no patients waiting for him or her, the BHC might even intentionally deviate and take a few extra minutes for history-gathering. This can be a helpful contribution to the patient's future healthcare and PCPs appreciate it. But hopefully more often than not the BHC will have a busy schedule and will need to stay focused on the referral problem in order to stay on time. (When spare time occurs, it can also be used to work on educational presentations for PCPs, design a program service, or follow-up with a PCP about a patient issue.) Limiting exploration of responses to life context questions is, frankly, one of the most difficult skills for a new BHC to learn but one of the most critical.

For children, the same template can be used, but with some slight modifications. The following are commonly asked about school and social life:

- grade in school
- attitude toward school and teacher
- favorite subject
- number of friends
- favorite activities
- participation in sports or clubs
- whether classes are special or regular
- grades.

Depending on the answers, possible follow-up questions about school might include:

- the number of times the patient has been sent to the office for behavior problems in the past few months
- academic skills problems and/or homework completion habits.

Also commonly asked are questions about home life, family relationships, and activities:

- who lives in the home with the patient
- the patient's sibling position
- his or her relationships with the people in the home
- recreational and relaxation activities at home
- the level of physical activity
- the number of hours spent with a computer/TV/videogames on a daily basis
- difficulties with sleep or eating.

With teenagers, asking about use of tobacco products, alcohol, and illegal drugs is a good idea. Follow-up questions about sexual activity can also be important.

When posing life context questions to patients of any age, listen for strengths and resources. Does the child with a behavior problem at school have a strong relationship with his or her parents? Does the patient with diabetes who is struggling with diet change have a history of successful work (which would suggest the ability to tolerate frustration and persevere)? Does the teenager who is experimenting with drugs have a specific occupational goal? The BHC can use identified strengths and resources to design interventions and, in some occasions, to build the patient's sense of hope and self-efficacy. For example, the patient referred for help with smoking cessation who has successfully quit drugs might be able to reflect on his drug recovery experience to gain ideas for how to stop smoking.

Functional Analysis Questions. After completing life context questions, the focus turns to a functional analysis of the referral issue and target behavior. In the PCBH model, this is done in place of the diagnostic assessment used in specialty MH models. Understanding how to conduct a functional analysis is central to the work of a BHC. However, for those with little background in behavioral assessment and treatment, it might be a new concept. At the risk of giving just enough information to confuse the reader new to this area, a bit of background is provided here. For those seeking more on this topic, a classic book that offers an excellent description of behavioral assessment is *Clinical Behavior Therapy* (Goldfried & Davison, 1994).

The term "functional analysis" implies two parts. The "functional" part refers to the functions of a behavior, or the purposes it seems to serve in the environment. Perhaps, for example, the pain behavior displayed by a patient with chronic back pain serves a function of getting him excused from household chores. The "analysis" part refers to careful assessment of contextual factors that perpetuate this and of other factors that control the behavior (Kazdin, 2001). Central to the functional analysis is the notion that behavior may be maintained through a variety of reinforcers and/or environmental conditions (i.e., modeling, operant and/or classical conditioning). Thus, determining what those reinforcers or environmental conditions are allows one to develop an intervention uniquely tailored to the individual and his or her context.

A typical functional analysis has three components, including problem specification, hypothesis generation, and identification/teaching of alternative behaviors. In problem specification, the goal is to identify a target behavior to focus on. Often, the link between the referral concern (expressed by the PCP or the patient) and the target behavior is direct, as in the case of a specific referral for "poor sleep" or "headache pain." Other times, one may need to tease out a target behavior, as in the case of a referral for the rather vague "behavior problems at home." Unless the focus of vague referrals is narrowed to a specific target behavior, a clear treatment plan will be hard to develop. Continuing with the example of "behavior problems at home," helpful questions for the BHC to ask might be which behaviors the parent tolerates least well and/or which are most problematic for the parent. Follow-up questions may help the BHC decide whether it is more realistic to target a specific behavior (for example, swearing when asked to turn off the television) or a response class (for example, consistently complying with parental requests without swearing). Another example of a referral concern that may require some problem specification work is "depression." This is a common referral in primary care but is very nonspecific. Consider asking the patient referred for this about the most troubling aspects of his or her functioning. Possible answers could include fatigue, concentration problems, sleep disturbance, or social isolation, among others. With this type of questioning, a more specific and observable behavior to work on will emerge.

After identifying one or two target behaviors, the next step is to gather more specifics regarding it/them and its/their context. For example, when did the swearing or oppositionality begin at home? Or, when did the sleep disturbance or fatigue begin? With only a few questions, a BHC may learn that fatigue began after the death of a parent three months ago, that it is worse after talking with a sibling with whom there is an acrimonious relationship, and that it is better when seeing a friend and/or going for a walk outside. For a child with headaches, assessment may reveal that they occur after school and improve after rest, relaxation and eating, but worsen when pushed to do chores or homework. Figure 7.5 presents a list of areas to explore when assessing a target behavior.

Problem specification questions help define a problem clearly and open the door for understanding possible relationships between behavior and context/environment. Generating hypotheses about such relationships is the next step in the functional analysis. In the case of the child who swears when being asked to do something at home, might the lecture given by the parents afterward be reinforcing the swearing? Might hypersomnia and/or fatigue function to help the depressed patient avoid the full experience of grief? Does a headache complaint help the child obtain positive, nurturing attention from busy parents? Consider the case of a seven-year-old child recently referred to one of us for the referral concern of "sleep disturbance." Problem specification questioning revealed the child had never slept in her own bed, and her mother and father wanted this to change. Hypothesis generation questions revealed that the child feared being alone in her room, where she often recalled images from horror movies. This led to the hypotheses that the child lacked skills for responding to these images and for relaxing in her room, particularly when alone, and that the relief of escaping to her parents' bed was reinforcing avoidance of her own bed.

In the third part of a functional analysis, the patient is taught more adaptive and health-protective behaviors, the rationale for which stems directly from hypotheses generated earlier. For the child with sleep problems described in the previous paragraph, this involved asking the parents to stop exposure to images of horror and violence and teaching both the mother and child a new set of skills. Both were taught a relaxation procedure (diaphragmatic breathing) to be used first in the context of being held by the mother and then in the context of lying in the bedroom alone. Additionally, the patient's mother agreed to return the patient to her room in a quiet, efficient, and caring manner should she go to the parents' room after having gone to bed. The patient and her mother returned for a follow-up consultation and reported that the patient was sleeping in her room, and was even showing less of a fear response to the family dog as well. Quite often, this type of generalization occurs with a successful intervention, which means that even if there are initially many areas of concern, a well-formulated intervention for just one target behavior can end up affecting many others as well.

Functional analysis tends to fit well in the primary care environment, where PCPs are usually focused on functioning (whether they realize and label it as such or not). It allows the BHC to offer the patient a clear plan that can be supported well by a PCP, and it fits the time constraints of the primary care setting. Admittedly, though, for those unaccustomed to behavioral assessment processes, some practice and outside reading may be needed.

Putting it all Together. As mentioned earlier, most primary care clinics use the "SOAP" format for charting services delivered to patients. This format, developed by Lawrence Weed, M.D., in the 1960s, provides a logical structure for medical record documentation. Many specialty MH clinics also utilize a SOAP format so this will not be a difficult part of care for many BHCs. The "O" and "P" sections in particular tend to be similar in the PCBH and specialty MH models. In the SOAP format the "Subjective" information (here consisting of life context and functional analysis questions) is followed by "Objective" information, such as mental status findings and test results. Rarely is a comprehensive mental status evaluation conducted, but the core elements of one may be documented.

These first two sections are followed by the "Assessment" summary. In specialty MH the "A" is usually a diagnosis, and might be displayed as Axis I, Axis II, etc. However, in the PCBH model the hypothesis resulting from the functional analysis is listed instead. The primary physical health diagnosis from the PCP is noted here as well (recall the discussion of this in Chapter 4). In cases where a psychiatric diagnosis is clear (e.g., if one has done an extensive ADHD work-up), many BHCs do list it. Other times a PCP will specifically ask for a diagnostic impression, in which case one can be provided. (Often we use qualifier terms such as "*Likely* bipolar disorder" if we have been unable to do a comprehensive diagnostic workup during our brief visit.) However, as much as possible, use the "A" section for the physical health problem and functional analysis hypotheses.

The "P" section details the "Plan." Some clinicians combine the "A" and "P" sections while others list them separately. Combining them may help

PCPs better understand how the plan developed from the assessment. Many BHCs divide the plan into two sections, one containing recommendations for the patient and the other recommendations for the PCP. The reality is that many PCPs will not have or take the time to read an entire BHC note, even if it's brief, but they may glance at the plan. They are often particularly likely to get into this habit if there is a separate section with clear and specific recommendations for them. Table 7.1 displays the basic contents of SOAP notes as they are applied in the PCBH model.

In Chapters 9 and 10, we provide examples of BHC SOAP notes for initial and follow-up consultations with children and adults. As a rule, chart notes should be under one page in length and completed immediately after ending contact with the patient. Quality and efficiency in charting drop considerably the longer one waits to do it.

Questions Not to Ask

Throughout the initial consult, and consistent with a focus on functional analysis, avoid asking questions not directly related to the referral problem. Although specialty MH providers may explore and probe during a history, this practice in PCBH can quickly place a BHC behind in the

Table 7.1. SOAP note contents

Subjective:	Patient age and sex; referring provider and referral issue; patient's responses to life context questions; data from the functional analysis
Objective:	Behavioral observations of the patient and any others present; pertinent mental status issues (e.g., alertness, cognitive organization, suicidal ideation, etc.); test results (e.g., health-related quality of life assessment scores);
Assessment and Plan:	Hypotheses from the functional analysis; physical diagnosis from the PCP; plan, including recommendations for the patient (e.g., psychoeducation, skill-building, referral to outside agency, goals) and for the PCP (e.g., support newly learned skills/goals or referral to a clinical pathway or outside agency, focus on educating or reassuring patient on a particular topic); any further planned assessment or follow-up with the BHC

patient schedule. Sometimes significant information does come up during a visit that simply must be explored (e.g., a patient being started on an SSRI for depression reveals a history of manic symptoms, or a patient referred for sleep problems divulges current domestic violence). In such situations, rigid adherence to an agenda would not be in anyone's best interest. Yet, routinely deviating from the referral issue comes with many of its own problems. After some initial experience, the new BHC will probably be surprised at how much can be accomplished and how well patients respond to this more limited visit structure.

Questions geared toward establishing a psychiatric diagnosis also are not generally recommended. There is simply not enough time to do this well and to also complete an effective functional analysis and plan. Further, most will find that producing a specific diagnosis lends little to a treatment plan beyond what a functional analysis can offer. That said, sometimes PCPs will ask a BHC specifically for help with a diagnosis, usually because he or she is considering a medication trial and has been trained to dispense medications according to diagnosis. If this happens, use of the specific self-report tools discussed in Chapter 6 may augment the usual initial assessment routine.

FOLLOW-UP CONSULTS

At first glance, distinguishing a follow-up from an initial visit seems simple enough. However, as mentioned early in the discussion of initial visits, sometimes the line between the two is not so clear. Patients will sometimes be referred for one problem, only to return a few weeks later with an entirely new problem. Alternatively, patients might be referred back to the BHC numerous times over the course of a few years, always for the same problem. Deciding whether to schedule a patient as an initial or follow-up consult deserves some discussion, because the length and structure of the consult will vary depending on how the visit is classified.

Consider two criteria, time elapsed and reason for referral, when deciding whether to make a visit an initial or a follow-up. If the patient is returning within six months of an initial visit with the BHC and the reason for referral remains the same, the visit is usually best classified as a follow-up. In these visits, the BHC does not necessarily need to spend time updating life context. Instead, questions should focus on the patient's progress with the initial plan and problem-solving of any barriers to fulfilling the plan. If the patient comes to the BHC with an entirely new reason for referral, regardless of the time that has elapsed since the initial consultation, this is usually best treated as an initial consultation. In these cases, the BHC will need to define the target behavior in relation to the new referral reason and conduct a new functional analysis and plan. Patients returning after an absence of six months or greater are probably best scheduled as initial consults, even when the reason for referral is the same. For such patients, more time should be devoted to updating life context and development of a new plan based on a new functional analysis.

Although over half of primary care consultations will be single consults, a significant number of patients will come for planned follow-up visits with the BHC. Most planned follow-ups will occur within one to two months of the initial consultation (and may be much sooner, if the patient is high-risk). Other follow-up visits will be with patients for whom there was no planned follow-up. These patients generally divide into three groups: those with worsening stress that is interfering with implementing the initial plan; those who have relapsed with a behavior previously improved after the initial BHC visit(s); those with a new reason for referral.

During follow-up visits of any sort, the main focus will be on assessing progress with the initial plan and formation of a new plan. Listen for any parts of the plan the patient was able to implement and be sure to recognize and support these. If the patient had difficulty implementing the plan, the focus of the follow-up might be problem-solving barriers. Keep in mind also that in some cases the target behavior may not be the same as for the initial consult, thereby requiring a new functional analysis.

Length and Frequency of Follow-Up Consults

Typically, follow-up appointments are briefer than initial consultations and less frequent and fewer in number than in outpatient MH or chemical dependency treatment. When a patient reports success with the planned intervention, the consult may be as brief as fifteen minutes. If the BHC had reserved twenty to thirty minutes, the extra time can be applied to providing PCP feedback, or may be needed to catch up after going longer than planned with an earlier patient. Examples of PCP feedback include talking with the PCP about a successful intervention, leaving a written message, or (in the case of particularly successful or unique interventions) summarizing the case for a five-minute presentation at a provider meeting or an article in a PCBH newsletter.

Most patients who come for a follow-up consultation come for only one or two, but a few do come for more. For example, high-risk or multiproblem patients may come for numerous appointments spaced out over time. This approach allows for the BHC to influence the primary care plan for patients over a longer period, as well as to perhaps take some of the visit load off of the PCP.

Playing Ping Pong with the Primary Care Provider

Playing ping pong is a metaphor that describes the process of shouldering some of the PCP's visit load for high stakes patients or intensifying PCP/BHC coordination for certain patients. The PCP starts the rally by referring the patient to the BHC, who then returns the ball by having the patient follow-up with the PCP prior to the next BHC follow-up. In the initial consultation, the BHC typically recommends the ping-pong strategy and suggests specific content for the follow-up visit with the PCP. For example, the BHC might determine during an initial consult that a patient with chronic pain is avoiding physical therapy sessions because he or she misinterprets postsession pain flare-ups as a sign of reinjury. Thus, the BHC might send the patient back to the PCP and ask the PCP to focus specifically on reassuring the patient that acute pain episodes do not mean reinjury. The PCP could then, in turn, have the patient return to the BHC to further discuss pain management. Another example might be a patient with paranoid schizophrenia who visits her PCP frequently to refill medicine or to discuss a perceived conflict with neighbors. Because the patient's visits are so frequently psychosocial in nature, the BHC might alternate visits with the PCP and simply schedule PCP visits for dates when medications are due for refill.

Ping pong can continue for two or more iterations, depending on the patient and the target behavior. In a small number of cases it may continue indefinitely, but prior to each volley the BHC should check-in with the PCP to ensure that he or she understands and supports the recommended content for the follow-up. Played well, each volley offers an opportunity for the BHC to help the PCP help the patient, while also assuming some of the follow-up visit load from the PCP. Though this extended contact might seem more like a specialty MH model, visits remain brief and focused and always produce a recommendation for the PCP.

Venues for Follow-Up Contact

Not all follow-ups need to be face to face with the BHC. Often, patients benefit from a brief phone call follow-up. The phone call follow-up is particularly useful for the patient who wants to implement a behavior change (e.g., starting a medication, beginning a walking plan) but has limited confidence in her or his ability to get started. The BHC may suggest a follow-up call within twenty-four to forty-eight hours to assure that the patient made a start or to assist in developing an alternative plan if the original plan was not viable. Another alternative follow-up venue is e-mail. For confidentiality and practice management reasons e-mail is not always feasible. However, some clinics have implemented a formal system for secure PCP-provider e-mails, and some patients can actually be more easily contacted via e-mail than phone (especially homeless patients, who often have a free e-mail account but no phone). Land mail can also be a helpful method of follow-up, as it can be written and read at times that are convenient for both parties. Land mail is often used to notify patients of resources in which they have expressed interest. For example, the BHC might maintain a list of patients interested in parenting groups and send out letters of notification when one is starting.

Decisions About Continuing Care

The main thrust of a planned follow-up is to assess the effect(s) of the initial intervention and, if it was successful, to discuss ways to continue it. As in initial consults, patients returning for follow-up should complete a standard health-related quality of life measure prior to the visit. Results might be shared with the patient and compared with the initial consult score(s) as one way of continuing the functional analysis to help determine the need for further visits. The goal, of course, is to back out of planned care as soon as possible and have the patient simply follow-up with his or her PCP, who can continue to support the behavior plan. The best time to do this is when the patient has embarked on a clear plan that he or she seems to understand and has the motivation and confidence to continue. In the case of an ineffective intervention, the BHC might further assess the function of the target behavior and refine the functional analysis to hopefully generate a more effective intervention.

The BHC also should note whether the patient had contact with the PCP during the last six months regarding the referral question. If this has not occurred, it should be scheduled as part of the planned intervention. Some patients may struggle with developing a working relationship with their PCP and may seek continuing care from the BHC instead. The BHC needs to always support development of a strong PCP–patient relationship and to avoid becoming a substitute for the PCP.

Making Sense of Advanced Access

One of the first things a new BHC will probably notice is that scheduling is done quite differently in primary care than in specialty MH. In the latter setting, most all visits are considered routine and only emergency (i.e., suicidal or homicidal) patients are given same-day appointments. However, in primary care, patients commonly expect same-day appointments, and the acrobatics required to accommodate them can overload the system and push routine visits well into the future. Appointment demand often seems to far outstrip the supply of PCPs. However, a practice management approach called "Advanced Access" aims to improve this mess, and because of its proliferation no discussion of visit scheduling in primary care would be complete without discussing it. As introduced in a recent JAMA article (Murray & Berwick, 2003), Advanced Access is a strategy for scheduling medical visits that can reduce wait times for appointments without adding staff or providers. BH providers have a significant role to play in the successful implementation of Advanced Access, but also can utilize the concept with their own scheduling.

In traditional scheduling approaches, patients are often sorted according to urgency of need (i.e., urgent patients are squeezed into a same-day appointment or sent to the emergency room while nonurgent are pushed off into the future), or a clinic might carve-out time each day to accommodate urgent patients. For a variety of reasons, both approaches actually perpetuate scheduling headaches. For example, to decide if a patient has an "urgent" need, the patient must be triaged by a nurse, who then must consult with a PCP. If the patient is designated "urgent" but no appointments can be found, the patient is sent to the emergency department, where the follow-up plan usually includes returning to the PCP to track progress. In this scenario, one urgent patient required the time of the nurse, the scheduler, and the PCP, only to return later to follow-up with the PCP for the same problem (not to mention the unnecessary utilization of the emergency department).

In clinics using an Advanced Access model, the goal would be to have that patient seen the same day by his or her personal PCP. In fact, the goal is for all patients desiring a same-day appointment to be given one. The motto of Advanced Access is, "Do today's work today" (Murray & Berwick, 2003), meaning the system design gives patients appointments essentially on demand. (One important assumption is that the number of PCPs is adequate for meeting patient demand.) Each PCP has a percentage of appointment time each day, ideally 50 percent, available for same-day care. This allows most patients to see their usual PCP at the time of their request. Only patients who decline a same-day appointment or who are seen same-day and need a follow-up at some definite time in the future are scheduled out. By providing same-day appointments, the triage nurse and scheduler are freed to do other tasks, and the PCP avoids being interrupted by the triage nurse or having to coordinate follow-up with the emergency room provider.

There are many more details to Advanced Access than can be covered here. Most important is for the BHC to have a basic idea of the concept and how he or she can participate in or apply it. One way a BHC can participate and help is to be present on high-volume days (usually Mondays and Fridays) and times of the year (e.g., back-to-school time and the day after thanksgiving). This enables the BHC to take some of the demand load off the PCP when it is most needed. For example, some patients desiring a PCP appointment might be redirected to the BHC, or the BHC might at least see the patient immediately prior to the PCP to obtain a history and help make the PCP's visit more efficient. Another way to help is by organizing group medical visits (see Chapter 12). These can help reduce demand and are a wonderful activity for a BHC to be involved with. The "ping-pong" strategy described in the previous section also fits well with Advanced Access, because it reduces demand on the PCP.

As a BHC service grows, many of the same scheduling problems that PCPs encounter may also happen to the BHC. However, several practices can put Advanced Access to work for the BHC. For one, patients needing follow-up might be asked to call for an appointment on either the day before or the day of desired follow-up, rather than scheduling an appointment date immediately after the initial consult. This can help decrease the rate of no-shows and last-minute cancellations and thereby ensure a more open schedule for same-day patients. Patients can be given a card with call-in information and a desired follow-up interval. Some patients, such as those with suicidal ideation, might need to be scheduled, but the majority will probably not need to be. Some BHCs (especially those with a BHA for administrative support) maintain a list of patients needing follow-up and send a letter to those patients reminding them to call for follow-up.

Another Advanced Access technique is to extend the interval between return visits. Most follow-up intervals have been taught and passed-on through generations of providers without any empirical evidence of an optimal interval (Schwartz, Woloshin, Wasson, Renfrew, & Welch, 1999). Many BHCs are in the habit of scheduling follow-ups for one or two weeks later, when in fact three or four weeks might be adequate or even better. A third technique, also mentioned in the previous paragraph, is the formation of group visits. Just as these can reduce demand for a PCP they can also help with a BHC's demand problems. Advanced Access may require some getting used to, but it holds great promise for optimizing BHC time and for highlighting the role of BHCs as primary care team members.

CHARTING AND MEDICAL RECORDS

Though it comes as a surprise to some, BHC consultation notes are primary care records and should not be treated any differently from other primary care notes. They are placed in the medical chart and look like primary care notes in all respects. This is true whether the official medical record is a paper one or, as is the case more often these days, electronic.

Chart Note Location

The PCBH consultation note belongs in the section of the medical record where all routine visit notes are placed (often labeled the "chronology" section or, in the Electronic Medical Record, the "clinical information" section). This helps ensure that other primary care team members will read the note and follow its recommendations, as a note placed in a separate section will rarely be viewed. Some clinics using paper charts place a sticker at the bottom of the BHC note page so it can be more easily found and referred to by interested team members.

Electronic Medical Records

The Electronic Medical Record (EMR) offers a great deal of support to the work of the BHC and PCP and to their collaboration. Most larger primary care clinics have plans to transition to an EMR or already have done so. This trend is not just a reflection of an increasingly technology-based world; it is a central strategy for empowering primary care to better manage chronic conditions. As summarized by Bodenheimer, Wagner, and Grumbach (2002a,b), the EMR fills three important roles: (1) establishment of registries that coordinate and track care for patients with chronic conditions; (2) provision of feedback to providers regarding patient status on various health indices, and (3) development of reminder systems that help providers follow practice guidelines.

In the case of diabetes, for example, clinic staff may enter every diagnosed patient into a registry or database. Staff members update database information whenever a patient in the registry for a specific condition comes for service. Specific data fields typically include a wide array of information, such as lab tests, referrals (e.g., a retinal exam), patient counseling (e.g., smoking cessation counseling), and patient–PCP establishment of self-management goals. Registries provide PCPs with feedback on the extent to which patients on their panel are obtaining services recommended by guidelines. One PCP might learn that she needs to improve her foot check rates, while another might notice his patients' blood pressures are higher than the patients of other PCPs. Tracking data in this manner helps providers find areas where their performance has been weak, and provides subtle peer pressure to improve. During the actual patient visit, the reminder feature of EMR comes into play. When the PCP enters the patient's particulars into the system, he or she might be reminded to place the patient on aspirin therapy, start the patient on a statin, or to follow some other practice guideline. The EMR can support registries, reminders, and PCP comparisons for any number of chronic conditions in addition to diabetes, such as depression, chronic pain, asthma, ADHD, and others.

The BHC can use the EMR to influence care and improve PCP practice in a number of ways. For example, the BHC can advocate for inclusion of reminders that prompt PCPs to refer specific patients that might be otherwise overlooked (e.g., patients with tension headaches or irritable bowel syndrome). Templates, which are used by most EMR systems, can include health-related quality of life scores in the laboratory section, which may improve PCP use of them in planning medical treatments. The BHC might also spearhead development of registries for a variety of conditions in the EMR. Most clinics will plan to create a diabetes registry, but building one for, say, depression or ADHD might require BHC help. This allows the BHC to influence how care is delivered for depression and/or ADHD and increases the likelihood of more referrals of individual patients. Such registries might also compare PCP performance on the percentage of patients referred to the BHC or the percentage of patients taking narcotics who are referred to a chronic pain pathway.

Another helpful aspect of EMR is that the BHC can provide same-day feedback to PCPs without moving charts around or worrying that the post-it note stuck on top of the chart will be lost. Most EMR programs even have integrated e-mail services in which BHC and PCP communications are automatically entered into the EMR. These are some of the most readily apparent ways the EMR can help the BHC to do his or her part to improve healthcare, but we are optimistic that as the technology develops even more uses will become clear.

SUMMARY

1. Initial patient visits in the PCBH model consist of life context and functional analysis questions. The former is much more limited than its counterpart in specialty MH evaluations and the latter might not be familiar to some new BHCs. Both may require significant practice in the early stages of a service.

2. The SOAP format used by most clinics provides a structured approach to charting, and one that will be easily read by PCPs.

3. Notes pertaining to patient care are placed in the medical record. They are not given a separate section in the chart, though they may be marked in some way to help PCPs and others find needed information.

4. Follow-up is limited for most patients, but some high-impact patients may be seen more frequently. Often this is done through alternative venues to the in-person visit or involves alternating visits with the PCP.

5. Electronic medical records can help tremendously with implementing the PCBH model. They allow for more immediate feedback to and frequent communications with PCPs, and provide new opportunities for influencing PCP behavior.

6. Advanced Access, a strategy used by many clinics to optimize appointment availability, contains important roles for a BHC. Its principles can also be applied to the BHC's own scheduling practices.

8

START-UP:
WHAT TO DO AND
HOW TO INFLUENCE PCPS

"I have learned that success is to be measured not so much by the posi-
tion that one has reached in life as by the obstacles which he has had to
overcome while trying to succeed."

—Booker T. Washington

There are obstacles related to our history of separating behavioral and physical health treatment that can only be overcome through day-to-day delivery of integrated services. To succeed in starting a truly integrated service, new BHCs need clear guidance to avoid old pitfalls and to change how PCPs perceive their services. This chapter offers a step-by-step approach to starting up a new service, along with specific strategies for influencing provider behavior. It also gives the new BHC suggestions for responding to administrator and staff requests for various types of help. Finally, an approach and specific tools for monitoring and overcoming obstacles to PCP referrals is detailed.

A START-UP CHECKLIST

Starting a new job is difficult enough but starting a new job with a new model of care that is new to a system is an especially daunting task. What should be done first? Who should be involved in helping? The BHC Start-Up Checklist (see Table 8.1) offers a structure for the new BHC who needs

Table 8.1. Start-up checklist for behavioral health consultants

Week 1: Be visible and get the lay of the land
- Tour clinic, get keys, order business cards
- Set up voice mail, e-mail
- Obtain and learn to use pager or cell phone, have your number added to the provider roster
- Post list of staff and PCP contact numbers at your work station
- Meet or talk by phone with a BHC working in a similar primary care setting
- Meet or schedule meetings with senior leadership
- Develop or clarify the billing plan
- Shadow every willing PCP for part of a day
- Stay late one day
- Ask PCPs what problems they most desire help with
- Obtain list of clinic meetings and determine which to attend regularly
- Attend at least one of each of the clinical team meetings
- Form a Behavioral Health Team
- Begin work on (or read) the BHC program manual
- Visit or call important social service organizations that you are likely to utilize

Week 2: Begin patient care and continue service planning
- Meet with scheduling staff to discuss how to schedule BHC appointments (especially same-day appointments)
- Develop a role introduction and initial visit template
- Learn how to use dictation services
- Recruit and train a BHC assistant (BHA)
- Talk with interpreters about BHC services
- Research and select brief self-report measures to aid assessment
- Review the clinic's risk management policies and procedures
- Shadow more experienced BHC for 2 days
- Distribute handout to staff and/or talk at a staff meeting to introduce yourself and the BHC service
- Speak at a provider's meeting to introduce yourself and the service
- Talk with referral manager and visit affiliated specialty MH service (if applicable)
- Begin seeing patients (see every patient referred, keep the door open unless with a patient, remind PCPs to interrupt as needed for same-day appointments)
- Walk through the halls every hour when not busy with a patient

Week 3 and beyond: Expand and be guided by outcomes
- Ask to preview schedules with PCPs to identify possible same-day patients, particularly PCPs who have referred few or no patients
- Offer to debrief patients
- Administer the referral barriers questionnaire and use results to increase referrals
- Develop needed or requested brochures, patient education materials
- Develop psychoeducational classes or group visits
- Schedule standing time in provider and staff meetings
- Develop a BH newsletter to distribute regularly to staff and PCPs
- Establish processes for evaluating the program (Chapter 15)
- Conduct pilot studies of a proposed clinical pathway
- Spend another day with an experienced BHC with a plan of observing a class or clinical pathway activity

answers to these questions. The checklist contains activities that most often need to be attended to in the early stages of a service. After perusing the table, we recommend referring back to it from time to time to ensure ongoing attention to important activities. The following paragraphs elaborate on the checklist's contents.

Week One: Be Visible and Get the Lay of the Land

An old Chinese proverb will prove useful in your first week: If you wish to succeed, consult three old people. Who are the old people that the BHC needs to meet? These include senior providers, particularly those with strong interests in behavioral health, and senior leaders in the clinic or health care system (e.g., the CEO, CFO, and/or other administrators). Relationships with the clinic medical director, the clinic manager, and the director of nursing are also pivotal to success, and should be formed early. During the first week, try to schedule time with as many of these individuals as possible to introduce yourself and your new service. These are the individuals who will need to be consulted when developing or clarifying the billing plan, an important first week activity. Also important is to locate a more experienced BHC and plan to meet or talk by phone. Note that finding someone actually working out of an integrated model of the type described here is crucial. Simply finding a MH professional in a primary care setting might not be too difficult, but if that person is utilizing a co-located or other type of model, he or she will probably have a very different approach and philosophy.

Day one of the new job will probably involve a tour of the clinic and introductions to staff, but don't expect anyone to be able to talk long. Afterward, activities will usually focus on basic orientating. Many clinics will have a provider orientation process established but not all will. The processes of those that do will probably be geared toward physicians, and so will have many parts that do not apply to a BHC. Practice patience as you explain repeatedly that you are not a physician (assuming you are not). During orientation, be sure to acquire a list of staff contact numbers, set up e-mail and voice mail, get keys, order business cards, and learn to use the phones. Obtain a list of regular clinic meetings from the medical director and/or manager and ask their opinion on which ones to attend. Attending at least one of each of the clinical team meetings during the first week or two (e.g., the diabetes team, depression team, or whatever other clinical groups the clinic might have) can be very helpful. Also consider staying late one day, as providers are most likely to have time to talk at the end of the day (this also shows one's willingness to work hard, like his or her PCP colleagues, for whom staying late is almost a daily occurrence).

Also important is to shadow every willing PCP for half-a-day or a couple of hours during the first week. Shadowing involves sitting in on every patient visit. The reasons for shadowing are to learn about the types of problems the providers see, the nature of PCP–patient interactions in the clinic, patient flow issues, and ways a new BHC service can be of help. There is also much to be learned from watching PCPs in action. When shadowing, most people simply listen, observe, and make note of what the PCP might need in order to be more effective (e.g., a new screening tool, help with history-gathering, knowledge of some simple coping techniques to teach patients, etc.). Because providers vary greatly in their interests, different objectives will become clear for different providers. Some may be eager to learn specific cognitive behavioral interventions, while others will be much less interested in psychosocial issues. For the latter group, one might set an initial goal of simply shaping them to consistently make same-day referrals.

If a behavioral issue arises when shadowing, be prepared to provide input; but avoid jumping into discussions if not invited. Talking with PCPs beforehand about how active they want you to be during visits can help you decide when to chime in. Somewhat surprisingly, some PCPs will feel anxious being observed, so be sure to mention that the purpose of shadowing is not for judging performance. Take notes as needed between patients, discuss any questions or observations with the PCPs at day's end, and of course thank those who are willing to be shadowed.

Form a Behavioral Health (BH) Team. Laying the groundwork for a BH Team should also be done during the first week. The purpose of this team is to help achieve the mission of the PCBH model, as described in Chapter 3. The best BH team members will be those that support this mission and have a history of working effectively as team members. As with Noah's Ark, try to bring aboard a variety of players. The clinic manager is a critical member, as he or she will know how to best support new projects. In cases where the clinic manager supervises the BHC, the team experience will also generate good information for performance reviews. While the medical director is also a good team member, he or she may decline due to lack of time. In such cases, ask if he or she can recommend another provider who has strong interests in BH issues. Having a PCP "champion" on the team is crucial for PCP–BHC communications and the development of PCP-friendly services. Nursing staff can also be a useful and critical part of the team. Again, if the Nursing Director is reluctant due to time or other constraints, ask that he or she designate an alternative nursing staff member. If a BHA is hired, he or she should definitely be a team member. If there is no BHA support, a nursing assistant with interests in BH issues is a good option. Nursing and nursing assistant members can help ensure all layers of staff know about BHC services and they are crucial for figuring out the nuts and bolts of program implementation.

During the first two to three months, the team should meet weekly if possible. If this is not possible, try to meet with each team member briefly on a weekly basis. The meetings do not need to be long; fifteen minutes may be adequate. In the beginning, greater frequency is important because many questions will emerge and these may need quick answers in order to stay on track. However, after the first three months, the team may meet less frequently. Meetings may become monthly, quarterly, or simply as needed once the service seems to be running smoothly. Table 8.2 presents common topics for BH Team meetings.

While not all topics need to be covered at every meeting, the team needs to look at all areas at least quarterly. Even in the first few months, we recommend that the BHC discuss clinical pathways with team members, as these offer potent strategies for extending BHC services to a large

Table 8.2. Common topics for BHC meetings

1. Administrative issues (including space, supplies, equipment, billing, development of a program manual, interface with other clinic staff, etc.)
2. Performance (including feedback from patients and providers, efforts to provide educational presentations or documents to providers)
3. Clinical issues (including number of referrals from each provider, the ratio of same-day to scheduled visits, the diversity of referral issues, the BHC's ability to stay on time)
4. Clinical pathway issues (including identification of potential target problems, pilot studies to evaluate elements of a pathway, etc.)

number of patients. Chapters 9–12 offer specific suggestions for development of pathways.

Finally, if time permits during the first week, make a point of visiting local social service organizations. Government and nonprofit agencies that help patients find housing, food, transportation, and other basics are extremely important to know about. Understanding a bit about the extent of their services, which patients will be eligible, and how their services can be accessed will pay off when faced with a patient in need. Making personal connections with staff in these organizations can also help tremendously when needing to advocate for patients. If there is no time for visiting organizations during the first week, prioritize it during the second.

What About Seeing Patients? If entering an established BHC service, patient care might begin after just a day or two of orientation. However, if starting up a new BHC service, there will usually be no expectations for seeing patients in the first week. The pressure will almost certainly be on to begin clinical work in the second week, though.

Week Two:
Begin Patient Care and Continue Service Planning

The beginning of the second week is the time to complete final organizing work for seeing patients. Have an introductory discussion with the interpreter(s), develop your role introduction and initial visit template, and learn how to use dictation services. If the clinic plans to hire a BHA, devote some time to recruiting and training this person this week. Also meet with scheduling staff to ensure the schedule is set up and that they understand how to schedule all types of BHC visits. Some discussion will likely be needed about how to best work same-day patients into the schedule. Schedulers might also be able to explain how to make time-off requests and schedule changes.

At some point this week, spend two or more days shadowing a more experienced BHC, if possible. A BHC mentor will most likely share hand-outs, readings, and other materials. Discuss options for self-report measures with this person, or do some self-guided research on this topic (see Chapter 6). Opportunities for trying out different measures will emerge as soon as patient care begins. Also try to get time to introduce the PCBH model at a provider meeting (if one is scheduled) and make and distribute a handout to providers to solicit same-day referrals. In the next section of this chapter, "Influencing PCPs," we offer materials to use as handouts or as flyers. The goal of these efforts is to help providers understand the differences between specialty care and PCBH services and to give them tools for describing the BHC service to patients.

After getting the basics organized, proclaim the service open to patients this week. Remember to be accessible. Keep the office door open and/or walk the halls each hour in search of referrals when not with a patient. Post a work schedule on the office door or in a common area where other provider schedules are displayed. On the schedule, include contact information such as a pager or cell phone number, and a reminder for PCPs to knock if the door is closed. Although one might expect to be overwhelmed with patients from the outset, rarely does this actually happen. There will be plenty of time to continue service planning while seeing patients, so avoid the temptation to block out time for "administrative work" or "catch up." Though this is sometimes a practice in specialty MH, it is a cardinal sin in the PCBH model! It gives the wrong impression about accessibility and may alienate some PCP colleagues who will not have the luxury of blocking time in their schedules. Referrals to a BHC service will almost certainly grow over time, but during the first few months the pace will be slow enough to allow for service planning activities.

At some point this week, also take time to learn about the process for referring patients to specialty psychology and psychiatry services. This might involve talking with the referral manager or visiting the affiliated specialty MH service, if the clinic has one. The goal of these visits is to learn what types of specialty MH services exist and what the common barriers are to patients accessing them. If visiting an affiliated service, one topic of discussion should be coordination of care for shared patients (i.e., those patients referred to the BHC who are also being followed in MH).

Week Three and Beyond: Expand and be Guided by Outcomes

By this point relationships have often begun to form with PCPs, so it can be a good time to ask to preview schedules with them. The goal of this is to identify possible same-day patients for referral. Some clinics have "team huddles" at the beginning of each day, in which the PCP and his or her support staff survey the day's schedule to prepare, and this is an ideal activity for the BHC to participate in. Schedule previews are an excellent time to educate and/or remind the team that many common "medical" symptoms and conditions, such as hypertension, diabetes, enuresis, insomnia, etc., may make good referrals. If the clinic does not do morning huddles, the best option is to ask each PCP for a minute of time to preview the schedule. However, if a PCP seems exceptionally busy, simply reviewing a paper copy of his or her schedule and writing "BHC referral?" next to select patients can work.

Another possible activity for this week involves "debriefing" patients. Usually this is done for a half-day at a time and focuses on just one PCP's patients at a time. In debriefings, the BHC meets with patients for a few minutes after they finish the PCP visit. They might be asked about satisfaction with the visit or about psychosocial issues not mentioned in the visit. Obviously, one needs to get the permission of the PCP beforehand to do this and patients should be allowed to opt out as desired. The PCP might have his or her nursing assistant escort patients to the BHC after finishing the visit. Feedback from patient debriefings may help PCPs better recognize patients to refer in the future. When combined with shadowing, they also can help a BHC to set priorities for program development. Learning more about the patient populations of greatest concern to PCPs and the issues of greatest need in the clinic can inform the development of clinical pathways, written educational materials, etc.

Looking beyond the first few weeks, many activities will be important for stimulating growth in a new BHC service. As data are collected formally and informally (from debriefings, shadowing, program evaluation, etc.), the best avenues for expansion start to materialize. Most BHCs will find the first year of a service to be full of challenges, stimulation, and personal and professional growth. Keep the following in mind as the first year progresses.

Additional Visits with a BHC Mentor. If attempts to find an experienced BHC mentor have been successful, make additional visits to him or her and continue to search out other mentors. Actual visits (rather than phone calls) are preferred, as few activities are more helpful for learning this model than observing a BHC in practice. Visits on days when the senior BHC is conducting a class or workshop or facilitating a BH Team meeting may prove especially helpful. During standing time in provider and staff meetings, summarize what was learned in visits with other BHCs, particularly as it applies to specific PCP concerns or ideas for service expansion.

Using Outcomes to Guide Program Development. A good deal of data will begin to accumulate during the first year of a BHC service, in both qualitative and quantitative forms, and this can be used to help grow a service. Informal or formal analysis of the conditions that seem to occur most often in the clinic, take the most PCP time, or cause the most PCP headaches can help inform development of targeted services. If, for example, chronic pain is a frequently seen and frequently complained about problem in the clinic, developing a clinical pathway to improve chronic pain care processes would be an excellent initiative. If PCPs seem to struggle with "noncompliant patients," writing a Behavioral Health Newsletter column (see Figures 8.3 and 8.4) on motivational interviewing techniques would make sense and might lead to teaching opportunities with PCPs. Data might also be collected on the number of BHC referrals from each PCP and on barriers to PCP referral. This, in turn, might lead one to talk with a nonreferring PCP about how the BHC can help more, or to development of strategies for overcoming common referral barriers in the clinic (discussed in the last section of this chapter).

Other relevant data, such as clinical outcome scores on self-report measures, PCP and patient satisfaction with BHC services, chart and performance reviews, and self-assessment of one's core competencies can also be used to promote service growth. Perhaps, for example, an analysis of BHC patient demographics shows a smaller proportion of Spanish-speaking patients than is typical of the greater clinic population. In this scenario, a prudent strategy might be to develop passive screening posters in Spanish or group visits specifically targeting Spanish-speakers. Processes for program evaluation, discussed in detail in Chapter 15, should be established early in a service so growth of the service can be tracked.

EDUCATING PROVIDERS ABOUT THE BHC SERVICE

The most important aspect of BHC work is influencing the practice of PCPs. Methods for influencing PCPs vary widely and include presentations at provider meetings or lunch hour workshops, written communications (e.g., e-mails, newsletters, and brief handouts) and "professional detailing." Detailing involves brief individual meetings with a PCP to discuss some topic identified a priori by the BHC (e.g., how to use or score the PHQ-9). In this section, we suggest critical messages for the BHC to convey in the first year, along with materials to support these efforts.

Teaching the PCBH Model to PCPs

In some cases, a behavioral health service will not be new to the primary care clinic or a new concept to PCPs. Some health care systems across the United States began employing behavioral health providers on-site in the 1970s and 1980s. However, these systems usually utilized a co-location model of care rather than the PCBH model. In the co-located model, traditional specialty MH policies and procedures are followed, meaning intake procedures are usually extensive and diagnosis-focused, and regular therapy visits are used. Providers in these services usually focus their resources on "mental health" problems rather than the broader range of problems seen in the PCBH model. A BHC taking a position in a system accustomed to using a co-located model may need to work doubly hard to orient staff and patients to the PCBH model. The PCPs might have a limited notion of how to utilize the BHC, might expect him or her to provide intensive therapy and evaluation, and will probably expect to have to go through a formal referral process. They will probably also expect problems with accessing the BHC's services and struggle with the concept of interrupting the BHC when needed.

In clinics that have never had a behavioral health provider on site, providers may tune into descriptions of the PCBH model more readily. Still, many will make assumptions about BHC services based on their training and their professional experiences with specialty MH providers.

They may see the BHC as a precious resource, a therapist that must be reserved for the most disabled and symptomatic of their patients with mental disorders. A few PCPs may also have ambivalent feelings toward the BHC after having been thwarted in past efforts to obtain specialty MH care. Table 8.3 provides a summary of the differences between PCBH services and specialty behavioral services. This can be used as a handout for a

Table 8.3. PCBH services and specialty mental health services

Dimension	BHC services	Specialty services
What?	Consultation focused on PCP question or concern (15–40 minute visits)	Comprehensive evaluation and treatment (1-hour visits)
For whom?	Any patient with a behaviorally influenced problem(s)	Moderately to severely impaired patients with mental health concerns
When?	Immediately after PCP visit (same-day patients preferred)	Scheduled appointments with variable (usually limited) access
Why?	Functional assessment and treatment plan to enhance the PCP's care plan; population-health model	Diagnostic assessment, symptom alleviation, improved functioning; focus on individual care delivered by specialist
Where?	Primary care (notes placed directly into medical chart)	External (copies of notes obtained with patient permission)
Cost to patients?	Less (free in some clinics)	More
What Else?	Episodic, longitudinal care (over the lifespan)	Treatment discontinued when symptoms alleviated
	Brief intensive or programmatic care (consultation-focused)	Regular (weekly or every other week) therapy visits
	Referral to community resources	Case management (some clinics)
	Group medical visits and classes for chronic medical problems	Support/Therapy groups focused on mental health issues
	Efforts to improve healthcare delivery in general	Focused on mental health care specifically
	Probably less stigma	Probably more stigma

provider meeting or simply as a reference point when engaged in professional detailing with individual PCPs. It should also be distributed over time to new PCPs as they enter the system.

Consultant Versus Therapist

Especially during the first year, repeated efforts will likely be needed to explain one's role as a consultant (as opposed to a therapist). This includes explaining that the PCP is the BHC's principal customer, for whom the goal is to provide practical care recommendations. The irony is that PCPs consult everyday with specialists, and clearly understand the role consultations play in care. Yet, they have been so indoctrinated into the specialty MH model that they often have a great deal of difficulty perceiving a behavioral health provider as a consultant. Periodic reminders will be needed to explain that the BHC does not conduct ongoing care but rather teaches patients new skills that hopefully will be discussed, reinforced, and perhaps even expanded upon during subsequent PCP visits. Consistent with the consultant role, PCPs should also be encouraged to consult on general behavioral issues and on patient-specific issues for patients not seen by the BHC.

Referring Patients to BHC Services

Most PCPs will welcome and use ideas about how to refer patients to the BHC. While PCPs vary a great deal, most have a practiced approach to referring patients for specialty MH care, but this habit may cause problems when making BHC referrals. For example, some PCPs may talk about the BHC as a MH provider who does therapy, or as a case manager who can check in with the patient every week. The PCP's choice of words can influence patient expectations and affect the patient's willingness to be referred. At the same time, PCPs who struggle with how to refer patients are usually less likely to do so. For these reasons, consider offering a handout with phrases for a referring PCP to use, such as the one in Table 8.4.

Notice that the script encourages PCPs to find a referral problem the patient is concerned about in cases where the patient resists the initial referral reason. For example, if a PCP's main concern is smoking cessation but the patient is not willing to see the BHC for that, there is probably little point in trying to convince the patient to do otherwise. However, if the

Table 8.4. Scripted components of successful referrals

Component	Referral behavior
Reason for referral	Identify specific reason for consultation with BHC (if patient is resistant, find a problem he or she is concerned about)
	Examples:
	"I want you to see Dr. Reiter, as I think he can help us develop a plan for quitting cigarettes."
	"I want you to see Dr. Robinson, as she is an expert on stress and I think stress is affecting your diabetes management."
Role of BHC	Emphasize consultative relationship ("He or she helps me to help patients with these types of problems.")
	Examples:
	"Dr. Reiter is a psychologist, but he does not offer therapy. He is a consultant, and he'll provide ideas we can work on together to improve your hypertension self-care."
	"Dr. Robinson is my colleague. Her job is to help me improve my treatment plan for parents having problems with a child."
Positive regard	Display confidence in the BHC
	Examples:
	"Dr. Reiter is just down the hall, and he often sees my patients right away. I always find his ideas useful."
	"Dr. Robinson is a warm and caring person, and my patients give me very good feedback about her."

patient *is* concerned about weight loss, this can make for a perfectly acceptable referral reason (even if the PCP is less concerned about it). Quite frankly, health and behavior are so intertwined that tussling over whether to pursue a referral for "this" problem versus "that" problem is usually needless. Many patients who resist a referral for one reason but engage with the BHC for another ultimately end up making changes in the problem of initial concern.

Some PCPs have difficulty encouraging patients to see the BHC if the patient is resistant. Encourage these PCPs to treat a referral to the BHC in the same way they treat referrals to other consultants. Most have no problem being assertive with patients who are reluctant to pursue a referral to an ophthalmologist or a diabetes educator, yet they become passive when a patient resists a BHC referral. Helping PCPs to reflect on how they handle patients who resist referrals to other specialties may result in them summoning up those same skills when patients resist seeing the BHC.

The most common barriers to referrals, along with strategies to overcome them, are discussed later in this chapter.

A Few Words about Written Strategies for Influencing Providers

While PCP meetings, curbside consultations, and professional detailing are useful, supplementing these with written materials is also important. Two strategies that work well are the quarter-/half-/full-sheet approach and the PCBH newsletter. The quarter sheet is an educational message that can be communicated on a quarter sheet of paper; the half on a half sheet; etc. These require little time to construct and work well when the goal is to influence specific PCP behaviors, such as making same-day referrals or referring specific types of patients.

The Quarter-/Half-/Full-Sheet Message. In the first year, these messages can be particularly useful, since they can be used numerous times for different problems. Only a quarter sheet is needed to provide important reminders, such as "SAME DAY BEHAVIORAL HEALTH CONSULTATIONS AVAILABLE EVERY DAY—CALL 3075444 FOR PATIENT TRIAGE NOW OR BRING YOUR PATIENT TO ROOM 237." Figure 8.1 provides an example of a quarter-sheet announcement designed to highlight a problem PCPs might not think of referring, while Figure 8.2 presents an example of a full-sheet approach. As a rule of thumb, the more information packed into an announcement, the more important it is to follow the message with a discussion, either in a PCP meeting or in professional detailing encounters. Half-sheets are also useful for announcing the start of behavioral health classes in primary care and parenting classes in the community. Distributing these brief messages by e-mail is acceptable, but hard copies should also be used. They can be placed at PCP work stations, on common-use bulletin boards, in mailboxes, or taped onto computer screens.

From your BHC, ___:
One in five patients presenting to primary care settings has persistent insomnia. There are a number of effective behavioral strategies for improving sleep. Please consider referring your patients with chronic sleep disturbance for a consultation!

(Perhaps add a clip art picture here.)

Figure 8.1. A quarter-sheet on insomnia.

Develop a PCBH Newsletter. In a study conducted in primary care, over 50% of providers described PCBH newsletters, such as those presented in Figures 8.3 and 8.4, as very useful (Robinson et al., 1997). These can be created weekly in the first month or two, and then may need to become monthly or quarterly as the rate of referral builds. Newsletters offer an excellent way to address staff concerns and questions and to provide on-going training for providers. Planning regular sections for the newsletter is a good idea, and these can change as the service matures. During the first year, one might write a regular column that introduces basic behavior change concepts and how to apply them to common problems. In the second year, a regular column might be "Primary Care Pathway News," a "Caring for Children" column, or a "Chronic Disease and Self-Management" column. A "What's New?" column that summarizes a recent study pertinent to PCBH practice is always worth writing. Many PCPs will read a brief summary and even apply an idea from it during a subsequent patient visit. Some PCPs will see a newsletter as an invitation for interaction and bring the BHC articles from medical journals.

Newsletters are best kept to one page. They can be distributed via e-mail, but again hard copies should also be used. In contrast to the messages discussed, newsletters should go out to staff as well as PCPs, because they contain information relevant to all. They might also be tacked up in common staff areas such as the lunchroom or bathroom. More than once,

ONES YOU MIGHT NOT HAVE THOUGHT OF ...

OFTEN APPROPRIATE BUT LESS COMMON BHC REFERRAL PROBLEMS

- Temporomandibular disorder (TMD)

Successful treatments include habit-reversal and stress management education

- Habit-reversal (Thumb-sucking, fingernail-biting, hair-pulling)
- Acute post-trauma problems

Early intervention may help prevent PTSD

- Irritable bowel syndrome

Behavioral intervention may help even when there is no psychiatric co-morbidity

- Some dermatological problems (urticarias, alopecia, hyperhydrosis)

Skin problems often worsen when stress is high

- Chronic dizziness

2001 study showed 2/3 had panic attacks

- Lifestyle change for cholesterol, blood pressure problems
- Patients currently doing well, but at a high risk of relapse (based on history)

Patient may use BHC instead of PCP in a future crisis or for case management

- Every newly diagnosed diabetes patient

BHC will screen for potential problems, intervene before problem develops

WAYS TO USE THE BHC THAT YOU MIGHT NOT HAVE THOUGHT OF ...

- Information-gathering calls (e.g., to school, other health care providers)

Such persons often will call BHC for future needs because of easier access and thus decrease PCP phone call load

Figure 8.2. A full sheet on uncommon referrals.

> - Complete medication agreements with patients
> - Gather history for you on a same-day patient with likely psychological problems
> - Gather history on a scheduled patient with psychological problems when you are behind
> - Return phone call to patient with psychological complaints

Figure 8.2.—*Cont'd*

a nurse or PCP will probably tell the BHC that they passed along a copy of a newsletter to a patient.

RESPONDING TO COMMON ADMINISTRATOR AND STAFF REQUESTS

Multiple staff members, ranging from the clinic manager to nursing assistants, may have questions about the extent to which they can utilize BHC services. They may approach the BHC with requests for personal assistance, or for help with nonclinical, organizational issues. Having a basic plan for responding to such requests will be important.

Services for Staff

Shortly after starting a BHC service, one or more members of the staff will almost certainly approach the BHC with a request for help, sometimes for communication problems within a work group and sometimes regarding a personal problem. Occasionally, the clinic manager will also ask the BHC to consult with a staff member who is having job performance problems, or a PCP will refer a patient who happens to be a staff member. These situations provide an opportunity to improve the health and functioning of the clinic, but they also can pose ethical and interpersonal challenges. Consider the suggestions below for handling or even preventing such situations, and talk with the clinic manager to develop a plan before problems arise.

Primary Care Behavioral Health News	
Issue 1	October 18, 2002

We're up and running!
Jeff Reiter, PhD
Behavioral Health Consultant

Today marks the end of the fourth week of the brand spanking new ECHC Behavioral Health Service! It's been a busy month, with plenty of administrative and organizational work to do (and even some patients thrown into the mix!). From what I've seen thus far, ECHC has a great bunch of people to work with, and I appreciate the total support you've given me and this service. I'll be publishing a newsletter roughly every month to keep you informed of BHC issues. I'll highlight a behavioral health issue each month, so if you'd like me to write on a specific topic, feel free to let me know. Here's to a bright future for us!

Hot News!

A weekly **Relaxation Training Class** is now in place. The class is held every **Wednesday from 2:30 to 3:30** in the Garibaldi Room, and is available on a drop-in basis. That is, no appointment is necessary. However, providers wishing to refer patients need to talk to Dr Reiter first. Patients should check in at the front desk by 2:20. In conjunction with Julie Miller (nutritionist), a **Weight Management class** will also be beginning in November. Class time is being determined but will probably be Thursdays 4–5. No prior sign-up is required; drop-ins will always be welcome. Please ask interested patients to call back later this month for the class time.

Handouts Now Available

If you'd like to give patients handouts on sleep hygiene, brief relaxation strategies, making lifestyle changes, or progressive muscle relaxation...just ask! I'll offer other handouts as I develop them.

Problem of the Month:
Insomnia

Most of us have experienced insomnia at one point. In fact, 1/3 of Americans report having insomina at a given time, and half of these people consider the problem serious. It's a common problem, and one behavioral health can often help with.

There are four possible etiologies of insomina. Determining the primary cause is crucial to deciding on a treatment, as insomnia is more a symptom than a disease itself.

Possible causes of insomnia include *medical problems* (pain, respiratory problems, and some medications); *psychological problems* (depression, anxiety); *lifestyle* (drinking alcohol or caffeine or smoking or exercising close to bedtime); *poor sleep hygiene* (arguing/worrying in bed, lying awake long hours in bed). Insomnia is most commonly an acute problem due to one of the above, and typically resolves as the causal problem resolves. However, it can also become a chronic condition that makes daily life difficult.

If you have a patient with insomnia, try recommending the following:

- Avoid alcohol within 2 hours of bedtime; it may help sleep onset, but it will fragment sleep.
- Avoid caffeine within 2–3 hours of bedtime.
- Avoid smoking/dipping within 2–3 hours of bed
- Avoid activities that will raise body temperature close to bedtime, such as exercise and hot showers. However, do exercise (and shower!) regularly.
- Use the bed only for sleeping (and sex). If awake in bed for >15 minutes, leave the room to do something relaxing, then return when very drowsy.
- Avoid frequent or prolonged (>20 minute) naps during the day.

I've developed handouts for patients, and you can also refer them to a great self-help book: Hauri, P. & Linde, S. (1996). No More Sleepless Nights. John Wiley & Sons. It's $12 on Amazon. A good review of the literature can be found at:
Kupfer, D. & Reynolds, C. (1997). Management of insomnia. N Engl J Med 336:341-6.

Figure 8.3. An example of a primary care behavioral health newsletter.

A Pilot Study of a Primary Care Chronic Pain Pathway: Early Outcomes at the Toppenish Clinic

Last summer, Family Practice providers started building a clinical pathway for patients with chronic pain. The pathway includes service from the clinic's Behavioral Health Consultant (BHC), Dr. Patti Robinson. In the pathway, patients receive

- ❏ monthly assessments of Quality of Life (QOL),
- ❏ instruction in skills for accepting pain, including mindfulness techniques,
- ❏ opportunities for clarifying important values about life, and
- ❏ instruction in skills for making commitments to behavior change.

Comparison of surveys from patients before starting in the pathway and at 4-month follow-up suggests that their satisfaction with care is improving.

These are the processes in the pathway:

1. Provider explains the program (named the Pain and Quality of Life Program) and asks the patient to sign an agreement concerning participation.
2. The BHC evaluates the patient's baseline quality of life and helps the patient start work on a Values Plan (and this plan goes into the medical record, so that the provider can support it during routine medical visits).
3. Patient attends monthly class meetings, where she or he completes QOL assessments, works on the Values Plan, and learns new strategies for improving quality of life. (Patients receive pain medication prescriptions at end of the class meeting—if the patient does not attend, the patient is given a tapering prescription for any narcotic pain medication at the time of the next contact with the clinic.) Class attendance is very good.
4. Providers see patients 1:1 according to need and usually separate from the class visit.

Provider and nurse satisfaction with caring for patients with chronic pain is improving, as shown in the graph below. The questionnaire has nine items, and the score range is from 0 (lowest) to 45 (highest). E-mail Dr. Robinson for a copy of the survey at pattir@yvfwc.org.

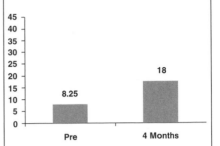

BHC Suggestions for Providers:

➢ Continue to ask patients if they use **tobacco products** and if they are interested in talking with someone about reducing or stopping use of tobacco products. The nicotine patch and nicotine chewing gum significantly increase nicotine abstinence rates. Many of your patients may qualify for free tobacco cessation aids. Give them the number for the Tobacco Quite Line—

877-270-STOP.

Also ask if anyone smokes inside the home. Your BHC can help patients learn to intervene effectively with people smoking in their homes. Your BHC may also provide highly effective motivational interviewing and cognitive behavioral interventions for smokers.

➢ Refer patients who complain of **excessive daytime sleepiness** to your BHC. These patients are often getting insufficient sleep at night. There are many possible causes—use of alcohol, poor sleep hygiene, sleep apnea, etc. Your BHC will teach your patients skills for sleeping well.

Figure 8.4. Another example of a primary care behavioral health newsletter.

Efforts to Improve Staff Functioning. Some organizational problems might be prevented or calmed by teaching staff skills for resolving conflict, managing stress, or promoting teamwork. Meetings of the BH team are a good place to generate ideas for such trainings. The clinic manager and the director of nursing often know which departments are experiencing the most stress and staff turnover and are often the ones to ask for training. Sometimes trainings are brief, one-time offerings during staff meetings, while other times they can become a regular part of staff meetings or an ongoing offering during lunch.

Changes to the work environment can also sometimes prevent or calm problems. For example, if clinic reception staff is stressed from frequent conflicts with patients, they may benefit from more variety in their daily work or more control over their break times. One need not be an expert in organizational psychology to be able to help. Applying functional analysis skills to an organizational problem will often generate very useful ideas.

Most BHCs do not seek out this type of work; rather, the problems tend to find them. Though one's regular focus should be first and foremost on patient care, to the extent organizational problems are influencing patient care it is justifiable to try to help. Whatever the service provided, be sure to develop a survey to evaluate participant satisfaction, as positive feedback helps justify this use of time and adds to one's job performance evaluation. An evaluative report to clinic leaders summarizing the project and its outcome is also good to do.

Brief Consultation for Staff with Personal Problems. When individual staff members seek out the BHC, there can be ethical challenges to getting involved. If there is an urgent and significant problem with no other assistance readily available, the BHC may offer a single consultation, assuming this has administrative support. In such situations, the interview will usually be more limited and the focus will be on providing support, risk assessment, giving ideas for coping, and making a referral(s). Some BHCs have a policy of not seeing staff members and instead simply providing a referral to the employee assistance program. This might often be sufficient, but if there is a significant acute need in a staff person the ethics of this practice could be questioned.

If the staff person is a patient of the clinic (some staff are), and if the BHC agrees to see him or her, the staff member should first talk to his or her PCP. This allows the BHC to practice within the PCBH model and to have a PCP ready for supporting any recommendations from the BHC.

Minimal charting is usually adequate and desirable, as more personal information may be shared verbally with the referring provider as necessary. If the staff person is not a patient at the clinic, the best option for documentation is probably to make him or her a patient so a chart can be made to note the visit. Be sure to have written information about the clinic's employee assistance program readily available and to address with the staff person/patient any barriers to use of these services. Keep in mind also that information from the visit must not be shared with other staff, such as the clinic manager, without the written consent of the staff person/patient.

Services to Administrators/Managers

Administrators will definitely request BHC help at some point and their requests are diverse and interesting. They may seek advice on topics ranging from handling a difficult employee to dealing with a demanding patient to developing a patient satisfaction survey. Keeping in mind that managers are trained to handle these problems, the BHC should not rush in with advice every time a problem occurs. However, if asked, there is usually advice that can be given.

In the case of patients who are frequently threatening or disruptive or otherwise problematic, for example, the BHC might help develop a behavioral agreement between the clinic and the patient. Such agreements usually specify how the patient is expected to behave in various areas of the clinic, accommodations the clinic will make to serve the patient, and consequences for violating the agreement. Using one's behavioral training can help to devise an agreement that has realistic expectations of both patient and staff, and clearly defined behaviors and consequences. These are also situations where the BHC might need to advocate for a patient. The idea of "firing" a bothersome patient (i.e., disallowing him or her from returning to the clinic) will undoubtedly be raised by someone, but this should always be avoided. This is especially true at community health centers where patients may have no other care options. Encourage staff to view the patient's behavior problems as health problems that require their help, while at the same time empathizing with their fears and supporting steps to keep them safe. Involving the clinic's risk manager is also suggested for these types of situations, as he or she usually is trained for them.

The skills most BHCs have in program development and evaluation may also be sought out by administrators. They might ask for help developing surveys to identify systems problems or to evaluate the outcome of a recent systems change. They might also ask for assistance with clinical pathway development, participation in various work groups, and membership on collaborative teams. Because of the relevance of behavioral issues to so many problems, there are seemingly limitless opportunities to help. Participation in these types of efforts is an excellent way to influence the workings of the primary care clinic, but too much time out of the clinic for meetings will inevitably harm a BHC service. When asked to help with an optional activity, balance the pros of being involved (i.e., how much potential is there to change delivery of care in the system) against the cons that may result from time out of the clinic.

ASSESSING AND OVERCOMING REFERRAL BARRIERS

No matter one's enthusiasm or knowledge base, there will undoubtedly be barriers to the success of a BHC service. One commonly encountered problem, especially in a service's early days, is a lack of referrals. This might seem odd given the ubiquitous nature of behaviorally-based problems in primary care, yet it happens. Success depends on referrals from PCPs, but given the newness of the PCBH model, they might not comprehend how to fully utilize the service. Simple problems, such as a poorly located BHC office, can inhibit referrals and prevent a service from achieving its potential. The Referral Barriers Questionnaire (RBQ) (see Figure 8.5) is an approach to obtaining information about the many cultural, attitudinal, logistical, and other barriers that may inhibit a service's success. The RBQ provides a list of the most common obstacles to BHC referrals, compiled from the literature on PCBH and the authors' own experiences. Respondents (i.e., PCPs) identify which items are barriers and the frequency of their occurrence, and the BHC can then look for patterns in the responses. The questionnaire is not standardized but instead can be used qualitatively to develop a plan for overcoming barriers.

	Not a barrier (0)	Occasionally a barrier (1)	Often a barrier (2)
A. When you have considered referring to the BHC or a BHC class, which factors have *deterred* you from referring? Check the column that best describes your experience.			
1. Patient is already seeing a therapist			
2. No time to find the BHC and make the referral			
3. Forgot by the end of the visit			
4. Patient refused the referral			
5. Patient has seen BHC before for same problem, isn't likely to benefit from another referral			
6. Worry about alienating patient by recommending a behavioral health referral			
7. Not sure how to make the referral			
8. BHC is unavailable or seems busy			
9. BHC doesn't speak patient's primary language			

Figure 8.5. The Referral Barriers Questionnaire.

10. Patient is responding well to medications alone; no need for referral			
11. Don't want to overwhelm the BHC			
12. Not sure what to say about cost of BHC visit			
13. Unlikely BHC could help with this type of problem			

What was/were the problem(s)?
Other barrier (Please explain):

B. Overall, how helpful is the BHC service *for your patients*? (Circle the number)

    0   1   2   3   4   5   6   7   8   9   10

no apparent benefit   extremely helpful,

                              excellent patient feedback

C. Overall, how helpful is the BHC service *to you* (i.e., helps you better serve patients, etc.)? (Circle the number)

    0   1   2   3   4   5   6   7   8   9   10

not helpful   extremely helpful

D. What change(s) could result in a higher rating from you?

Figure 8.5.—*Cont'd*

Information from the RBQ can be summarized for use in three ways (Reiter, Berghuis & Robinson, manuscript in preparation). First, items A1 through A13 may be assigned a score of 0 (Not a Barrier), 1 (Occasionally a Barrier), or 2 (Often a Barrier). The sum of individual scores on items A1 through A13 provides an indication of the overall level of barriers to referral. If providers are willing to include names, the BHC can make specific plans to address barriers identified by each provider. If not, the responses in aggregate are useful for understanding the relative impact of various barriers and for designing interventions that may effectively address perceived barriers (See Table 8.5). The second and third scores available from the RBQ are the individual scores from questions B and C. The primary purpose for including these satisfaction ratings on the RBQ is to compare them to the number of barriers identified. Hopefully, as the number of identified referral barriers decreases over time, satisfaction and perceived usefulness of the service will increase. We must reiterate, though, that this measure is still in experimental status and has not been validated or standardized yet, so be cautious when using it to make quantitative comparisons. At this point the best use is probably for assessing which barriers are present at any given time.

After administering the RBQ, be sure to summarize the feedback and review it with PCPs during a provider meeting. Ideas can be exchanged about how to overcome referral barriers and improve provider satisfaction. Consider asking the PCPs to identify the two or three barriers that warrant priority for change in the next six or twelve months, and then develop a plan and report progress on it during BH Team or provider meetings.

Tips for Overcoming Barriers

There are specific activities worth exploring for each of the thirteen specific barriers on the RBQ (Reiter et al., manuscript in preparation). For example, in response to provider perception that item #1 ("Patient is already seeing a therapist") is a barrier to referral, the BHC can explain that in fact such patients are good referrals because (1) the BHC can help coordinate specialty and primary care by calling therapists and/or procuring records, (2) having an established relationship with the BHC may be important in the event that therapy ends prematurely or a crisis occurs when the therapist is unavailable, and (3) the BHC might address health

Table 8.5. Common referral barriers in primary care and strategies for reducing them

Barrier[a]	BHC counter-strategies
1. Patient is already seeing a therapist	Offer to coordinate care (call the therapist, procure records). Emphasize establishing a relationship with the patient, in case therapy ends prematurely (crisis visits may be needed) or relapse occurs. Consider seeing the patient for problems not addressed in therapy (e.g., headaches or obesity).
2. No time to find the BHC and make the referral	Try communicators (walkie-talkies, pagers). Locate the BHC office in a convenient spot. Work with each PCP to find an efficient referral strategy. Keep handoff time to a minimum by avoiding lengthy discussion. Demonstrate long-term time saving to PCPs by assuming management tasks (phone calls to schools, letter-writing, completing disability forms, etc.). Do not require a written referral.
3. Forgot by the end of the visit	Place passive behavioral health screening posters in exam rooms and waiting areas (and change often). Develop signs to advertise your service. Increase visibility by coming out of your office or charting in the PCP office. Begin each day by meeting with each PCP to review potential referrals on the schedule. (If appropriate, offer to see patients *before* or *instead of* the PCP.) Empower nurses or nursing/medical assistants to remind PCPs to refer. Make a BHC referral part of the clinical pathway for appropriate conditions.
4. Patient refused the referral	Be willing to see a patient very briefly, if limited time is the problem. Train

Table 8.5.—*Cont'd*

Barrier[a]	BHC counter-strategies
	PCPs to say, "It would help me help you." Demystify your service by talking in classes, posting signs, being visible, and friendly.
5. Patient has seen BHC before for same problem, isn't likely to benefit from another referral	Provide trainings on readiness for change (via BHC Newsletters or Drop-in lunch hour classes using case illustrations). Remind the PCPs to view you as a routine part of care. ("Anytime the treatment plan needs changed have the patient see me.")
6. Worry about alienating patient by recommending a BH referral	Train PCPs to phrase referrals using terms like "lifestyle change," "stress," and "consultation." Present the BHC as a PCP and part of usual care, and emphasize the consultative role.
7. Not sure how to make the referral	Discern specific questions PCPs have. Train them to interrupt you as needed; to find a referral issue the patient is concerned about (even if it's not the PCP's primary concern); and to describe you as a "consultant" or "team member."
8. BHC is unavailable or seems busy	Use this feedback to seek increased hours, if needed. Keep your door open when alone. Let PCPs know if you're not busy. Post work hours on your door. Welcome interruptions. Wear a pager or use walkie-talkies. *Be flexible*; if short on time, a ten-minute initial visit is better than no visit. Avoid complaining about your workload.
9. BHC doesn't speak patient's primary language	Train to work with an interpreter. Teach interpreters common interventions. Develop picture-based patient education materials. Translate handouts into the most commonly encountered languages. Demonstrate cultural competence to staff via case discussions and newsletters.

Table 8.5.—*Cont'd*

Barrier[a]	BHC counter-strategies
10. Patient is responding well to medications alone; no need for referral	Educate PCPs about relapse potential and the benefits of relapse prevention training. Leave study abstracts on these topics in the PCPs' office.
11. Don't want to overwhelm the BHC	If overwhelmed, seek more hours or investigate group visits or ways to be more efficient. Reassure PCPs. Avoid comments or behaviors suggesting you're overwhelmed.
12. Not sure what to say about cost of BHC visit	Train PCPs to use motivational techniques to overcome patient concerns. Develop fee structures that reduce resistance. Ensure PCPs have a clear understanding of the billing plan.
13. Unlikely BHC could help with this type of problem. What was/were the problem(s)?	Encourage PCPs to refer freely. Accept all referrals. Distinguish BHC care from MH care. Use newsletters, talks, shadowing to educate PCPs about psychosocial factors and the variety of problems seen.
14. Other barriers:	Identify specific barriers and talk with PCPs and staff regarding how to overcome them.

[a]Items in this column are from the Referral Barriers Questionnaire (RBQ).

risk behaviors (e.g., smoking or obesity) that are not a focus in therapy. Table 8.5 lists potential barriers from the RBQ, along with a summary of ideas for overcoming each. Review this table after analyzing RBQ data, to generate ideas for solutions that can be discussed with PCPs.

Because providers come and go and situations change, we recommend repeating the RBQ at least annually, even if the referral rate is strong. Like checking one's cholesterol each year, it can be helpful to know if there are problems looming on the horizon. One might also discover issues that are preventing a good service from becoming a great one.

SUMMARY

1. Knowing what activities to prioritize when starting a new BHC service can be difficult. Following the Start-Up Checklist will allow one to have a structured approach to the first weeks and months.

2. Helping PCPs understand how to utilize the BHC service completely and teaching them how to refer patients are crucial undertakings. A variety of strategies illustrated in this chapter can be used for this, ranging from talks to newsletters to brief handouts.

3. Administrators and staff will undoubtedly ask for the BHC's help with non-clinical activities. These might include consulting on organizational issues, intervening with troubled staff members, and participating in work groups, among others. Though these can be powerful ways to contribute and change system functioning, they can also present ethical challenges and are not always the best use of a BHC's time.

4. Despite the overwhelming presence of behaviorally-based problems in PC, the frequency of referrals to a BHC service is sometimes low. Assessing the barriers to referral using the Referral Barriers Questionnaire and applying counter-strategies suggested in this chapter can help maintain a healthy and growing service.

PART V

CONSULTING WITH PATIENTS AND PROVIDERS

This section is the heart of this book. Just like the heart, it is of huge importance, and this is reflected by its long length! Therefore, we suggest that readers take a moment to consider how to approach it. It is meant to be a compendium full of examples and ideas to help with day-to-day clinical practice in the PCBH model. While some people would read an encyclopedia from front to end, others would only delve into it when they need information on a specific topic. Readers in the second category may want to scan Chapters 9 to 11, and use the List of Tables at the front of the book to help with locating case examples at the time of need.

While the heart pumps blood, consulting with patients pumps interaction with PCPs. Without patients to see and effective interventions to offer them, the BHC cannot hope to deliver the potent services of the PCBH model to the primary care clinic. This section is about patients, interventions, and interactions with PCPs. Given the size of the job, the BHC needs to work from a strong heart and to employ what Strosahl (1997) has called horizontal and vertical intervention philosophies. Horizontal interventions refer to the day-to-day, take-all-comers, consultation model where the BHC formulates plans with patients and works in collaboration with the PCP to support them over time. Vertical interventions involve clinical programs that target specific patient populations (e.g., patients with ADHD, patients with chronic pain, or patients over age sixty-five). Vertical interventions employ the tools of clinical pathways, may involve group services, and support the goal of improving the health of most members of a specific population.

This section includes chapters that focus on how to conduct consultations with children and youth, adults, and older adults. Each chapter includes multiple case examples, ideas for vertical integration programs, and strategies for consulting with and teaching PCPs. The case examples are drawn from real life experience working in the primary care milieu. BHCs, on average, will spend 30 to 40 percent of their time with children, 50 to 60 percent with adults between eighteen and sixty years of age, and 10 to 20 percent with adults over age sixty years old. The organization of Chapters 9 to 11 is rather like the "clinical monograph" model that is so popular in general medicine circles. It gives the reader the opportunity to watch an experienced BHC in day-to-day practice and to "pick his or her brains" after each patient interaction. In Chapters 9 to 11, we describe twenty-three such patients. That's about how many patients a BHC will see in two clinic days. For every patient seen individually, there are dozens more that would benefit from BHC services. To reach them, the BHC will need to work smarter, not harder. Chapter 12 describes a range of group services that empower "smarter" strategies for responding to the needs of primary care patients seen more than one at a time.

While the interventions described in this section are derivatives of treatments with an empirical basis (as established by various bodies including the American Psychological Association and the Society for Behavioral Medicine), the PCBH model of consultation is a very pragmatic approach. The interventions selected by a BHC for any given patient are the result of many influences, some of which are not under the BHC's control. Factors influencing intervention design include the results of the functional analysis, patient expectations and preferences, and the actual amount of time that the BHC and patient have for a particular encounter. In the PCBH model, the assumption is that even a ten minute interaction with a patient who is at a "teachable moment" can produce a lasting impact in that patient's life. The population health philosophy evident throughout this book is that it is far better to give someone twenty minutes of help than to give them no help at all. We do what we can, given the constraints of the situation, and we try to help as many people as possible.

Many of the interventions described in the case examples reflect a behavioral treatment approach known as Acceptance and Commitment Therapy (ACT). Space precludes anything resembling an in-depth description of ACT; the interested reader is advised to pick up the major texts describing this approach (Hayes, Strosahl, & Wilson, 1999; Hayes & Strosahl, 2004). We chose to highlight use of these newer technologies in order to provide readers with greater awareness of their potential value in the primary care context. We also recognize that many more traditional cognitive behavior therapy interventions might work as well. Our purpose is not to promote the use of one treatment approach over the other, but rather to focus on producing interventions that work in this setting. If we have achieved that objective for the majority of our readers, our vision in writing this book will have been fulfilled.

9

EXAMPLES OF CONSULTATIONS WITH YOUTH AND THEIR FAMILIES

"The proper time to influence the character of a child is about a hundred years before he is born."

—William Ralph Inge

Pediatricians spend 25 percent to 60 percent of their time in well child care visits, which typically include screening and assessment of developmental issues, anticipatory guidance, and identification and treatment of behavior problems. Therefore, pediatricians and their family medicine colleagues are in an ideal position to detect and address the psychosocial problems affecting the health of children and youth. However, there are numerous barriers, including time, difficulties communicating psychosocial concerns clearly, an overly biomedical orientation within PC, the lack of effective screening processes and, historically, the absence of integrated behavioral health services in the clinic. In the PCBH model, BHC services have the potential for reducing these impediments, and this chapter aims to show how.

As many as a quarter of primary care pediatric patients present with significant psychosocial dysfunction (Costello et al., 1988; Horwitz, Leaf, Leventhal, Forsyth, & Speechley, 1992; National Institute of Mental Health, 1990; United States Public Health Service, 2000). Most are living their childhood years in contexts that include a plethora of adverse experiences, and, without detection and intervention, these experiences function in an additive fashion to harm the child's health as an adult. The Adverse Childhood Experiences (ACE) study (Felitti, 2002; Felitti et al., 1998), interviewed over 17,000 adults to determine the prevalence of events in five categories of household dysfunction and three categories of abuse during childhood. Participants received ACE scores based on the number of events experienced, with scores ranging from 0 to 8 events. Many adult health problems proved to have a strong, linear relationship to ACE scores, including heart disease, fractures, diabetes, obesity, unintended pregnancy, sexually transmitted diseases, and alcoholism. As ACE scores increased, job performance worsened progressively as did the probability of problematic health and health risk behaviors. For example, a person with an ACE Score of 4 was 260 percent more likely to have chronic obstructive pulmonary disease (COPD) than a person with an ACE Score of 0. A person with an ACE score of 6 was 600 times more likely to be an intravenous drug user than a person with a score of 0. Additionally, results indicated that adverse events occur more frequently in childhood than most people imagine. For example, almost one in four of the ACE subjects reported some form of childhood abuse.

This chapter will look at opportunities the BHC has everyday for responding to the often significant healthcare needs of children and adolescents. Come in, sit down, jump up, and walk down the halls with a BHC on a Monday morning as we consult on six patients. For some case examples, we provide examples of documentation (e.g., a SOAP note) and suggest use of patient education materials. Also, Appendix B offers a reading list for BHCs to use to increase their skill base for developing interventions for children, adolescents and their families, along with a book list for children and parents. Appendix D offers a compact disc that includes patient handouts (e.g., Enuresis Plan, Designing Reward Plans, Great Reward Ideas, and Using Time-Out with Your Child). Table 9.1 provides an overview of the chapter, along with the BHC schedule and the reasons for referral. We encourage you to slow your reading momentarily after each patient and ask, "What are the prevention opportunities here?" Perhaps, as Ralph William Inge's quote reminds us, your answers will improve the character of children who come into the world long after this book is written.

So let your imagination take over—you are in a primary care clinic looking over the shoulder of a BHC. Since most clinic days bring a variety

Table 9.1. A morning in the life of a BHC (providing care to children)

Chapter section	BHC # 1442	Referral reason
Young children with behavior problems	8:15 Lucille	Annoying behaviors, irritability
Overweight and obese children	8:45 Juan	Weight gain, sadness
Children with aches and pains	9:15 Rita	Abdominal pain
Children with social problems	9:45 Paul	School problems
Children recovering from trauma	10:15 Mary	Unplanned pregnancy
Children with ADHD	11:00 Samuel	School problems

of child and adult patients, let's pretend it's a school holiday and the morning schedule involves only children and adolescents.

YOUNG CHILDREN WITH BEHAVIOR PROBLEMS

Behavior problems are common with young children, and many are detectable by age two or three. It is quite possible that BHCs could help PCPs identify children at risk by screening parents at the 1-year physical. We, in fact, know of at least one PCBH program where every well-child visit starts with a brief BHC screening interaction. With integrated behavioral health services, there's no need to wait until children, like Lucille, come to the clinic with annoying behaviors.

My Daughter (Lucille) is Annoying Me

Dr. Chan referred this three-year-old patient for a consultation concerning development of parenting skills, after the patient's mother complained that her daughter was annoying to her a great deal of the time. At the consultation, the mother, who was pregnant with a second child, reported that she worried about Lucille's relationship with her father, as she was developing a pattern of saying no to many of his requests and the father felt hurt by this. The BHC inquired about the mother's interest in learning more about parenting, and she agreed. After providing basic information about positive reinforcement strategies, the BHC explored the mother's concern about the father's responses to Lucille's no–no–no behavior (an example of a behavior that annoyed the mother) and explained that this demonstrates how unwanted behaviors increase if the response is increased parental attention. The BHC helped the mother to develop a program involving the father using a star chart to positively reinforce Lucille for saying "yes." Additionally, they planned for the father to ignore Lucille's no–no–no behavior or turn it into a game of no, no, no, yes, yes, no—engaging her in a guessing game about when the father would switch from no to yes. The BHC explained that such games help to take the provocative meaning out of the word "no," and place it in a new context (in this case, the context of play which supports a positive father–daughter relationship).

At the end of the visit, Lucille's mother voiced a desire to reduce the frequency of her daughter's requests for nursing at night. The BHC helped mother plan a program for this, involving the mother asking Lucille to try to refrain from making the requests, so that the mother would be rested and ready to have a special morning play time with her. When Lucille made the request, the mother would give her a choice between having a snack and getting a "smiley face" sticker or nursing. Additionally, she would remind Lucille that she could put the sticker beside Mom's bed if she wanted to exchange it for fifteen minutes of reading and cuddling with Mom the next morning in her bed.

Since Lucille's mother and father wanted to read a book on parenting and to attend a class, the BHC suggested a book and provided information about an upcoming class in the community. The BHC asked patient's mother to follow-up with Dr. Chan within a month and to return for a follow-up with the BHC if she did not obtain desired results within a few weeks. In follow-up with Dr. Chan, the mother reported that she had implemented the plans and that both concerns were resolved. She did not attend the parenting class due to time conflicts, but was watching a program on parenting on television.

Intervention Possibilities for Young Children with Behavior Problems. The case example of Lucille demonstrates the importance of a good functional analysis. The BHC's plan focused on improving Lucille's relationships with her mother and father, as it was stress in these relationships that made her vulnerable to the reported behavior problems. Parents often lack the perspective to perceive the evolution of these circumstances, and the PCP often lacks the time (and skill) to complete a functional analysis.

Table 9.2 suggests possible approaches for BHCs to use to increase basic parenting strategies and apply specific behavior change techniques to common behavior problems, which often arise at family transition points. The BHC can teach behavior change and parenting strategies by integrating them with programs developed through a functional analysis of a target behavior, as was done with Lucille and her mother. Additionally, the BHC may recommend specific reading and/or provide opportunities to practice skills. Many parents will read pamphlets, articles, or books and/or watch videos about parenting, with or without BHC consultation visits. There are many good books related to parenting, and we provide a list of possibilities in Appendix B.

The BHC might also provide information about The Home Chip System, which is an excellent program for parents of three- to seven-year-olds that have behavior problems (Christophersen & Mortweet, 2003). The procedures in The Home Chip System have been used in families with parents whose education ranged from less than high school to postgraduate studies and with income levels ranging from poverty to upper-income professional. This approach has also been used with families from a variety of ethnic and racial backgrounds.

Another possibility involves networking with community-based parenting class teachers, posting notices about upcoming series, and providing reminders to parents and PCPs about start dates. Unfortunately, many, if not most, parents will not participate for a variety of reasons, such as work schedules and lack of resources for childcare. For parents who prefer to learn parenting skills in consultation visits with a BHC, the

Table 9.2. BHC intervention possibilities for young children with behavior problems

1. Integrate instruction in parenting with behavioral programs resulting from a functional analysis.
2. Provide pamphlets or articles on common behavior problems and parenting strategies.
3. Recommend specific books on parenting and/or The Home Chip System.
4. Notify PCPs and patients of parenting class resources in the community.
5. Develop a PCBH parenting protocol that the BHC can deliver efficiently over time, perhaps in tandem with the child's medical visits.

use of a protocol often improves consistency and time-effectiveness. Table 9.3 offers an example of a parenting protocol that a BHC can deliver in a series of one-to-one consultation visits, in classes or in a one day workshop. This protocol entails a minimum of three consultations and an optional fourth visit. When parents are in conflict about numerous issues related to parenting, we suggest that the second contact focus on teaching skills related to effective conflict resolution and ways to present a united front. Then, the second visit in the protocol becomes the third and the third the fourth.

In the initial visit, the BHC helps the parent(s) develop a plan to improve their relationship with the child. Content includes information about modeling and planning and engaging in playful activities that improve communication and respect. The BHC may help the parent(s) develop a value statement concerning the qualities of parenting and the lifestyle behaviors that he or she wants to model for the child (children). Parents may set small goals (e.g., spending fifteen minutes each day with each child engaged in active listening or exercising for fifteen minutes daily) to improve the consistency between daily activities and valued styles of parenting (e.g., being a good listener, modeling healthy lifestyle behaviors).

In the three-contact model, the second and third contacts provide the parent(s) with a variety of skills. The second consult includes instruction

Table 9.3. Teaching parenting skills: a protocol for the BHC

BHC consult visit	Skill focus	Handout topics
Initial	Improving the parent–child relationship	Positive parenting
Second	Building skills for setting limits and using incentive programs	Setting limits and using incentives and consequences
Third	Building skills for using ignoring and time-out and working as a team	The power of your attention and a united front
Fourth (optional)	How to model effective conflict resolution and present a united front	No handout

about providing clear commands, setting limits, and the details of using incentives and consequences. The BHC can explain and model strategies such as the "when–then" command in five or ten minutes. This involves the parent deciding exactly what they want the child to do and then determining what incentives are available to reinforce compliance with the request. Once the parent has these two elements in mind, he or she can explain to the child, "When you do "X" (i.e., put your backpack in your room; finish the dishes), then you can do "Y" (i.e., continue with your play; go to the store with me)." The third contact involves more training concerning the use of positive attention to influence the child's behavior, including procedures for ignoring unwanted behaviors and establishing time-out as a contingency. This consult also includes a brief discussion of the importance of both parents presenting a united front to the child.

After the series, the BHC asks the patient and his or her parents to follow-up with the PCP. At follow-up, the PCP needs to assess parental confidence in implementing their newly learned skills and devise a support plan that is adequate for solidifying skill gains over the next six months. BHCs may develop parent education handouts for specific visits in a parenting protocol, and these may be shared with the PCP so that they can provide informed support to parents over time. The content of this recommended protocol is consistent with empirically supported programs detailed elsewhere (see Webster-Stratton & Reid, 2004). It is a good option for parents who are unable to attend community classes, as it can be delivered to them in a series of same-day visits over time.

PCP Teaching Points Concerning Young Children with Behavior Problems. Many PCPs were not exposed to basic principles of behavior modification in medical school. The context of teaching parenting strategies is a great one for introducing PCPs to the ubiquitous and useful concepts of positive reinforcement, extinction, negative reinforcement, and schedules of reinforcement. As suggested in Table 9.4, the BHC can use PCBH newsletters as well as articles to provide information about managing behavior problems and positive parenting strategies, such as star charts, time out procedures, and differential reinforcement of other behavior (DRO) schedules. Individual consultations provide an opportunity for the BHC to demonstrate techniques presented in written materials and/or workshops for providers. Keep in mind that providers vary in their level of interest in behavior change technology.

Table 9.4. PCP teaching points concerning young children with behavior problems

1. Teach the method of functional analysis when giving feedback on the development of a behavior modification program.
2. Use PCBH newsletters to reinforce specific behavior change and parenting strategies.
3. Invite PCPs to attend classes and workshops on parenting that the BHC teaches.
4. Provide copies of articles about management of common behavior problems on the BHC's door (or other highly accessible areas).
5. Teach providers how to talk with parents and young children about their values and how to help them set small goals for change that are consistent with their values (e.g., pursuing the value of being a kind parent by setting a goal of giving descriptive praise statements for a specific behavior twice hourly).
6. Teach providers to teach parents to play with words with children in order to avoid needless power struggles (e.g., the no–no–no game).

Some will order and read a book on parenting and schedule a time with the BHC to discuss the book. At the low interest end of the continuum, a few will simply continue charting when the BHC talks about negative reinforcement. Most will be somewhere in between. Offering on-going parenting classes or workshops is another way to further disseminate behavioral strategies focused on parenting and child behavior problems, as providers may be able to attend classes that are offered at the end of the patient care day or on weekends. Additionally, a BHC may provide copies of brief articles on common parent–child issues and parenting skills (e.g., lying, emotion regulation, praise, etc.) in a wall hanger near his or her office.

PCPs will also respond positively to BHC efforts to introduce concepts related to modeling, identifying values, setting small goals that increase consistency between daily activities and values, and turning power struggles into word games. The best way to convey these ideas is through case discussions. While some of these strategies derive from Acceptance and Commitment Therapy, the BHC need not pass along any psychobabble in order to relay their essence. Strategies such as value directed behavior change and diffusion are new tools that may be of use when older tools are inadequate or require more time. Often, these newer approaches enhance the impact of tried and true behavioral parenting strategies. The BHC could use the consultation with Lucille to teach the PCP about the process of fusion and the strategy of diffusion. Lucille had "no" in a response class that included refusing to cooperate, being stubborn, and perhaps being independent. "No" fused with negative emotional states (her own and her fathers), including anger and sadness. The father perhaps had his own fusion problem, with his daughter's refusal behavior pulling forth a response class, or group of associations, that included being disliked, unloved, and perhaps inadequate. The diffusion technique involved repeating the word "no", with variations in volume and speed and with unpredictable interjections of yes, and the result was the loss of problematic properties of "no." The word "no" would continue to appear in their interactions, but its function was changed, and the father and daughter could now play and enjoy each other.

OVERWEIGHT AND OBESE CHILDREN

In the U. S., 10 percent of two- to five-year olds and 15 percent of six- to nineteen-year-olds are overweight (Ogden, Flegal, Carroll, & Johnson, 2002). Children that are overweight or obese face many social challenges and are at risk for developing additional health problems as they grow into adulthood. Many of these youngsters, like Juan, seek comfort in food and eating, as it provides a respite from adverse events in their dysfunctional homes.

The Doctor Says He (Juan) Weighs Too Much

Dr. Funk referred this fourteen-year-old patient for a consultation concerning weight gain, fatigue, and sad mood. At the consultation, Juan reported that he had followed Dr. Funk's recommended changes in diet and exercise regimens. He was eating more fruits and vegetables, walking with his step-father, and playing soccer with his brothers. He said that he hoped to lose forty pounds. The BHC provided educational information and written materials to help Juan distinguish between a diet and a healthy lifestyle and, based on the results of a functional analysis, focused planning around emotional eating. This was a potential a barrier to long-term establishment of a healthy lifestyle.

Juan indicated significant life stresses, including conflicts between his parents that had led to their recent separation. His description of his father's behavior suggested problems with emotional instability. Juan explained that his father had attempted suicide when he and his sister requested permission to live with their mother. While his grades were mostly C's, Juan wanted to make A and B grades and to grow up to be an artist. He agreed to continue his new healthy lifestyle behaviors, look for a recommended book on art and drawing, and return for follow-up with the BHC in two weeks. The BHC also asked Juan to notice when he felt upset or worried and what he did at those times. They planned to talk more about emotional triggers for eating and strategies for self-care when family members are upset and acting unpredictably.

Juan returned for follow-up three weeks later and reported some improvement in his family situation. He was continuing to eat smaller portions and to be physically active; he was avoiding fast foods and soda, and he was drinking one glass of water for every glass of juice. Juan was monitoring his weight and was pleased to report that he was not gaining weight. Juan told the BHC that he felt afraid when his father talked loud or said bad things about his mother and that he tended to use favorite foods to both calm and distract himself when these situations arose. He also reported that he would turn the TV on while overeating to further avoid the unpleasant home situation. The BHC taught Juan a strategy for breathing and focusing on the here and now, so that he could make room for fear and painful memories of his parents' arguments, while choosing to engage in healthy lifestyle behaviors. They also made a safety plan for Juan in the event his father's behavior became unusually erratic during a visit.

Juan returned for a third consult during the summer and indicated that his relationship with his father was improving. He was swimming and planned to join a swim team in the fall. He had continued to practice the breathing and mindfulness exercises and had lost six pounds. The BHC supported his gains, and helped Juan schedule a follow-up visit with his PCP in three months.

BHC Intervention Possibilities for Obese and Overweight Children. Children with weight control problems, as well their parents (who are often also overweight or obese) may lack both the information and skills necessary to change their behavior. In the case of Juan, the BHC provided handouts that reinforced some of the concepts that Juan had heard from other providers, including his PCP and the dietician. With these children, a team approach is critical as it increases the availability of social support as well as giving the child a consistent "message." The BHC can develop brief handouts that suggest guidelines for healthy eating, exercise, and sleep and share them with patients, PCPs, and dieticians. In this case, the functional analysis identified a pattern of dysfunctional eating that functioned in the service of regulating painful emotions, and the homework assignment included self-monitoring to gather further information about this link. The case also illustrates the value of broadening the focus on the child to include his or her development into adulthood where work is a part of their lives. Some overweight children may tend to avoid day dreams about their future, as this might have become associated with self-critical and rejecting thoughts about physical appearance and the likelihood of future success.

As can be seen in Table 9.5, we recommend that the BHC provide other educational services to these children. For example, the BHC may explain the impact of stress on health and one's ability to make healthy choices. Without skills for reducing various psychosocial stresses, one may be unable to generate energy and concentration for food preparation and instead rely on fast food and snack foods that are high in calories and low in nutrients. Turning on the television, of course, helps distance oneself from directly experiencing distressing emotions, as does emotionally triggered overeating and/or making poor food choices. Children and parents are often surprised to learn that the probability of being overweight as a child increases in proportion to the amount of time spent watching television.

The BHC may weave educational activities with motivational interviewing strategies in an effort to engage the child (and parent) in developing a plan that focuses on an area of lifestyle change where motivation is greatest. This approach also works well with prediabetic or diabetic children. For example, the BHC might read through a one-page handout offering three or four guidelines for healthy eating, exercise, and sleep and ask the child to choose one behavioral goal that interests him or her. Some children may like the idea of planning to eat breakfast daily while others prefer to make a plan of riding their bike everyday.

For some children, the functional analysis may center on behavior patterns linked to eating larger portion sizes or eating in the absence of

Table 9.5. BHC intervention possibilities for obese and overweight children

1. Provide guidelines for healthy lifestyle behaviors related to eating, exercise, and sleep.
2. Discuss the impact of stress on one's ability to make healthy choices and implement them (i.e., increasing levels of stress in the absence of skills for reducing it may provoke ineffective avoidant patterns of behavior involving food and sedentary activities).
3. Ask about the patient's rate of viewing television, playing video games, and engaging in other sedentary activities.
4. Ask about the patient's ideals concerning physical health and caring for his or her body and assist with planning specific goals that move the patient toward his or her own standard.
5. Use motivational interviewing to select the initial area of lifestyle change (e.g., diet versus exercise versus sleep) to stack the deck for enhancing self-efficacy.
6. Complete a functional analysis concerning any recurring pattern of eating larger portion sizes or eating in the absence of hunger sensations.
7. Address skill deficits that predispose the patient to dysfunctional eating behaviors (e.g., lack of mindfulness skills, relaxation strategies, and/or safety plans that address high risk family situations).
8. Address any problematic parental response to patient's eating behavior (e.g., attempting to over-control patient's access to food or denying the negative health consequences of being overweight or obese).
9. Offer workshops and classes for families that teach skills for adopting healthy lifestyle behaviors.

hunger sensations. This may help identify deficits in coping skills (which are often present in this behavior pattern) and help direct coping skills training. In addition to television viewing, overweight or obese children may have high rates of other sedentary behaviors (playing video games, reading), so the BHC may inquire about these as well. The function of the sedentary activity varies from child to child, but often includes avoiding emotionally or behaviorally challenging circumstances in their homes (e.g., loneliness, problematic parent–child relationships, domestic violence, etc.). Once overweight, children find sedentary activities even more attractive, as they provide entertainment that is free of the discomforts of peer teasing about weight as well as the pain and awkwardness of exercising when one is overweight. Mindfulness skills are empowering to children who are emotionally and/or behaviorally avoidant. A simultaneous focus on values related to taking care of one's body can enhance motivation and set the stage for development of a long term, resilient action plan that the child can implement with parent and PCP support.

BHC interventions need to also address the needs of parents, as they often struggle in a variety of ways. They may attempt to control patient access to food, which usually does not work well. Many children will rebel against perceived attempts to restrict access to food and may even eat more. Parents who are overweight may minimize the importance of changing eating patterns, and they may suggest to the BHC, "We like him the way he is—just a little heavy." Educating parents about calculation of the Body Mass Index and health consequences of obesity are useful, but even more empowering interventions are those that enhance the parents' level of motivation for modeling a healthy lifestyle and in engaging in healthy lifestyle behaviors together with the child.

Given the growing prevalence of overweight and obese children, BHCs need to support expansion of both prevention and intervention efforts on their behalf. Classes and workshops that empower development of a healthy lifestyle may be useful. For example, one of us (PR) works in a clinic that offers a six-session group program for children and their families that combines a weight management and diabetes prevention curriculum (Bienestar Health Program, see Trevino et al., 1998) with behavioral parent training.

Discussion: Teaching Points for Primary Care Providers. BHCs need to encourage medical providers to routinely refer overweight as well as obese children and their families. The addition of behavior change expertise enriches a lifestyle change plan and enhances the opportunities for generating motivation for change in the child. In some cases, it may prevent an escalation in conflict between child and parent(s). As suggested in Table 9.6, handouts may help PCPs remember to refer, and clinical pathways that suggest referral for dietician and BHC services may also help. Overtime, prevention workshops will probably become common in primary care centers, and this will support PCP efforts to learn interventions commonly used by BHCs.

Table 9.6. PCP teaching points concerning obese and overweight children

1. Provide handouts that offer guidelines for healthy lifestyle behaviors and suggest that PCPs provide such to the patient when referring.
2. Suggest use of a clinical pathway that directs the PCP to refer overweight and obese children and their families.
3. Invite PCPs to attend (or co-lead) workshops and classes provided by the BHC on the topic of healthy lifestyle behaviors.

CHILDREN WITH ACHES AND PAINS

The BHC will see many different types of children with pain complaints. For example, children with cancer, AIDS, sickle cell disease, and rheumatoid arthritis often report on-going pain. About 3 percent of children younger than age eighteen experience headaches (Newacheck & Taylor, 1992), while 9 percent to 17 percent of school-age or younger children experience recurrent abdominal pain (Zuckerman, Stevenson, & Bailey, 1987). Other children experience pain in conjunction with medical procedures. All of these children may benefit from BHC services. When seeing pediatric pain patients, the BHC needs to pay close attention to parental responses to pain (both the child's pain and the parent's pain). As the consultation with Rita demonstrates, this is often a significant factor in the development (and resolution) of problematic pain behaviors.

Rita: My tummy hurts

Dr. Moore referred this four-year-old girl for a consultation concerning abdominal pain. Rita's pain complaint had started eight months prior at about the same time that she began to occasionally fall on the floor and yell. These episodes tended to occur when her mother told her to stop or start something not to her liking. Rita's mother's response was to focus on the pain complaints and to shower her with comforting hugs and kisses. The stomach pain and tantrum events often escalated when Rita visited with her cousins and the mother insisted that she share her toys with them. Being an only child, Rita had limited opportunities for learning how to share, and her mother did not know that learning sharing behavior often required parental coaching. The mother was pregnant, and Rita was not eager to have a brother or sister that might try to take her toys away. Rita also thought that the baby might hurt her mother's tummy.

In the first of a series of three consultations (a total of one hour of service), the BHC helped Rita's mother develop a star chart program to reinforce compliance and a time out procedure for noncompliant and tantrum behaviors. The BHC also provided a few suggestions on how to set up a series of learning sessions concerning sharing behavior, which included having Rita select toys to take with her to share with her cousins and leaving toys she did not want to share at home. The BHC taught Rita and her mother to use belly breathing and a circle tummy massage to relax when their growing tummies growled or hurt. Mother agreed to use her hugs and kisses to reinforce compliant and sharing behavior and to prompt her child to engage in the breathing and self-massage activity when she made a pain complaint. The BHC also suggested a plan for strengthening their relationship in preparation for the addition of a new family member. This involved their making a list of all of the privileges and responsibilities accorded to a big sister and a second list of special mother–daughter and father–daughter activities that Rita would do alone with her parents starting now and continuing after the birth.

Though asked to return within two weeks, Rita and her mother returned two and one-half months later. At that time, the mother was less concerned about Rita's abdominal pain and more concerned about her behavior. The mother had used the star chart with some success, but stopped after the birth of the baby, who was now three weeks old. She had tried time out, but had not been able to follow through when Rita was not quiet in time out. She insisted that she had no time to spend one-to-one with Rita, who was of course very jealous of the attention the mother gave to the new baby. Rita was talking like a baby, and this was annoying for the mother. Rita continued to be slow to follow her mother's requests, but was following her father's requests most of the time.

The BHC reviewed the basics of creating a positive parent–child relationship, modeling, positive reinforcement, extinction, and time out. The mother agreed to target Rita's independent behavior for positive reinforcement. Additionally, she agreed to ask Rita's father to spend fifteen minutes alone with her on a daily basis and then to watch the new baby so that the mother could also consistently spend at least fifteen minutes alone each day with Rita. The BHC carefully described the qualities of play and its importance in building a strong parent–child relationship.

Though Rita's mother agreed to return for follow-up in two to three weeks, she came with her child for a third consult six weeks later. She reported spending more time alone with Rita and praising her frequently for independent and compliant behaviors. Rita was not having abdominal pain, was following her mother's commands more often, and was generally less irritable and more active. The mother agreed to go to a parenting class that offered day care and to follow-up with the BHC after the class if she felt it necessary.

BHC Intervention Possibilities for Children with Aches and Pains. This case example highlights several important aspects of treating childhood pain complaints and behavior problems. First, it is important that the BHC address the pain problem and teach a coping skill to the patient and the parent. An important aspect of this intervention is obtaining a commitment from the parent to model the coping skill and to prompt its use when the child complains of pain. Another important principle is that these families often are experiencing a great deal of stress. This may influence their ability to absorb information in a consult and to follow through on more complicated interventions. Rita's BHC worried about Rita's escalating behavior problems, given the mother's lack of skills and somewhat detached attitude toward her. In trying to give the mother the whole enchilada of parent training rather than a few manageable bites, the BHC may have overwhelmed the mother, as she clearly did not have a grip on how to implement a time-out procedure at the follow-up visit. BHCs face difficult choices in time-constrained settings, and we recommend erring in the direction of simplifying and limiting the intervention. Another important point concerns her mother's failure to return at the planned time. This happens fairly often with BHC patients, and the job of the BHC is to avoid a power struggle with the patient and simply evaluate how the plan has worked since the last visit, troubleshoot obstacles and modify the ensuing plan accordingly.

In terms of therapeutic interventions for pain, cognitive-behavioral therapy (CBT) is the best researched nonpharmacological intervention, and emerging research suggests that ACT interventions may augment clinical outcomes (Robinson, Wicksell, & Olssen, 2004). CBT strategies may include breathing exercises, distraction, imagery, relaxation training, modeling, behavioral rehearsal, and reinforcement. These strategies, along with other interventions listed in Table 9.7 are useful for children with many different pain problems. With parents who experience excessive levels of distress in response to a child's pain, the BHC will need to pay particular attention to assisting the parent. The response of well-intentioned parents may lead a sensitive child to fear that something—of a physical nature—is dangerously wrong with them. Children may be particularly vulnerable to this when someone in their immediate or extended family has been acutely ill or has had symptoms of illness over a prolonged period of time that could not be medically explained. In a worst case scenario, a parent experiences a child's pain as if it was his or her own pain and both see the pain as dangerous. In this scenario, both the child and the parents won't settle for anything less than complete elimination of the pain. The BHC can help them shift from the unachievable goal of eliminating pain to an acceptance of the fact that some level of pain will be present. The goal is to not allow pain to function as a barrier to activities and pursuits that are valued by

Table 9.7. BHC intervention possibilities for children with aches and pains

1. Complete a functional analysis on the pain or ache, being attentive to parental response and parental modeling.
2. Teach the child a method for coping with the pain.
3. Limit your intervention in each visit to one or two skills, even when the child and family seem to need a great deal of help.
4. When the child and parent see the pain as dangerous and insist that it be eliminated, help them shift to a goal of experiencing the pain in a less distressing context.
5. When the pain functions to help the child to obtain parental affection or avoid undesirable activities (e.g., chores), develop a program that modifies these contingencies.
6. Identify activities that the child values and help them set goals to bring activities of daily living closer to valued directions, even with pain sensations (e.g., the "draw what's in your heart" activity).
7. Help parents address the distress they feel when the child reports or displays pain.
8. Suggest a resource book for families to use for advice on common medical problems.

the child. This may involve helping the child and parent explore their elimination goal, the methods they've employed in pursuit of it, and the results obtained thus far.

Value-directed behavior change techniques (as discussed in earlier examples in this chapter) are helpful to children with pain. (See Robinson, Wicksell, & Olsson, 2004 for an in-depth discussion.) Children will often readily identify valued activities (e.g., having fun with Mom or Dad or being a good helper in the family for a younger child; going to school and doing cool things with friends for an older child). Greco and Dew (2005) developed a technique involving inviting the child to draw a picture of something that really matters to him or her inside the empty space of a heart (the "Draw What's in your Heart" exercise). The BHC can look at the heart and ask the child if she or he wants to do more things like those in the heart picture, even if there is pain involved. The BHC may also help the child defuse from the pain by suggesting that the pain sensations and thoughts sometimes act like bullies and try to boss the child around and that the BHC can help the child learn to cope with bullies without fighting them. The BHC can also coach the child to request parental support for not getting bullied by thoughts about pain and for doing more things like those in his or her heart. Some parents may need help with learning how to provide timely reinforcement when the child exhibits new behaviors. Various books may help children and parents cope more successfully with pain and other discomforts (e.g., fear, anger, etc.). Greco and Dew (2005) compiled a list of books to support better coping in children with pain and other complaints; these are provided in Appendix B. Many of these books can readily be integrated as part of the behavior change plan generated in the BHC consultation.

Another BHC intervention for this group concerns meeting the information needs of parents, particularly those who are new parents and lack both information about childhood pain and strategies for responding to pain behaviors. There are a number of books available that provide information on treating common minor health problems at home without medical assistance, and we recommend that the family purchase a resource book if they don't already have one. (See, for example, Smyth, Haas, & Jones, 1995.) These books usually help readers to decide if medical care is necessary. The BHC may suggest that parents develop a question that helps them talk with their child about whether or not medical care is necessary, such as "Do you think this is a case for Dr. Mommy (or Daddy) or for Dr. X (PCP)? If it's a Dr. Mommy case, this is what we will do …." We also advise parents to explain that if it is a Dr. X (PCP) case, and if medical care is sought during school hours and the child is too ill to return to school, the child will need to remain in bed with television and game devices off for the remainder of the day while the parent delivers the medically advised treatment. Having a planned way of communicating with a sick child can help parents avoid reinforcing somatic complaints and sick behavior and to instead provide support for healthy functioning.

PCP Teaching Points Concerning Young Children with Aches and Pains. PCPs are likely to experience more success with children with pain complaints and their parents when they include an evaluation of life stresses and apply the concepts of value-driven behavior change. One of our PCP colleagues recently participated in the making of a video about his experience with the PCBH model. When asked about the impact of BHC services on his clinic, he said that the greatest change had been in his practice style. He explained that, "When I see a child with headaches, my first set of questions include those about stress at home and school, and overall I am much less likely to refer for neurological or other specialty consults during the process of treating children with pain complaints." The idea of helping patients function with pain appeals to PCPs. They support it more heartily after patients learn (often from BHCs) active strategies for coping with pain (such as those suggested in Table 9.7) and even more when the BHC explains that behavior changes made in the service of values are more durable than those made outside of a values context. We also recommend that PCPs assess sleep when exploring routine pain complaints, as inadequate sleep is common (particularly among adolescents) and may predispose them to the experience of chronic, low grade pain.

Table 9.8. PCP teaching points concerning young children with aches and pains

1. Suggest that PCPs include questions about stress at home and school when exploring common pain complaints, such as headaches and stomachaches.
2. Suggest that PCPs also explore sleep when evaluating pain complaints.
3. Encourage PCPs to tell patients that some pain is normal and that it is important to find active coping strategies for addressing it (e.g., breathing techniques, self-massage or massage from others, exercise, relaxation activities, etc.).

CHILDREN WITH SOCIAL PROBLEMS

While there are empirically supported interventions for teaching young children how to be socially and emotionally competent, most children do not have the opportunity to participate in them. Therefore, BHCs see many children who lack social skills, including shy children, bullies, and their victims. When children like Paul come in with these types of social deficits, BHC interventions can help build better social skills to support improvements in overall functioning.

Paul: They're mean to me at school

Dr. Marks referred this ten-year-old, fourth-grader for a consultation concerning social problems at school. Paul's sister had come for a consultation with the BHC several months prior, and the parents asked to see the BHC for recommendations on how to respond to their son's current problems. The parents observed that Paul was experiencing more fatigue, irritability, and worry in response to the stress of being bullied at school. Figure 9.1 displays a copy of the "SOAP" note from the initial BHC consult and Figure 9.2 from the follow-up BHC consult. Reviewing them now should provide the reader with a feel for the intervention.

BHC Intervention Possibilities for Children with Social Problems. Paul's case example demonstrates the value of brief BHC services aimed at improving the child's flexibility in responding to challenging social circumstances. With a few more tools in his bag of social tricks, his distress level dropped and he actually made enemies into friends. This intervention focused on helping Paul develop some rudimentary social skills, and it probably served to allay some of his "parent's" concerns as well. As can be seen in Table 9.9, teaching social skills is a first order BHC intervention for children with any type of social problem. Additionally, practicing relaxation and mindfulness skills both in session and at home empowers the child to apply these skills successfully in real-life circumstances. Such skill training is also helpful to shy and socially anxious children.

While Paul required very little in the way of intervention, other children with social problems may benefit from brief co-management by the BHC and PCP. Children like Paul have relatively strong social skills and

SUBJECTIVE: Dr. Marks refers this ten-year-old, fourth grader for a consultation concerning school problems and related fatigue, irritability, and increased worry, which started after several bullying incidents at school. Patient indicated that he usually resists being bullied, and that the bullying tends to escalate when he resists. The two students bullying patient started this two years prior, and one recently threatened to slit patient's throat. The parents are working with school personnel on this issue. Patient is doing well in school academically and has a group of friends. He likes to play sports, ride his bike, and play computer games.

OBJECTIVE: Pediatric Symptom Profile total score is twelve, and this suggests psychosocial dysfunction for a Mexican American child.

ASSESSMENT/PLAN: Patient wants to learn more about self-discipline and making intentional choices when responding to stressful interpersonal exchanges. We talked about an image of letting balls go by versus trying to catch all of the balls and return them. Additionally, we generated a list of ways to respond to bullying (e.g., walking away, ignoring, looking for win-win solutions, etc.). Patient's mother agreed to explore his participation on a football team and/or a karate class over the coming summer, as he would like to be more physically active. I recommend that Dr. Marks support patient's efforts to learn new ways to respond to bullying. Patient will come for one additional follow-up with me in 2 to 3 weeks.

Figure 9.1. SOAP Note on Paul's Initial BHC Consult.

SUBJECTIVE: This Dr. Marks patient returns with his mother for follow-up of his consultation concerning fatigue, irritability, and worry in relation to school social problems. Patient has been experimenting with new ways to respond to bullying, and his relationships with the students that were bullying him are much better. In fact, some of the bullies are now his friends. He plans to go to Boy Scout Camp this summer and to work on his swimming badge.

OBJECTIVE: Pediatric Symptom Profile score is 11, which is below the cut-off of 12 for significant psychosocial dysfunction for a Mexican American child.

ASSESSMENT/PLAN: All symptoms targeted in the consultation are improving. Patient plans to continue using a variety of strategies to address bullying and making and maintaining friends. Patient will see Dr. Marks in two months for support of these behavior changes.

Figure 9.2. SOAP Note on Paul's Follow-up Consult.

Table 9.9. BHC intervention possibilities for children with social problems

1. After completing a functional analysis on a social situation that illustrates the social problem, teach social skills to remediate deficits.
2. Teach mindfulness and relaxation skills so that the child is able to be present and choose a strategy for responding, rather than simply react.
3. Use role-playing to provide skill practice, and enlist parent support in home-based practice.
4. Enlist support from teachers, such as preparing bullied children to be seen as competent by teaching them a skill that they can demonstrate well before the class (e.g., how to build a model airplane or make an origami bird).
5. Start a workshop or series of classes that draws from materials such as the Incredible Years Dinosaur Social Skills and Problem-Solving Child Training Program.

are more resilient to bullying. Children with less developed social skills, particularly those with learning disabilities, may experience more harm from bullying and may respond by withdrawal, isolation, and loneliness (Asher & Paquette, 2003). For these children, the BHC will need to provide more skill training in concert with the PCP and to consider placement in social skills training groups in the community. Additionally, teachers may be willing to work with the BHC and PCPs to improve the social status of these children in the classroom. This may involve giving the child a socially desirable asset outside of the class situation (e.g., demonstrating the steps in a planned science or art project) that the child can use to generate social approval in the classroom. For example, the child might learn the steps of a "cool" science experiment and lead the class in the experiment, or simply pass some type of reward, such as candies or tokens.

The BHC may develop primary care workshops and classes that foster social competence, as the lack of remediation of social skills early in a child's school experience puts him or her at risk academically and psychosocially. Socially anxious and bullied children may be more at risk for developing symptoms of depression, and young bullies may blossom into children with conduct disorders. The Incredible Years Dinosaur Social Skills and Problem-Solving Child Training Program (Webster-Stratton, 2001) offers a curriculum for teaching young children how to work with their emotions, take perspective, make friends, communicate, manage anger, solve interpersonal problems, and succeed at school. This excellent program has been adapted for use by preschool and elementary teachers as a prevention curriculum, and it could certainly be adapted for primary care implementation. (See Webster-Stratton & Reid, 2004, for information about this curriculum and its efficacy.)

PCP Teaching Points Concerning Young Children with Social Problems. PCPs, particularly those with a more biomedical orientation, may not routinely ask about a child's social situation when the child presents with symptoms of anxiety and/or depression. However, most children with symptoms of anxiety and depression do have social problems and coming up with solutions may improve symptoms. As suggested in Table 9.10, teaching PCPs to assess for social problems is an effective strategy for identifying children with social skill deficits. Many PCPs are

Table 9.10. PCP teaching points concerning children with social problems

1. Teach PCPs to explore social concerns when children present with possible symptoms of depression and anxiety, such as fatigue, sleep problems, and excessive worry.
2. Invite PCPs to co-lead or sit-in on workshops or class series on social skills led by the BHC.
3. Provide a list of children's books that address common social skill topics.

quite savvy regarding the importance of social skills, so the BHC will need to formulate an individual plan of attack for each PCP. Inviting a PCP with less training to observe a workshop or class series on social skills provides an "innocuous" learning opportunity, as does sharing a list of children's books that address common issues related to social skills (e.g., sharing, bullying, being friendly, etc.). Having a list of books to pass along to parents may help PCPs to consistently ask about social skills.

CHILDREN RECOVERING FROM TRAUMA

The BHC will receive many referrals that involve helping children and their families recover from trauma. In these consults, the primary focus is on helping the child and family increase their general functioning, and the BHC will need to listen to the child and family members carefully to hear exactly how this needs to happen. Mary's case example illustrates this process of strategic listening that then puts the BHC in a position to support a rapid return to functioning.

Mary: I am going to have a baby

Dr. Rose referred this thirteen-year-old patient and her parents for a consultation concerning an unplanned pregnancy. Mary was seven months pregnant, and the pregnancy was the result of rape by a cousin that was no longer in the area. He had threatened Mary's life if she told anyone about the rape, so she had not revealed the trauma or her pregnancy until her parents sought medical care for her in the seventh month of her pregnancy. Mary told the BHC that she wanted to have the baby, be a good mother, and return to school full time as soon as possible. She was afraid that she might be too small to give birth and feared the pain of childbirth. She hoped that she could grow up and study to become a doctor, like Dr. Rose, as her care had been very helpful to Mary. She had a strong academic background, and the BHC encouraged her aspiration and told her about job-shadowing opportunities for high school students in the clinic. The initial consultation focused on Mary's main concerns: preparation for birth (the reason for referral) and being able to return to school. The BHC taught her a breathing technique to practice to improve her relaxation skills and answered specific questions concerning the process of giving birth.

At the end of the visit, she briefly mentioned that she worried about how her problems affected her parents, and the BHC offered to speak with each of them to provide ideas for coping. The BHC saw Mary's mother alone for a few minutes and explained the breathing technique she had taught Mary. The mother agreed to attend birthing classes with Mary and to support her expeditious return to school by caring for the baby while Mary attended classes. The mother explained that she felt sad and also voiced concern about how angry and frustrated her husband felt. The BHC saw the father alone for a few minutes, and he said he felt that he had failed to protect Mary. The BHC listened and suggested that he had done many things right as a father and that most parents want to offer their children more protection than they often actually can. The BHC asked him how he thought he could protect Mary now, and he indicated that he could take care of her and the baby and support her return to school. He also indicated that he would take the lead in working with law enforcement officials. During the remainder of the visit, the BHC helped the father plan how he could take a central, protective role in helping Mary and others in the family recover from this painful event. He left with a plan to talk with his daughter, wife, and other children about his desire to protect and care for them now and in the future. He also agreed to be a leader in helping the family care for Mary and her baby as the birth approached and afterwards.

The BHC discussed the plan with Dr. Rose and emphasized the extent to which Mary saw her as helpful. The relationship between Mary and Dr. Rose, already strong, grew stronger, and this further enabled Mary to face childbirth with confidence. After birth, Mary maintained contact with her

PCP, who had become not only her PCP but her role model. Mary came for two follow-up visits with the BHC, and at these visits, the BHC discussed approach versus avoidance coping styles and coached her on problem solving skills. The BHC focused on strategies to increase her attachment to the baby and helped her make a plan that allowed her to continue nursing while attending school part-time. Lastly, the BHC helped her to address hurtful comments from classmates concerning her being sexually active and being an unwed mother.

BHC Intervention Possibilities for Children Recovering from Trauma. There are a variety of interventions that are useful to children recovering from trauma, including efforts to bolster child and family resources for coping after a traumatic event. Mary's case example illustrates how important it is for the BHC to focus on the referral question first, and then move onto other behavioral goals if they seem indicated. Mary wanted information to allay her fears, skills for preparing for birth, and support for returning to normal childhood activities, such as attending school. The BHC addressed these needs immediately and then incorporated Mary's values to create a long-term life plan that was big enough and desirable enough (i.e., becoming a doctor) to justify her current struggles. Mary knew that her parents were upset; she asked the BHC to help them. The BHC's rapid response helped build Mary's sense of being able to cope with her circumstance. The BHC also taught Mary problem-solving methods in follow-up appointments, which she applied to social situations at school and to issues related to sorting out being a teenage parent.

It is important to highlight what the BHC did not do with Mary or her parents, as this reflects the pragmatic and practical side of BHC work. The BHC did not engage Mary or her parents in clinical interactions about the repeated instances of assault that she had experienced (when her parents were away from home). Beyond uncovering enough information to know that the patient and her family were safe and that law enforcement officials were involved, there was no exploration of the trauma per se. The BHC did ask the father to continue to take the lead in working with police, as this functioned to protect Mary and to provide a sense of vindication to the father.

As indicated in Table 9.11, a top priority in using the tools of functional analysis with trauma victims is that of identifying the child's concerns. Mary's concern was that she was physically small, that she was not moving

Table 9.11. BHC intervention possibilities for children recovering from trauma

1. Identify patient's current need and center the functional analysis on ways to meet this need.
2. Emphasize child (and parent) strengths and resources in planning.
3. Help the child (and parents) sort out roles that may become confused by the trauma.
4. Teach problem-solving skills to use in addressing current and future problems (that may relate to the consequences of the trauma).

along in her school curriculum with her friends, and that her parents were upset. She was not concerned about intrusive images, nightmares, etc. The plan resulting from the initial consultation addressed her immediate concerns and directed support to her parents. The BHC helped the parents sort out their post-trauma roles so that they could offer maximum support. The mother came to terms with being a mother for and with her daughter, and the father developed a strong stance for being a protective father in the present moment and in the future. Numerous cognitive behavioral techniques may be helpful to traumatized children, and the choice to use them revolves around their relevance to the goal of helping the child and family recover optimal functioning. Possibilities include interventions such as relaxation training, anger management, personal assertion, developing an observer self, learning to focus on the present moment, and problem-solving skills.

PCP Teaching Points Concerning Children Recovering from Trauma. Many PCPs feel overwhelmed when learning that a child has experienced trauma. PCPs may want to offer patients comprehensive specialty treatment, and, for most trauma victims, this is not—for a myriad of reasons—feasible. Crisis services are strained by lack of funding, and geographical and economic barriers loom large for many children and their families. PCPs may also struggle with blaming themselves for not detecting ongoing traumatic experiences earlier, particularly in the case of sexual or physical abuse by a family member. As suggested in Table 9.12, the BHC may need to explain the process of dissociation to PCPs and the survival value of blocking recall or denying the trauma. PCPs may assume that trauma patients always need to discuss the trauma in detail in order to recover. In contrast, many victims don't want to delve into the trauma and instead

Table 9.12. PCP teaching points concerning children recovering from trauma

1. Encourage PCPs to refer children recovering from trauma to the BHC for consultation, as this may be the only BH service they receive.
2. Listen for "hints" that the PCP blames himself or herself for failure to detect trauma resulting from on-going abuse and provide reassurance.
3. Explain the process of dissociation and the survival value of a child's being able to block recall or deny the trauma.
4. Inform PCPs that simply rehashing a trauma, as in defriefings, does not prevent onset of post-traumatic stress disorder nor reduce psychological distress and in fact may put the patient more at risk.
5. Encourage the PCP to see the child trauma victim as resilient (and not as "damaged goods").

want to regain a sense of being in control of their lives. Available evidence suggests that a single session of individual debriefing post trauma is not associated with a subsequent reduction in the likelihood of post-traumatic stress disorder (PTSD), nor does debriefing reduce self-reported psychological distress. In fact, one year follow-up data suggest that the risk of PTSD may be significantly greater for individuals who receive such service (Rose, Bisson, Churchill, & Wessely, 2005). Finally, it is important that the PCP understand the potential inherent in a strong patient–PCP relationship. Many child trauma victims identify strongly with the PCPs that help them. This identification process is best supported by PCPs who see the child as resilient and capable, rather than damaged and "broken" by virtue of exposure to the traumatic event(s).

CHILDREN WITH ADHD

While children may have disabilities (such as ADHD, learning disabilities, and speech delays), their lives remain workable when they have the skills to make and maintain friendships and illicit positive regard from their parents and teachers. Estimates suggest three to six percent of children are affected by ADHD nationwide (Hibbs & Jensen, 1996), and since most receive care exclusively in primary care settings, BHCs will have many opportunities to assist them. Samuel's case example illustrates the potential role the BHC can play in supporting diagnosis, bringing behavioral interventions to the youth and his or her family, and evaluating treatment response.

Samuel: He's intelligent, but ... he interrupts ... argues....

Dr. Davis referred this thirteen-year-old, seventh-grader for a consultation concerning academic attention and interpersonal problems. Historically, Samuel had struggled academically, as he had been slow to develop writing skills. Now in sixth grade, he was failing all classes and having social problems. His parents came with him to the initial consultation, bringing a note from his teacher that stated, "... very intelligent ... always full of information and willing to contribute to discussions, but interrupts other students ... rarely turns in written work ... argues quite a bit with other students ... recently crawled under his desk and cried after receiving his grade on a test."

In the initial consult, Samuel indicated that he enjoyed learning about computers, science, and math and that he wanted to play a sport, such as soccer, but could not due to his grades. The BHC initiated an objective assessment for ADHD by giving his parents a questionnaire for them to complete and a second one for them to ask the teacher to complete. Additionally, the BHC encouraged the parents to locate a sports team for Samuel that week and to support his efforts to complete homework by staying in the same room with him while he worked (his request) and allowing him to listen to rock music as he worked. The parents also agreed to stay in touch with teachers about homework assignments through e-mails.

The BHC saw Samuel and his parents for three follow-up consultations over a two-month period, and Figure 9.3 shows a graph of his Pediatric Symptom Checklist (PSC) Scores at the initial and follow-up visits. His parents returned the ADHD questionnaires at the initial follow-up and results supported a diagnosis ADHD was warranted. The BHC worked with Dr. Smith during the consult with Samuel, and he initiated a medication trial, as Dr. Davis was out of the clinic. Samuel reported that he planned to wait to join a sports team until he had practiced for a while with his Dad. At the second follow-up, Samuel and his parents indicated significant improvement, and this was consistent with data provided by his teachers. However, reports indicated Sam continued to have problems

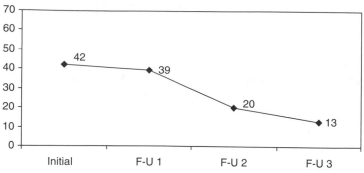

Note: PSC total scores range from 0 to 70; a score of 28 suggests significant psychosocial dysfunction

Figure 9.3. Graph of Samuel's Pediatric Symptom Checklist Scores.

with interrupting and talking excessively so the BHC conducted a functional analysis on these behaviors and helped him develop a self-control program. Specifically, Samuel agreed to monitor his urges to speak out in his first period class and to experiment with using a breathing technique on every other urge. This involved using "belly" breathing and stating "here" on the inhalation and "now" on the exhalation. To remember to use five here and now cycles for every other urge, he would keep his left hand under his left leg, and when the hand came up he would remember to start the breathing exercise. Samuel identified this as his breathing cue as he tended to use his hands to gesture when he spoke. Dr. Davis was not in the clinic at the second follow-up, so Dr. Jones provided a medication refill. The BHC recommended a follow-up visit with Dr. Davis to discuss medication issues, including making a decision about whether to continue medication use over the upcoming summer.

At Samuel's last follow-up visit with the BHC, his mother reported very positive feedback from his school counselor concerning his grades, which were now in the A, B, and C range. He had made some head-way with curbing his interrupting behavior and excessive talking in his first period, and it seemed to be generalizing some to other classes. His parents saw improvement at home, even though they did not have him take the medicine on weekends. The BHC encouraged the father to help Samuel improve his skills for playing a team sport over the summer and to become involved as a volunteer for Sam's team. This would allow the father to detect social skill training needs and later coach Sam on specific skills needed to work successfully in a group.

BHC Intervention Possibilities for Children with ADHD. Sam's case example demonstrates the important role the BHC plays in making a diagnosis and evaluating a medication trial based on objective information from parents and teachers. Additionally, the BHC checked on side effects, supported activities that strengthened relationships between the child and parents, and helped Sam develop skills for inhibiting urges to interrupt others in class. This example also illustrates the important role that the primary care team plays. Since Dr. Davis, Samuel's PCP was out of the clinic at the time of his second and third contacts with the BHC, another PCP covered for him. As a rule of thumb, the BHC should seek advice from the PCP that is covering for an absent PCP when there is a question concerning use of medication, rather than making the patient return later to see the PCP. If doing this, consider the potential benefit of a PCP starting or changing a medicine now (such as when a child is having serious problems in school) versus the risks of not having the patient's own PCP directly involved in medication decisions. The risks associated with starting or changing medicines without the direct involvement of patient's PCP are substantial when either the child or parents are ambivalent about using medications. In those cases, it may be best to have the child and his family schedule with the child's PCP, even though changes involving medication are delayed.

As can be seen in Table 9.13, there are many possible interventions that a BHC can offer beyond assessment and evaluation of medication trials. BHC interventions may address social skill deficits and relationship problems with parents and other family members. One of us (JR) offers group visits for ADHD children and their parents in which he provides parenting instruction specific for ADHD children. Materials are also available for the BHC to use in developing ADHD specific parent training programs for group visits, classes, or workshops (see Anastopoulos, Barkley, & Shelton, 1996). There are also numerous books that may help parents be effective social coaches for children with ADHD, as well as with learning disabilities (cf. Giler, 1998).

Other possibilities for BHC interventions involve use of resources outside the clinic. For example, many children benefit when the BHC helps teachers and parents start a daily report card program. The Vanderbilt

Table 9.13. BHC intervention possibilities for children with ADHD

1. Assist the PCP with administering and interpreting questionnaires that help establish the diagnosis and that evaluate medication trials (when medicines are started).
2. Evaluate medication side effects.
3. Assess social skills and social status and provide remediation as needed.
4. Assess relationship with parents and plan activities to improve relationship quality if indicated.
5. Teach parents to function as social skill coaches.
6. Recommend books to parents concerning parenting children with ADHD.
7. Co-lead group visits for children with ADHD and their parents.
8. Facilitate development of daily report card programs to improve home-work completion and/or other behaviors important to academic and social success.
9. Advocate for educational testing if a child appears to need a special education program.
10. Refer children to ADHD summer camp programs.

Tool Kit website offers an excellent handout to support this type of program. Some children will continue to make exceptionally slow progress in acquiring academic skills after a medication is started, and some will have specific deficits (e.g., difficulties with writing, reading, or math). The BHC can work with the PCP in making a decision concerning whether to write a letter to the school recommending that the patient receive individualized testing to assess the need for a special educational program. Additionally, various universities offer summer camp programs for children with ADHD, and we recommend that the BHC stay informed about these, as they offer children with ADHD unique opportunities for social and academic skill remediation.

PCP Teaching Points Concerning Children with ADHD. PCPs will readily adopt a consistent approach to assessment and monitoring of core ADHD symptoms, if the BHC does the "leg work" and provides the evidence base for using these assessment systems. Most PCPs will also pass along a reading list to parents. Over time, some PCPs will learn some of the interventions used by BHCs to remediate social skills and improve parent and child relationships, particularly when they participate in a group visit approach to caring for children with ADHD. As suggested in Table 9.14, the BHC may encourage PCPs to begin group visits in order to

Table 9.14. PCP teaching points concerning children with ADHD

1. Encourage PCPs to use ADHD questionnaires for assessment.
2. Explain the group visit approach to providing services to ADHD children.
3. Suggest that PCPs refer children with ADHD to the BHC for a discussion of developmental transition issues at the end of middle childhood and again toward the end of high school years.
4. Suggest that PCPs use the BHC to assist adolescents with ADHD who refuse to take medication.

improve their skills with this population (as well as other reasons, which we discuss in Chapter 12). Most PCPs want to see children with ADHD every three months, and the group visit makes this feasible.

Finally, BHCs may encourage PCPs to refer children with ADHD for visits focused on preparing them and their families for transitions, such as graduation into middle school. The BHC can help parents adjust their communication and problem-solving styles to accommodate the child's growing need for autonomy while continuing to provide adequate structure and support. Some children refuse to take medications at some point in adolescence, and this can also make for a good referral. The BHC can teach strategies for focusing and organizing study time and experiment with these behavioral strategies in lieu of using medicines. Data from parents, teacher and the patient may help the patient review his or her medication decision.

SUMMARY

1. BHCs see many children at a brisk pace in primary care. In fact, 20 to 40 percent of a BHC's contacts may be with children and teenagers, depending on the clinic. For most consults, the BHC will also need to work with the patient's family.
2. Many parents lack skills for parenting, and the ideal time to address their needs is probably when their children are between two and seven. BHCs may use a PCBH parenting protocol to teach basic skills in a three-session series, provide workshops or classes, or refer to parenting classes in the community.
3. Many children are overweight or obese, and the BHC needs to assist these children and their families with behavior change. Serving these

children and teenagers provides the BHC with opportunities to work closely with other members of the PC team, such as dieticians and diabetes educators.

4. Pediatric pain is a common reason for referral, and one that requires skillful use of the tools of functional analysis in the context of the family. ACT, along with other CBT strategies, offers potent interventions for improving functioning. Appendix B includes a reading list for parents and children.

5. Many BHC referrals will concern social problems, which can predispose children to development of more significant psychosocial dysfunction. Social skill training works well in the context of PCBH consultation.

6. Primary care is the safety net for victims of trauma, and this is no less true for children than for adults. BHCs can target victim's concerns and use identified strengths to help children and their families resume meaningful lives. Trauma victims should not be forced to "debrief."

7. Two-thirds of children with ADHD have significant problems with functioning in adulthood. BHCs can help change this statistic by assisting PCPs with diagnosis and interventions, teaching social skills and helping parents be more effective.

10

EXAMPLES OF CONSULTATIONS WITH ADULTS

"To find out what one is fitted to do, and to secure an opportunity to do it, is the key to happiness."

—John Dewey

Many adults in the U.S. have a person in their lives who they consider to be their primary care provider. Most hope that this special person, the PCP, will see them as a whole person and provide helpful advice and support over the course of a lifetime. Most want guidance on how to maintain their health and care for health problems when they develop. Most of all, patients hope that their PCP will provide good counsel when they are going through a challenging period of life.

General medicine has always been based on the belief that a collaborative, mutually respectful, life span relationship provides the best opportunity for good health care. The biopsychosocial model of general medicine (Engel, 1977) is the center piece of this philosophy. However, it is one thing to talk about the goal of biopsychosocial care, while it is an entirely different matter to deliver care in this framework. Any objective review of the U.S. primary care system would conclude that biopsychosocial medicine is a much talked about, seldom delivered form of care. The integration of primary care and behavioral health services and providers is one obvious step toward resolving this conundrum.

The BHC, as the newest addition to the PC team, is well-equipped to support the whole-person perspective, bring fresh ideas to the team, and provide interventions that strengthen the PCP–patient relationship. The demands of primary care practice are unforgiving. Many patients with problems are seen on any given day, and they must generally have their full medical and psychological needs addressed in less than ten minutes. For this reason, the addition of a BHC to the medical team is a "dream come true."

This chapter offers the reader a chance to join a day of BHC practice in an adult medicine team. We have a very busy schedule today, but that is nothing new. Everyday is a busy day. Today, you will shadow a BHC who provides consultations to eleven patients. In some consultations, readers will view graphs of assessment data and learn how to use these in providing services. In other consultations, readers will learn about practice tools (e.g., behavioral prescription pads). After a day in practice, the reader will have a much better idea of what he or she needs to learn to be a competent BHC. To this end, we have compiled Appendix C as a reading list for BHCs who want to increase their intervention skills with adults. Also, as is the case for working with children and families, patient education materials are a basic part of the BHC tool kit. Thus, we have included a compact disc that includes core patient handouts. So, let your imagination take over and let's get to work. Table 10.1 describes the day (and provides an overview of this chapter).

VAGUE PAIN COMPLAINTS AND DOMESTIC VIOLENCE

Vague pain complaints are very common in primary care, and functional analysis is an excellent tool for addressing them. Clinic visits by women involving vague pain complaints are commonly related to marital problems. Some of these women are victims of domestic violence, and their visit offers an opportunity to address safety issues, as well as relationship skill deficits. Maria's case example provides a demonstration of the services BHCs can offer women with vague pain complaints and marital problems.

Maria: My neck hurts

Dr. Sims scheduled Maria to see the BHC for neck pain and stress management after her medical appointment. When the BHC explored the neck

Table 10.1. A day in the life of a BHC (providing care to adults)

Chapter section	BHC # 1442	Referral reason
Vague pain complaints/ domestic violence	8:15 Maria	Neck pain
Chronic pain	8:45 David	Back pain
Medical adherence	9:15 Bud	Hypertension
Somatization	9:45 May	Dizziness
Chest pain (panic)	10:15 Ralph	Chest pain
Chronic conditions	1:00 Patty	Weight gain, chronic disease management
Learning disabilities	1:30 Penny	Dizziness, fatigue
Symptoms of trauma and depression	2:00 Leslie	Fatigue, sleep disturbance, depression
Suicidal ideation	2:30 Jose	Thoughts of suicide, new diagnosis of diabetes
Drug and alcohol problems	3:00 Ed	Alcohol problems
Serious mental illness	3:30 Elizabeth	Hearing voices, sleep problems

pain, Maria began to cry and said that it had started several months earlier after she was laid off from her job. She and her husband had been arguing more, and their youngest child was having problems in school. She was considering leaving her husband because of his verbal abuse, but had no place to live if she left. Walking and taking a shower seemed to help relieve her pain, and being with friends improved her outlook. However, she explained that her husband was jealous and that he did not like for her to see her friends. She admitted to feeling afraid of him and explained that he had hit her early in the marriage, but had stopped after she separated from him briefly. Maria explained to the BHC that she wanted to improve her marriage and to stay with her husband, as she had young children and wanted them to have a father in the home. She was also dependent financially on her husband.

The functional analysis suggested that Maria had responded to the increased stress in her relationship by isolating herself from friends at church and in her local community. As is true for many patients in unpleasant stressful family environments, she believed that her friends would soon "get tired" of hearing her talk about her stress and low life satisfaction. The net effect was that she was becoming more and more reliant on her husband to provide social support, even though he was the source of stress in the first place. This, combined with his jealousy at her being out of the house, resulted in a very clear pattern of withdrawal and social avoidance.

The BHC and Maria developed a plan that addressed both her pain and her desire to reduce stress and improve marital satisfaction. She agreed to resume regular attendance at her local church and to rejoin a group of women friends who took walks on a daily basis in her neighborhood. The BHC also explained the relationship between stress and pain and suggested that the pain would probably continue at some level as it was related to muscle tension in the neck and shoulders, which often increases with conflict. The BHC taught her an exercise involving diaphragmatic breathing combined with rhythmic gentle stretching of muscles in the neck, shoulders, and back. The BHC also mentioned that regular walks of thirty to forty-five minutes would probably help her feel more relaxed and ready to solve problems at home. This made sense to her as she often felt more optimistic when she occasionally took a walk to meet her children at their school. The BHC gave her a pamphlet that described services from a domestic violence agency in the community, explaining that they supported women in problem-solving and that she did not need to be planning to leave her husband in order to call them.

At follow-up, Maria reported that she was attending her church group and had talked with her sister several times about her marriage and her life direction. She was practicing the suggested breathing exercise daily and walking to and from her children's school on weekdays. She felt better about her marriage, as her husband was staying home more and treating her more respectfully. She had not called the domestic violence agency, but wanted to know more about their services and agreed to possibly call them in the future. The BHC taught her another breathing exercise to promote relaxation and reviewed the Stress Awareness Handout (see Appendix D) with her, and they talked about Maria's values concerning friendship and ways to bring more friends into her life. The BHC explained that Dr. Sims would support her behavior change goals and her plans for the future.

Figure 10.1 depicts a graph of Maria's Duke Health Profile Scores at her initial and follow-up visits with the BHC. As explained in Chapter

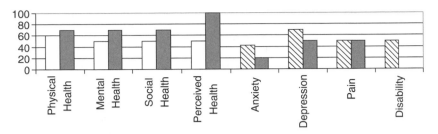

Figure 10.1. Maria's Duke Health Profile Scores at the Initial and Follow-up Consultations. (Scores range from 0 to 100. On Physical, Mental, Social, and Perceived Health Scales, higher Scores indicate better functioning. On Anxiety, Depression, Pain, and Disability Scales, higher scores indicate more severe symptoms.)

5, Duke Scores range from 0 to 100. Higher Scores suggest better health on Function Scales (Physical Health, Mental Health, Social Health, and Perceived Health, which are represented by white columns for the initial visit). The scoring is the opposite for Dysfunction Scales, where higher Scores suggest more severe symptoms (related to Anxiety, Depression, Pain, and Disability, which are represented by striped columns for the initial visit). Her follow-up scores confirmed her reported improvement, and are represented by shaded columns.

BHC Intervention Possibilities for Patients Reporting Pain and Domestic Violence. The interventions used with Maria are typical for patients with pain complaints and marital problems. As indicated in Table 10.2, the BHC accepted Maria's pain complaint and used it as the basis for a functional analysis. The results of functional analysis suggested a link to marital problems, and they worked together to plan interventions that might improve both. The functional analysis also suggested that pain was less troubling and marital conflict less problematic when Maria had more social outings, so the BHC supported her in efforts to improve her rate of socializing. The BHC accepted Maria's plan of staying in her marriage and, at the same time, offered her information on community services for victims of domestic violence. At follow-up, the BHC taught Maria to stay aware of her stress level and to practice relaxation skills to lower pain sensations related to muscle tension.

Table 10.2. BHC intervention possibilities for patients reporting pain and domestic violence

1. Accept the pain complaint and center the functional analysis on it.
2. Look for a link between pain and marital dissatisfaction and use it to inform the plan.
3. Accept the patient's preference to stay or leave the marriage or her or his lack of a determined direction and attempt to interject information and experiences that will enhance the patient's flexibility in choosing and pursuing a direction.
4. Help the patient clarify her or his values concerning intimate relationships.
5. Teach the patient about the value of using cognitive rather than emotion-focused coping strategies in addressing marital problems.
6. Devise a safety plan and collaborate, as appropriate, with police, domestic violence organizations, children's protective services, shelters, etc.
7. Help the patient determine a focus for skill development (self-care, improving her or his social network, personal assertion).
8. Use health-related quality of life scores to evaluate patient change, and return the patient to the PCP when the patient reports behavior change and scores suggest improvement.
9. Co-lead classes with a representative from the local domestic violence organization.

At follow-up, the BHC again evaluated Maria's functioning using the Duke, and, as both patient report and Duke Scores suggested improvement, the BHC returned her back to the PCP for ongoing follow up. The BHC had planted seeds that might grow over time, including use of the domestic violence program and increased social support. The BHC briefed the referring PCP on the present and future behavior change plan, with an emphasis on having the PCP actively query the patient about progress.

Patients involved in abusive relationships often need help to clarify their values concerning intimate relationships and to look at the viability of their marriage or partnership in the context of these values. Values clarified this way can provide a back drop for behavior change planning and for teaching specific coping skills. Most patients also benefit from learning the difference between problem-focused versus emotion-focused coping strategies, as well as the distinction between approach and avoidance oriented coping. In this case, the BHC also needed to be mindful of Maria's readiness to change in regards to her dysfunctional marriage and to encourage her continued contact with the clinic by matching the intervention to her level of readiness. Many patients benefit from first rebuilding their social supports and focusing on tension reduction and related self-care strategies.

Classes that help patients clarify values with respect to abusive relationships offer a way to intensify the treatment response to a large and troublesome group of primary care patients. Some PCPs tend to address violent, abusive, and dysfunctional relationships from a moralistic, advice heavy perspective. These authority based interventions seldom have a positive impact and may drive the patient out of care altogether. In some venues, the BHC may be able to involve a representative of the local domestic violence agency in group visits, so that a warm hand-off is possible.

The BHC also needs to address safety issues. Patients should be advised to stay out of the kitchen and bathroom during times of escalated conflict, as these are high risk areas. BHCs also need to inquire about factors that tend to be associated with serious or lethal injury, including an increase in frequency or severity of abuse, threats of homicide or suicide by the partner, presence or availability of a firearm, and whether the abuser is aware of a victim's plan to leave.

PCP Teaching Points Concerning Patients Reporting Pain and Domestic Violence

As suggested in Table 10.3, BHCs need to teach PCPs to routinely ask patients with vague pain complaints about recent stressful circumstances—"So, how are things going for you day-to-day?—How is your marriage going?—Are your children well?" These help the PCP lead into an explanation of the relationship between stress and pain (and often a referral to the BHC). The purpose of this line of inquiry is not to talk the patient out of being in pain, but to increase the context for understanding suffering in the patient's life.

When patients indicate marital problems, we encourage PCPs to ask one or more screening questions to help determine the likelihood of domestic violence (see Chapter 6 for examples.) When a patient answers affirmatively, we recommend that the PCP encourage the patient to see the BHC on a same-day basis. We also recommend that BHCs teach PCPs to consider the possibility of domestic violence when he or she notices any of

Table 10.3. PCP Teaching points concerning adult patients possibly affected by domestic violence

1. Encourage use of questions about stress, including marital stress, when patients report vague pain complaints.
2. When patients admit to marital problems, suggest use of a screening question (see chapter 6 for examples) to determine the need for a same-day consultation with the BHC.
3. Provide information about the types of findings in a physical exam that need to trigger exploration of domestic violence.
4. Show a film on the PCP's role in providing care to victims of domestic violence. (i.e., communicating concern, providing information, reviewing options, safety planning, and providing medical treatment).
5. Stock pamphlets describing services from local domestic violence agencies in a common area so that PCPs can access them easily.
6. Teach the basics of expressing concern and making safety plans.
7. Remind PCPs to photograph and document injuries.

the following findings during a physical exam: any injury to face, breast, genitals, or torso; bilateral or multiple injuries; delay between the injury event and presentation for care; explanation of injury inconsistent with injury pattern; prior use of emergency room services for trauma; chronic pain symptoms; psychological distress; evidence of rape or sexual assault; any injury in a pregnant woman, or, lastly, the presence of a partner who is overly protective, controlling, and/or refuses to leave the exam room. It is of course important for the PCP to document injuries, and most clinics have cameras available to assist with such efforts. The Family Violence Fund (www.endabuse.org) offers a good training video for PCPs on screening.

Once domestic violence has been identified, the PCP's role includes communicating concern, providing information, reviewing options, referring to the BHC, safety planning, and providing medical treatment. While many victims never leave abusing partners, their situation may improve when they talk about it. In our experience, patients who are victims of violence often do make significant changes, including leaving abusive relationships, when the PCP and BHC work together over a period of months or years and in collaboration with local domestic violence programs.

PATIENTS WITH CHRONIC PAIN

Patients with chronic pain have a high impact on primary care services. While they are not a large group, they are complex and difficult to serve as a group given the diversity of their medical problems and the variation in levels of psychosocial dysfunction among them. Clinical pathways (i.e., established programs that prescribe procedures implemented for every patient in a specific category) may improve relationships between patients with chronic pain and the providers that care for them. We provide information about a chronic pain pathway in Chapter 12. The following consultation with David exemplifies a clinical pathway for chronic pain patients called the "Pain and Quality of Life Program."

David: My back is killing me, and I need my pain medication refilled now

Dr. Clever referred this fifty-year-old man for enrollment in the Pain and Quality of Life Program. David was a new patient to the clinic and made a request for treatment of chronic back pain secondary to incomplete paraplegia and considerable spasticity. David also suffered from hypertension and diabetes. He had signed a clinical pathway agreement with Dr. Clever just prior to the consultation with the BHC. The agreement included the typical terms for use of opioid medications for pain (see Chapter 13 for a discussion of medication agreements), as well as additional terms concerning participation in the program.

In the initial visit with the BHC, David explained that his goal was to be free of pain. He had tried a variety of strategies for eliminating pain and, while none seemed to help him reach his goal of being pain-free, some worked better than others to reduce the pain. The BHC explained that the Pain and Quality of Life Program was designed to help patients with chronic pain improve their quality of life. David was given a patient education handout to help him begin the on-going process of pursuing value-based behavioral change. (See the Primary Care Patient Values Plan on the compact disc in Appendix D.) He chose to focus on his values concerning work and health, in particular being productive and creative. He took pride in his ability to write songs and poems. He played guitar, and most of his friends and family members enjoyed listening to him when he was willing to play.

David's initial responses to the Duke Health Profile suggested low Physical and Social Health Scores, while Mental Health was strong. The plan at the end of the initial consultation was that he would begin attending a monthly class associated with the Pain and Quality of Life Program and that failure to attend would result in his not receiving his pain medication prescription for the following month. Additionally, David agreed to plan at least two social activities weekly, as his mobility problems posed a barrier to socializing and he tended to feel worse when he was more isolated.

David did not come to the next class as planned, and someone called on his behalf several days later insisting that he would pick up David's pain prescription for him. This request was denied, and David came for an appointment with Dr. Clever later that week. At that contact, he received a tapering prescription for the month, and Dr. Clever reviewed his program agreement and referred him for a same-day consultation with the BHC. The BHC addressed barriers to David's successful participation in the program and reviewed psychoeducational material from the missed class. Over the following twelve months, David appeared for every class on time, completed assessments promptly, participated in class discussions and exercises, and picked up his prescription at the end of class. David's Physical and Social Health Scores on the Duke inched up over the course of the year, as he had become more active in a weight training program for his upper body, more productive in his writing, and more consistent in playing music for others.

BHC Intervention Possibilities for Patients with Chronic Pain. The BHC providing care to David worked within the structure of a clinical pathway designed to help patients make the transition from a focus on pain to a focus on improving quality of life. David received many of the interventions suggested in Table 10.4 over the course of the year following his enrollment in the pathway (and without requiring much individual contact with the BHC or PCP). When David did not hold to the terms of the signed agreement, the PCP delivered a consequence specified in the pain program agreement. David's subsequent adherence improved dramatically. As a part of the class, the BHC obtained health-related quality of life scores and included these in chart notes. These data provided the PCP with objective measures for gauging David's response to pathway treatment over time.

Table 10.4. BHC intervention possibilities for patients with chronic pain

1.	Provide information about chronic pain treatment strategies, the impact of stress on pain, and the chronic pain cycle of avoidance (See Managing Chronic Pain handout on compact disc on Appendix D).
2.	Help the patient shift from a goal of pain elimination to a goal of improving quality of life.
3.	Measure health related quality of life (or other indicator of functioning, such as results from the Healthy Days Questionnaire) at regular contacts and teach PCPs to use these to evaluate and plan treatment.
4.	Encourage daily physical exercise and stretching.
5.	Develop value-driven behavior change plans that the BHC and PCP can support in ping-pong visits with the patient (See Primary Care Patient Values Plan on compact disc in Appendix D).
6.	Work with others to create a pathway program for your clinic.
7.	Refer to community resources, such as yoga classes and fibromyalgia or chronic pain support groups.
8.	Suggest self-help books (See for example Jamison, 1996).

When BHCs do not have pathway programs for chronic pain, we recommend that they begin their intervention with information about the differences between acute and chronic pain treatment strategies, the impact of stress on pain, and the chronic pain cycle of avoidance. The Managing Chronic Pain handout in Appendix D provides patients with written information on these issues. BHC interventions with patients with chronic pain need to focus on activating the patient, because it is the avoidance of pain that leads to sedentary coping styles, greater muscle atrophy and uncomfortable stiffness, which can easily degenerate into a self perpetuating cycle. From an ACT perspective, the emphasis on pain elimination comes from the inability to detach from the experience of pain. Most such patients define themselves in terms of how much pain they are experiencing at any particular moment. Consequently, patients such as David will benefit from learning to monitor pain from an observer self or mindful stance. Once this skill is in place, the BHC can teach useful strategies such as pacing (which involves adjusting intensity, position, and other variables in physical activity to prolong function). The BHC may also teach distraction and relaxation skills and employ interventions involving de-catastrophizing pain and de-fusing from pain. Handouts such as the Primary Care Values Plan (see Appendix D) help the BHC and patient develop value-based behavior change plans that both the BHC and PCP can support in a series of ping-pong visits. The BHC may also suggest that chronic pain patients participate in community activities, such as yoga classes and support groups for individuals with fibromyalgia and chronic pain, as well as read books about coping with pain (see for example Jamison, 1996).

PCP Teaching Points Concerning Patients with Chronic Pain. To assist PCPs with effectively treating this challenging group of patients, the BHC needs to maintain a focus on training PCPs to conceptualize pain less from a biomedical perspective and more from a psychological acceptance point of view. Surveying providers as to their experiences with treating chronic pain patients may enhance their interest in exploring new treatment approaches. Figure 10.2 contains possible survey questions. In many cases, a discussion of the results may spur development of a work group charged with developing a pathway, along with educational programs and practice support tools.

As many PCPs did not receive training for treating chronic pain in medical school, they will be open to the ideas suggested in Table 10.5. Many want to avoid or stop prescribing opioids for chronic pain because the evidence for their long term effectiveness is poor. Nevertheless, PCPs may struggle with delivering a coherent explanation for shifting from medications to behavior change, and the BHC can help with this. Some patients are prone to thinking that the PCP sees their pain as "all in the head." The BHC can help PCPs engage these patients by teaching them to include statements such as the following in their standard explanation to patients: "We do not think that pain is in the heads of our patients. We know that pain is in the mind and the body, and we take a holistic approach." Most PCPs will also welcome presentations on behavioral techniques and use of quality of life measures to evaluate treatment and will use handouts, such as Managing Chronic Pain (available in Appendix D). While many PCPs use some type of medication agreement when prescribing longer term narcotic regimens, they will benefit from behaviorally sound strategies for responding to violations of the agreement. To support PCPs in shifting the focus of care from eliminating pain to improving functioning, BHCs may provide brief presentations on how to set exercise and social activity goals.

The purpose of this survey is to further understand the PCP experience in caring for chronic pain patients. I will ask these questions again periodically to assess the impact of educational activities and program development activities. Thank you for completing this survey.

Below you will find a list of statements. Please rate the truth of each statement as it applies to you. Use the following rating scale to make your choices. For instance, if you believe a statement is "Always true," you would write a 5 in the blank next to that statement.

0	1	2	3	4	5
Never true	Very rarely true	Some times true	Often true	Almost always true	Always true

1.	My training prepared me adequately for working with chronic pain patients.
2.	I enjoy working with chronic pain patients.
3.	I have all the skills I need to work effectively with chronic pain patients.
4.	I look forward to seeing chronic pain patients.
5.	I feel that I am successful with chronic pain patients.
6.	I want to specialize in treating chronic pain.
7.	I usually have a new idea about how to help my most difficult chronic pain patients.
8.	Pain medications are very helpful to my chronic pain patients.
9.	I am able to refer my chronic pain patients to accessible, effective programs.

Figure 10.2. PCP Experiences with Treating Patients with Chronic Pain.

Table 10.5. PCP Teaching points concerning patients with chronic pain

1. After surveying PCPs concerning their experiences with treating patients with chronic pain, ask to form a committee to develop a clinical pathway.
2. Teach PCPs to use patient education handouts promoting behavioral strategies for coping with pain (e.g., the Managing Chronic Pain handout in Appendix D).
3. Support consistent use of a medication agreement with chronic pain patients who use medications.
4. Help PCPs use language emphasizing that all pain is "real" and that pain is best understood as a body–mind experience.
5. Encourage PCPs to include increasing rates of socializing, exercising and stretching in care plans.
6. Help PCPs to identify patients who are at risk for developing chronic pain.
7. Teach PCPs to use strategies for preventing onset of chronic pain (e.g., use of a behavioral health prescription pad focused on functioning in lieu of a medication prescription pad).
8. Encourage use of BHC services for patients who voice strong fears of pain and report use of sedentary strategies two to four weeks after an acute injury.

BHCs should also teach PCPs about the opportunity to prevent chronic pain syndrome when treating patients with acute pain complaints. This involves teaching PCPs to detect patients at risk for development of chronic pain and ways to intervene meaningfully with them within weeks after an acute injury. Risk factors include job dissatisfaction, the ability to make as much money not working as when employed, history of or current symptoms of depression, a tendency toward somatization, a history of substance abuse, prior pain complaints, over-reliance on sedentary strategies for coping, and (when the injury occurred at work) failure of the employer to express concern about the patient's recovery in the weeks immediately following the injury. For acute pain patients with even moderate risk status, the PCP must be able to explain the difference between strategies for treating acute pain and chronic pain, to explain that pain is a normal part of the recovery process, to emphasize acceptance of the fact that pain may be present over time, to explain the concept of pacing, to encourage return to normal social activities as soon as possible, and to insist on some type of stretching and physical exercise regimen on a daily basis.

A behavioral health prescription pad such as the one in Figure 10.3 can help the provider curb the urge to prescribe medications when treating at-risk patients. This tool involves the Bull's Eye concept first developed by Tobias Lundgren of the University of Upsala in Sweden. This ACT tool supports behavior change plans based on valued directions in the areas of love, work, and play. When using the pad, the PCP can explain that recovery from an injury requires one to take stock of what's really important in life and to carefully plan ways to pursue these values. The PCP will also need to explain the difference between values and goals. Values (as globally constructed, abstract concepts) provide direction for behavior change, while goals (as specific attainable targets) provide an immediate target for changing behavior. The bull's eye represents a person's value in each of the three areas. He or she can draw a line from the bull's eye to the side and write down a few words representing what the patient reports as valued life directions (e.g., "kindness" for the love bull's eye or "dependability" for the work bull's eye). The PCP needs to point out that most people only sometimes behave in ways that represent their values, but that keeping one's values in mind helps one come closer to them over time. An injury or illness causing

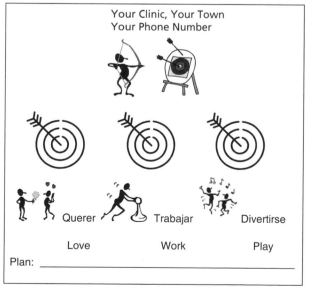

Note: Appendix D offers a different prescription pad (the ACT Behavioral Health Prescription Pad), along with directions for use

Figure 10.3. A Bull's Eye Behavioral Health Prescription Pad.

pain may make it difficult for one to think about values and personal meaning as the basis for making daily choices. While recognizing this, the PCP can invite the patient to form a goal in one or two areas (depending on time) that he or she believes would help him or her come closer to living in accordance with the bull's eye value over the next few weeks. For example, a patient might agree to spend fifteen minutes reading to her children in the evening (goal) in order to come closer to being a mother that puts her children first (value). It is also useful for the PCP to ask the patient to "throw the dart" or "shoot the arrow" into the target by making a dot with a pencil to show how close their behavior has been to the value for one or more areas (love, work, or play) over the past week. The PCP may wrap-up by suggesting, "I am thinking that your arrow will land closer to the bull's eye at our follow up visit. Let's see what happens." Many patients enjoy talking to a PCP about values. While we are suggesting this prescription pad for the purpose of teaching PCPs to prevent onset of chronic pain with high risk patients, it is also useful with patients with numerous other types of problems, such as difficulties with managing chronic disease.

MEDICAL ADHERENCE

Patients are most likely to adhere to plans that reflect their personal preferences, involve skills they can perform independently and with confidence, are supported by their family members or friends, and that fit within their perspective on health. Ann Fadiman's book, *The Spirit Catches You and You Fall Down: A Hmong Child, her American Doctors, and the Collision of Two Cultures* (Fadiman, 1997) providers an excellent demonstration of the tenacity that human beings are capable of demonstrating in interactions with medical providers. Ultimately, it is the patient who chooses what advice to heed, what procedures to tolerate, and what medical treatments to consume. Bud's case example demonstrates the important role the BHC can play in helping patients identify and overcome obstacles to medical adherence.

Bud: I don't like taking pills

Dr. Mason referred this forty-seven-year-old man for a consultation concerning hypertension, worry, and stress management. Bud explained that his worries were about his health and that they had started two months earlier when he was diagnosed with hypertension. Bud had made numerous behavior changes since the diagnosis, including starting a walking program and quitting smoking and drinking. He reported walking fourteen laps on a track six out of seven days weekly. He had lost twenty-five pounds, and people were complimenting him, as he had been overweight. Bud confessed that he had stopped taking the blood pressure medication when his prescription ran out after the first fourteen days. He explained that he took his blood pressure often and that it was usually normal.

In the initial consultation, the BHC helped Bud explore his worries and his values. His worries included health, dying and not being available to his children, and a fear of becoming manic, as his father had. The BHC provided corrective information about bipolar disorder, and Bud seemed somewhat reassured. As a part of the intervention, the BHC also used the Acceptance and Commitment Therapy (ACT) Behavioral Prescription Pad (see Appendix D) and explained that durable behavior change often requires that a person learn to experience feeling discouraged and/or afraid and worried—like pulling one's hair out (see two upper figures on pad). Additionally, the person needs to learn to experience these unwanted feelings while engaging in daily behaviors that are consistent with valued directions, which are suggested by figures on the bottom half of the page (e.g., walking at the track, avoiding salt, etc.). The BHC taught Bud a mindfulness technique for observing his thoughts and feelings (i.e., mentally placing them one-by-one onto the sides of imagined railroad cars.) She suggested that he use this technique during the first few laps of his walk and then switch to singing a few of his favorite songs and noticing appealing aspects of nature. He agreed to this modification to his walking program and to follow-up with the BHC in two weeks. He also agreed to learn progressive muscle relaxation in his planned follow-up visit with the BHC.

At follow-up, Duke Health Profile Scores suggested improvement, and all Function Scales were in the normal range. He reported that he was now walking nineteen laps on six out of seven days weekly and was spending the first part of his walk watching his worries and then switching to singing. He reported that he worried less at work and that he was more playful there, as he had been before his diagnosis. He reported that people at his job and in his family noticed this change. He wanted to talk about the way his parents treated him as an adolescent and his current struggle with his eighteen-year-old daughter. The BHC linked this discussion to a review of value driven behavior change, and Bud left with a plan of spending several hours weekly alone with his daughter in the service of promoting her ability to make decisions independently. As planned, the BHC taught Bud a five-minute version of progressive muscle relaxation (using the handout on the compact disc in Appendix D). He agreed to follow-up with his PCP and to recontact the BHC for support of behavior change if the need arose.

BHC Intervention Possibilities for Patients with Medical Adherence Problems. The case example illustrates commonly used interventions for behavioral treatment of hypertension (e.g., start of an exercise program, mastery of relaxation skills, support of dietary changes recommended by the PCP), as well as important interventions for addressing medical adherence. BHCs need to understand a patient's perspective on health and on the role of medical treatments to preserve health. This information can be used to facilitate better communication between the patient and PCP. The BHC told Dr. Mason about Bud stopping the medicine and starting the exercise program. Because Bud was monitoring his blood pressure and knew his program was working, Dr. Mason was pleased and the BHC conveyed this to Bud at his follow-up. Because Bud's new health promoting behaviors were still not "habits" and could reverse over time, the BHC asked that he follow-up with Dr. Mason in four to six weeks. While the BHC did offer to help with any bumps in the road, the planned follow-up was with the PCP. This is an important element of clinical practice with patients like Bud, who can easily get confused about the role of the BHC versus the PCP over time. In addition to the interventions suggested in Table 10.6, we suggest strategies for addressing medical adherence in an older adult in Chapter 11.

PCP Teaching Points. The best adherence comes from a strong patient–PCP relationship where both parties work diligently toward a common understanding of the patient's problem and an acceptable and effective attempt at solution. PCPs benefit from learning to ask questions that solicit information about the patient's view of a medical problem and the acceptability of medical treatments. Questions like this include: "Why do you think this (illness) happened to you? What do you think you should do to address it at this time? What are the things you can think of

Table 10.6. BHC intervention possibilities for patients with medical adherence problems

1. Attempt to understand patient's perspective on his or her illness, what caused it, the personal meaning of the condition for the person, and the treatments that make sense according to the unique world view of that specific patient.
2. Discuss values concerning health and concerns about dying.
3. Relate information to the PCP and consider ways to strengthen the relationship between the patient and the PCP.
4. Help the patient anticipate obstacles to maintaining newly established behaviors.
5. Make a plan for patient to the follow-up with his or her PCP.

that would get in the way of you following through with this treatment? Can you name some of these obstacles?" Patients are more likely to comply with treatments that are consistent with their values. When a patient's relationship with a PCP is at its beginning and there is a diagnosis of a disease, such as hypertension, the PCP may not know the patient well enough to anticipate a potential adherence problem. A consultation with the BHC can help the PCP better understand the patient's world view and link the treatment to important patient-centric values. Patients like Bud are a delight to PCPs because of their willingness to make behavior changes. However, PCPs will readily accept these changes as being a "done deal," not appreciating that new habits are unstable and that continued vigilance and reinforcement will be needed. This, of course, may be done through formats other than direct patient contact (e.g., brief letters of support, calls from a nurse, nursing assistant, or BHC), as suggested in Table 10.7.

SOMATIZATION

Some patients have learning histories that prepare them to be hypervigilant to even normal variations in bodily functions. Unlike the "normal" patient under stress, the somatizing patient is exquisitely sensitive to signs of physiological arousal, and attaches (fuses) to provocative, negative thoughts about their meaning. For example, a somatizing patient might interpret GI distress as a sign that a cancer is growing in the bowel; dizziness as a sign of a rare neurological disorder. Patients with a somatic

Table 10.7. PCP teaching points concerning patients with medical adherence problems

1. Encourage discussion of the patient's world view as it relates to a newly diagnosed health problem, along with their beliefs about viable treatments.
2. Encourage PCPs to see adherence as the result of a collaborative process and a good relationship.
3. Encourage PCPs to provide long term support to healthy behavior changes, using a variety of methods (e.g., nursing assistant phone calls, letters, etc.).

focus seek medical care on a more frequent basis even during the good times. During stressful periods, their medical visits can skyrocket to the point of frustrating and angering the PCP. Patients with somatization are renowned for their ability to elicit numerous, expensive and usually benign specialty tests and procedures. When the specialty test comes back negative, the PCP assumes the patient will drop the issue, while the patient concludes that the medical establishment has missed a diagnosis. ("After all, why would the doctor refer me for a test in the first place if he or she didn't secretly think that I have some type of life threatening problem?")

In general, PCPs find patients with somatization to be among the most difficult in a general practice. The case example of May demonstrates the dramatic impact the BHC can have on interrupting this ever expanding pattern of health care seeking.

May: I have problems with dizziness, and I want to be sure that I don't have …

Dr. West referred this thirty-seven-year-old married mother for a consultation concerning dizziness and weight loss. May explained that her problems with dizziness began in her twenties and agreed with the idea that stress made this problem worse. She also indicated a recurring fear that her dizziness was a sign of a brain aneurysm, explaining that this concern began after her father died of a brain aneurysm five years ago. May wanted to believe Dr. West's reassurances, but was troubled by her doubts and her continued dizziness. May had struggled with her weight since having children and had recently initiated a walking program and several dietary changes.

The BHC talked with May about the relationship between anxiety/worry, shallow-breathing and a myriad of physical symptoms including light headedness and dizziness. The more worried and anxious a person gets, the more there is a tendency to breathe rapidly and with a "shallow breath". Over time, this pattern can result in chronic problems with dizziness and light-headedness. The BHC taught May diaphragmatic breathing (using the Diaphragmatic Breathing Tips handout on the Compact Disc in Appendix D) and suggested that she practice it in the mornings by breathing in her thoughts of poor health and breathing out thoughts about poor health for a few minutes. Later, the same breathing pattern would be used to increase her skills for being present, even when having troubling thoughts about her health. The BHC instructed May to say "here" to herself as she breathed in slowly and "now" as she breathed out slowly. The cues of here and now might help her be present in the moment, where she was capable of changing her behavior and sustaining her efforts to eat well, exercise, and express love toward her husband and children—all activities of great importance to May.

Possible BHC Interventions Concerning Patients Who Somatisize. The case of May illustrates the potential for single BHC interventions to reinforce gains made by somatisizing patients during periods of relatively better functioning. The BHC taught her a skill that furthered her ability to function well with her long-standing pattern of worry. Additionally, the BHC supported the weight control behavior changes she had been making. Subsequent feedback from the PCP indicated that May was reporting significantly fewer periods of dizziness and did not seem as bothered by these symptoms when they did occur.

There are additional possibilities for intervening with patients that somatisize, including those in Table 10.8. With chronically somatisizing patients, it is often best to schedule regular follow-up appointments to reduce anxiety patients may have about being seen in a timely manner should they detect signs of a new medical problem. During periods of high stress, the PCP and BHC may want to see the somatically focused patient in a ping-pong fashion. These patients generally respond well to a biopsychosocial approach and are often open to improving stress management skills. Some patients with somatization may have symptoms of panic, as May did. Diaphragmatic breathing techniques and other relaxation exercises (see for example the CALM Exercise handout on the compact disc in Appendix D)

Table 10.8. Possible BHC interventions concerning patients who somatisize

1.	Encourage a plan of regular, scheduled, brief follow-up visits with the PCP or a series of ping-pong visits with the PCP and BHC.
2.	Explain the stress, coping, and vulnerability model to patient and possibly suggest a series of BHC consultation visits to learn stress reduction techniques.
3.	Clarify values about health and encourage adoption of healthy lifestyle behaviors.
4.	Teach relaxation, mindfulness, and acceptance strategies to help the patient detach from health related worries.
5.	Consider use of cognitive restructuring skill training to help the patient learn to identify and balance distorted interpretations.

are often helpful. Traditional cognitive restructuring strategies have also been used in the treatment of somatization. In this approach, one would list out the negative health related beliefs as examples of cognitive distortions, weigh the evidence pro and con, and then help the patient develop a more balanced interpretation of the physical symptom. In the ACT approach, the same process would trigger the use of mindfulness and acceptance strategies designed to help the patient learn to detach from negative health-related thoughts. Most patients who demonstrate a somatic focus do so because their learning history has reinforced this pattern, as was the case for the patient in this consultation example. The BHC needs to normalize the patient's worry and to express genuine compassion for the patient's experience—in this case the sudden loss of her father. At the same time, the BHC needs to encourage somatisizing patients to make choices about immediate and longer term life directions based upon personal values.

PCP Teaching Points. Some PCPs struggle with these patients, while others work skillfully with them. We've noticed that providers (like Dr. West) that focus on developing a trusting relationship often have the best outcomes. This is why most of the teaching points in Table 10.9 concern ways to develop this type of relationship. These providers tend to understand the patient's perspective and that allows them to help the patient develop a mindful or accepting perspective on the problem. In teaching providers how to do this, we have found that it helps to change the usual spatial configuration of the exam room. If the patient and provider sit side-by-side and look at the problem (in front of them) together, both may be more

Table 10.9. PCP teaching points concerning patients who somatisize

---

1. Encourage PCPs to schedule regular follow-ups with patients and to use a structured approach to monitoring various complaints.
2. Encourage PCPs to sit beside patients rather than across from them to support adoption of a more empathetic and less conflicted view of the patient's concerns.
3. Help PCPs develop ways of explaining that not all symptoms indicate disease and that most symptoms of concern increase with stress. Reinforce the importance of learning stress reduction techniques.
4. Help PCPs express compassion for the patient's on-going vulnerability and see it as an understandable position for the patient to take (given unique his or her personal history).

---

able to let it be there and not let the problem come between them. The PCP is less likely to get into a struggle with the patient who requests additional procedures and specialty consultations that are not warranted by medical findings. Many of the complaints made by somatizing patients cannot be solved or eradicated. However, they can be watched regularly, caringly, and confidently, especially when the patient and provider pursue this collaboratively.

CHEST PAIN (PANIC)

Many primary care patients present with medical complaints (e.g., shortness of breath, chest pain, rapid heart beat, dizziness, numbness or tingling, trembling, excessive sweating, etc.) that may be related to panic attacks rather than a dangerous medical condition. Behavioral treatments for panic are perhaps more effective than behavioral treatments for most conditions and indeed more effective than most medical treatments (Barlow, O'Leary, & Craske, 1992). The case example of Ralph shows the important role the BHC can play early in the course of a developing panic disorder to help suppress the disorder and forestall unnecessary medical tests and procedures.

Ralph: There's something wrong with my heart

Ms. Montemayor, R.N., referred this thirty-one-year-old Dr. Fine patient for a consultation concerning chest pain, shortness of breath, anxiety, and vomiting. In the initial consultation, Ralph described having an episode involving these symptoms, along with shaking and rapid heart beat, a week earlier. During the episode, Ralph feared that he was having a heart attack and sought urgent care. Ralph received a prescription for Lorazapam, and had experienced three similar episodes in the past week even while using the medication. Ralph had missed five days of work since the initial episode. He worked as an insurance agent and usually enjoyed going out with his girlfriend and being active in his church. Current stressors involved his attempts to forgive his mother's shortcomings during his childhood and forge a relationship with her, as well as trying to bring his older brothers into the process of repairing family relationships.

At the initial consultation, the BHC taught him the square breathing technique as a form of mindfulness training. This technique involves instructing the patient to imagine breathing slowly while imagining proceeding around the four sides of a square and counting slowly from one to four during the breath activity for each side. Side one is inhaling deeply; side two is holding the breath; side three is exhaling slowly and completely; side four is again holding the breath. During a practice period, patients should go around the square ten or more times. Ralph was instructed to "just notice" any sensations, thoughts, memories or feelings in a nonjudgmental way during the breathing practice. For psychoeducation, the BHC explained the impact of stress on breathing and the impact of shallow breathing on physiological functioning. The BHC encouraged him to begin a daily exercise program to reduce stress and suggested that he take a vacation from trying to solve his family of origin problems and consider what he might do to build a sociological family in his present community. He agreed to come for follow-up in one week. Figure 10.4 displays Ralph's Duke Health Profile Scores, which suggested significant problems with both physical and mental health at the initial consultation and normal functioning at the follow-up visit.

At the follow-up, Ralph reported that he had practiced the breathing-mindfulness exercise and had started a walking program. He had returned to work full time and had proposed marriage to his girlfriend of twelve months. Ralph had stopped trying to get his brothers to relate to his mother, but had continued his relationship activities with her. He reported no episodes of chest pain or shortness of breath over the prior week. The BHC recommended that he follow-up with Dr. Fine in one month to

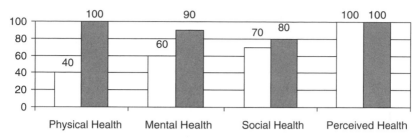

Figure 10.4. Ralph's Initial and Follow-up Function Scale Scores on the Duke Health Profile (Scores range from 0 to 100. On Physical, Mental, Social, and Perceived Health Scales, higher scores indicate better functioning).

discuss his progress with maintaining his walking program, breathing practice, and efforts to develop good family relationships.

Possible BHC Interventions Concerning Chest Pain and Other Symptoms of Panic. Ralph's case example demonstrates the potential helpfulness of early behavioral interventions with patients experiencing symptoms of panic. As a rule of thumb, earlier interventions mean less intensive treatment. Patients with symptoms of panic experience a great deal of relief when given a plausible explanation for their distressing symptoms. It is important for the BHC to take adequate time in providing this information and allow the patient time to ask questions. At times, it is useful to help the patient experience symptoms in the consult visit, as suggested in Table 10.10, so that he or she can use coping strategies while the BHC is available for immediate coaching. The BHC helped Ralph develop a behavior change plan to reduce stress, including starting an exercise program and reducing exposure to stressful family interactions. The BHC will often see these patients for one or two follow-ups, and then plan specific follow-up with the PCP. As with Ralph, it is important that the BHC chart specific recommendations to the PCP concerning the follow-up visit (e.g., I recommend that Dr. Fine support Ralph in continuing his walking program, practicing square breathing, and developing good relationships with his family members). As many of these patients have somewhat sensitive nervous systems, the BHC may help the patient anticipate and plan for future episodes of physical symptoms. Specifically, the BHC might suggest

Table 10.10. Possible BHC interventions concerning chest pain and other symptoms of panic

1. Educate the patient concerning the stress-coping-vulnerability model and the impact of shallow breathing on physiology (see compact disc in Appendix D for handout on Stress Awareness).
2. Teach diaphragmatic breathing instruction and/or mindfulness strategies supported by patient education handouts (See compact disc in Appendix D for handouts on the Calm Exercise, Progressive Muscle Relaxation, and Diaphragmatic Breathing Tips).
3. Expose the patient to symptoms and assist with application of new strategies.
4. Help the patient plan possible solutions to current stressful life circumstances.
5. Anticipate and plan for reoccurrence of panic symptoms.

that the patient intensify exercise, engage in targeted problem solving efforts, share relaxing activities with a good friend, or work with the PCP on these basic coping skills if symptoms become troubling in the future.

PCP Teaching Points for Patients with Chest Pain and Other Symptoms of Panic. Patients like Ralph commonly receive prescriptions for benzodiazepines and a nurse is often the first point of contact. Given this, the BHC would be wise to offer a presentation on diagnosis and treatment of panic to nursing staff, along with the PCPs, as suggested in Table 10.11. PCPs will often prescribe benzodiazepines prior to referring patients with panic to the BHC, but we strongly recommend that the BHC be involved at the time the medicine is prescribed. This strategy can short circuit the tendency of panic patients and prescribing providers to over utilize anxiolytic medicines, which the research shows are contraindicated in the long term treatment of panic. In addition, benzodiazepines have potential for abuse, dependence, and addiction. The BHC needs to assure that PCPs understand the research and that they can distinguish between addiction to and physical dependence on benzodiazepines. Regarding the latter point, patients with substance "abuse" problems use benzodiazepines most often to augment the high received from another drug or to offset the adverse effects of other drugs. Pharmacologic "dependence" is a predictable adaptation of a body system to a drug to which it becomes accustomed, and it may occur in patients taking therapeutic doses of benzodiazepines.

Table 10.11. PCP teaching points concerning patients with symptoms of panic

1. Help nursing staff and PCPs learn about behavioral treatment for symptoms related to panic through presentations at meetings.
2. Encourage PCPs to bring the BHC into the exam room for patients with panic symptoms prior to prescribing any medications, so that a solo behavioral intervention is an option.
3. Teach PCPs to promote lifestyle behaviors (e.g., engaging in daily cardiovascular exercise and relaxation activities) that enhance the patient's ability to prevent future episodes of troubling symptoms.
4. Plan a venue for discussing concerns about addiction, dependence, and rebound issues associated with use of benzodiazepines.

Symptoms of dependence occur with abrupt discontinuation of the medication, and the PCP may control these through dose tapering, medication switching, and/or medication augmentation. Pharmacologic dependence is not the same as "addiction," which is when aberrant behavior related to medication use results in problems for the patient. PCPs also need to understand the phenomenon of rebound, which is different from withdrawal. Rebound is the relative worsening of anxiety/panic symptoms at the point of discontinuation of anxiolytic medicine, regardless of the tapering schedule. When time allows, ask the PCP to remain in the room to observe BHC efforts to educate the patient concerning the stress-coping-vulnerability model, the role of medicines in treatment and core strategies for addressing panic inducing thoughts, sensations, and memories.

PATIENTS WITH CHRONIC CONDITIONS

The pace of primary care makes treatment of chronic medical conditions difficult. Unlike patients with acute conditions, patients with chronic conditions need to develop strong relationships with their PCPs to succeed in making changes to multiple self-management behaviors. While the addition of BHC services can enhance outcomes for this large and growing group, changes in the way medical care is delivered to this group are also needed. Patients with chronic medical conditions can benefit from a set of new approaches often referred to as chronic disease management programs, which include such strategies as the use of registries and the provision of services in group medical appointments (See Chapter 12). However, the first step with this group of patients is to engage them in the process of self-management of their medical condition. The case example of Patty demonstrates the important role the BHC can play in fostering this engagement.

Patty: I'm gaining weight, and my health just isn't very good

Dr. Forester referred this fifty-four-year-old married mother for a consultation concerning weight gain and diabetes. Patty had lived with diabetes for twenty-nine years, and her current level of control was generally good. However, Duke Health Profile Scores at the initial consult suggested she perceived her physical and mental health to be poor. A functional analysis suggested that Patty began overeating about a year prior to the consult when she left her job as a nursing assistant. She was forced to leave because of on-going vision problems related to diabetic complications. Patty had gained eighty pounds since leaving her job. A surgery on her eyes had been successful, and she could return to work if she lost weight. She had started controlling portion size, but was not exercising due to back pain and a sore on her foot. In the past she had lost a great deal of weight on three different occasions but always seemed to gain it back over time.

The BHC targeted Patty's motivation for change. She wanted help with developing a weight loss program. She had the requisite skills for making dietary changes but wanted to focus on starting an exercise program. The BHC asked Patty what would be different in her life if she lost weight, and she indicated that she would go back to work and would have a social life again. Patty agreed to a plan calling for her to walk to and from the mail box five to ten times daily and to invite her friends over to play cards with her two or three times per week. Patty returned two weeks later, and her Duke Scores suggested improvement in Social Health, which was the goal. She beamed when the BHC shared this good news with her, and she indicated that she was walking more, her foot sore was healing, and she was playing cards on a regular basis. The follow-up plan included having Patty maintain her dietary, exercise and social activities, and quarterly check-ins with the BHC for strategic adjustments to her plan. The PCP was advised to actively query Patty about these three behavior change goals at each diabetes exam and to reinforce their important role in her long term management of the disease.

BHC Interventions. The consultation with Patty demonstrates the potential for a BHC to fine tune programs started by the patient and PCP by further engaging the patient in the process of behavior change. The BHC helped Patty focus on her long-term goals of working and seeing her friends more often, and this perspective helped to dignify the process of losing weight. Her success in implementing the plan to increase social activities probably enhanced her sense of self-efficacy for other behavior changes. The BHC also offered to remain in contact with Patty as an auxiliary care team member focusing on maintaining behavior change. The BHC can be available for quarterly check-ins when a clinic does not have programs such as registries and/or group visits for patients with chronic diseases. Table 10.12 summarizes interventions BHCs may offer to patients like Patty who are struggling to live well with chronic conditions.

Patients with chronic conditions often experience discouragement and symptoms of depression, along with medical problems. The BHC can help the patient generate hope for a better future by taking a specific step that is feasible and that fits with their world view. Factors listed in Table 10.13 are important to the process of engagement needed to improve outcomes for patients living with chronic conditions. Patty believed she could lose weight, and she needed a medical provider to affirm this ability and help her continue in the direction she had already started. She needed problem solving and affirmation, not information and not admonition. The BHC took the role of being a player on the patient's team rather than a coach giving instructions, and the BHC suggested this perspective to the PCP. This is not an easy thing to do, as most providers experience a certain level

Table 10.12. Possible BHC interventions for patients living with chronic conditions

1.	Use value-based behavior change and motivational interviewing strategies.
2.	Focus on small, specific behavior change goals to help build self-efficacy for making more widespread behavior changes.
3.	Employ a team-member versus coach perspective.
4.	Offer quarterly consults (particularly when registry and/or group visit services are not available at the clinic).
5.	Promote development of registries and group care clinics.

Table 10.13. Engaging patients living with chronic conditions

1. Explore and validate patient reactions and expectations (desired service, belief about what PCP has to offer).
2. Form a working alliance using the collaborative set (e.g., "We are facing this together; what can we do to improve your sense of health?")
3. Encourage attendance at all medical appointments (classes and other formats).
4. Obtain on-going assessment of patient satisfaction with medical care.

of irritation with patients who, in the past, have failed to follow medical advice concerning strategies for coping with chronic conditions.

BHCs can also help patients living with chronic conditions by supporting system changes that promote on-going collaboration between patients and providers. These might include the development of registries and related "tickler" systems that trigger appropriate follow-up with patients, whether by phone or mail, or through in-person visits with providers. Group medical appointments (see Chapter 12) can be used to provide medical/behavioral care to a group of patients that share some similarity, such as having diabetes or having multiple health problems and being over the age of seventy. These programs address elements critical to engaging patients in self-care, including making on-going support available and addressing patient expectations in a respectful manner. In fact, many patients living with chronic conditions prefer a group appointment because of the longer appointment time and opportunity to receive social support and advice from other patients with the same type of problem.

PCP Teaching Points. The BHC can empower the PCP to work with this large group of patients by helping the PCP to experience frustration with this group while acting in ways that are consistent with promoting health. It is not easy to believe that a patient who has coped poorly with diabetes for ten years can change at any moment, yet this may be a prerequisite for helping some patients change. As suggested in Table 10.14, the BHC may consider developing a series of lunch hour workshops describing strategies from Acceptance and Commitment Therapy and exercises for empowering acceptance and committed action with even the most frustrating patients. Additionally, the BHC may teach PCPs to use health-related

Table 10.14. PCP teaching points concerning patients living with chronic conditions

1. Help PCPs to allow feelings of frustration in response to patients who struggle with self-management, while acting in ways that promote behavioral change (i.e., expressing confidence in the patient's ability to change).
2. Suggest PCPs experiment with use of behavioral prescription pads (e.g., see Figure 10.3) to plan self-management goals with patients.
3. Teach PCPs to use health-related quality of life as the principal disease management outcome and to tie this goal to motivational interviewing strategies.
4. Encourage PCPs to experiment with newer formats for delivering medical care to patients with chronic diseases (e.g., group visits and/or registries).

quality of life measures and motivational interviewing (MI) strategies with this group of patients. (See Burke, Arkowitz, & Menchola, 2003 for evidence concerning MI.) Providing PCPs with information about group medical appointments and registries may also be helpful, as these approaches may help relieve the burden of care on PCPs while improving patient satisfaction overall.

LEARNING DISABILITIES

Numerous adults function with impairments stemming from learning disabilities and ADHD. In some cases, these disabilities may not have been diagnosed in childhood, and, in others, they will have been. Either way, it is important that the PCP know that a patient has this type of impairment, so that the process of providing medical care can be adapted to fit the individual's limitations. Penny's case example demonstrates how the BHC can help PCPs improve outcomes for this sizeable group of adults.

Penny: I am scared to death of losing my job

Dr. Monroe referred this sixty-year-old married mother for a consultation concerning dizziness, fatigue, and chest pain. He had prescribed atenolol and, while this was helpful, it made her feel sleepy. She was married with adult children living out of the house and was working full time.

At the initial consultation, Penny's Duke Health Profile Scores suggested poor physical and mental health. A functional analysis of her symptoms suggested that these developed in the context of increasing problems at her job and conflicts with her two adult children. Penny explained that she had a learning disability, and that she was being required to change from her familiar job on an assembly line to working as a shipping clerk. She worried that she would be unable to keep her figures straight and that it wouldn't be long until she had trouble with the "big cheese." Penny liked the idea of the BHC writing a letter to her employer recommending that she remain in her current position.

The BHC also taught Penny a breathing exercise named the Courage Breath to help her manage job and family stress better. The Courage Breath involves teaching diaphragmatic breathing and then helping the patient to integrate an inhalation and exhalation with three movements of the shoulders. The first is that of lifting the shoulders toward the ears on the inhalation; the second is bringing the shoulders back (squeezing the shoulder blades together) on the exhalation, and the third is bringing the shoulders down as the exhalation is completed. This exercise opens the chest so that diaphragmatic breathing can occur more easily. This exercise can be taught quickly, and it is particularly useful for a person who breathes in a shallow manner and who is currently struggling with an interpersonal situation that requires him or her to be courageous. Model this exercise and then provide feedback after watching the patient. Most often, patients find this exercise relaxing and their facial expressions become more pleasant. When this happens, it is helpful to point this out to the patient and ask how he or she thinks this might affect the way that people respond to him or her. The BHC recommended that Penny practice this exercise on an hourly basis for several breathing cycles and routinely prior to a planned entry into interpersonally challenging situations.

When Penny returned, her Duke Scores suggested improvements in Mental and Social Health. She had practiced the Courage Breath exercise and had cut her atenolol dosage. She was pleased with this, as she was no longer sleepy from the atenolol and enjoyed her work day more. Her employer had agreed to allow her to continue in her present position for the time being. While she no longer had problems with dizziness, she noted that she still had some problems with fatigue. The BHC provided information about the impact of exercise on energy, and Penny indicated that she would like to resume walking during her lunch hour to see if this improved her energy in the afternoons. The BHC also provided her with information about the Americans with Disabilities Act.

BHC Interventions for Patients with Learning Disabilities. Penny's case illustrates how patients with learning disabilities and other impairments such as ADHD may have more difficulties adapting to changes in both their work and home situations. When these patients are referred, the BHC often needs to help the patient acquire new coping skills. Skills may focus specifically on coping with the learning disability (e.g., a plan for developing cashier skills) and/or reducing the stress and anxiety associated with a specific situation. Interventions may also address development of general self-care skills and healthy lifestyle behaviors. Penny's request for a letter is not unusual. BHCs often receive these types of requests, as this is a service that PCPs often provide. We both routinely write letters for patients during a visit. This is often helpful to the patient, and it only requires a few minutes of BHC time. Lastly, patients with disabilities may not know their rights, and the BHC may provide useful information about this, as suggested in Table 10.15.

PCP Teaching Points Concerning Patients with Learning Disabilities. As suggested in Table 10.16, the BHC can teach PCPs to ask new patients about their education and to follow-up on any indication of problems with questions such as, "Did you attend special classes?" This only takes seconds, and it can help the PCP adjust his or her care to accommodate the patient's disability. For example, a patient with a learning disability may benefit from having all instructions written rather than only spoken. It is also helpful for the BHC to stock copies of screeners that PCPs can use in diagnosing common problems such as ADHD (see for example the ADHD Symptom Checklist Adult Version—Self Report and the ADHD Symptom Checklist Adult Version—Observer Report, both of which are easily accessed and free on the Internet). As these types of disabilities may predispose patients to more stress in adulthood, the PCP also needs to make an effort to develop a working relationship that encourages more frequent contact (perhaps with the BHC as well as the PCP), particularly when life stresses challenge the patient's coping skills.

Table 10.15. BHC interventions for patients with learning disabilities

1. Support appropriate adaptations required to ensure continued employment by writing a letter if needed or requested.
2. Teach problem solving, particularly regarding relationship issues.
3. Provide resource information (e.g., Americans with Disabilities Act, programs offering assistance with development of personal financial management skills).
4. BHC consultation services in series of one to three visits every three to five years may improve outcomes for this relatively large group.

Table 10.16. PCP teaching points concerning patients with learning disabilities

1. Suggest that PCPs routinely ask new patients about their education.
2. Encourage PCPs to provide a regular pattern of more frequent visits over time to promote better risk monitoring.
3. Let PCPs know that the BHC can provide patients with information about the Americans with Disabilities Act.

SYMPTOMS OF DEPRESSION AND TRAUMATIC STRESS

Many PCPs practice under the assumption that depression, and to some extent traumatic stress, is a biological condition that requires medication to suppress various symptoms, such as fatigue, sadness, sleep disturbance, loss of appetite, etc. Many patients with symptoms of depression and secondary trauma report numerous psychosocial problems which may in fact be "driving" the symptoms. Simply prescribing medicines to suppress symptoms is an empty exercise, if the underlying psychosocial concerns are not adequately addressed. When the medication is withdrawn in such situations, the patient is at high risk for relapse. Leslie's case example demonstrates the impact the BHC can have on sorting out what needs to be suppressed, accepted, and changed and, in so doing, broaden the PCP perspective on treating traumatized and depressed patients.

Leslie: I can't stop myself from thinking about it, and I'm so tired ...

Dr. Mason referred this twenty-five-year-old married mother of one for a consultation concerning fatigue, loss of appetite, sleep disturbance, and flashbacks. Leslie was six months pregnant with her second child, and her rate of weight gain was slower than expected. Her Duke Scores at the initial visit suggested poor physical and mental health. In the functional analysis, the BHC learned that Leslie's symptoms had started several months prior when she attended her father's trial concerning sexual molestation of a child. This experience had triggered painful memories about abuse Leslie experienced from her father as a child. She was disgusted by these memories, avoided anything that brought them up for her, and still was plagued by gnawing details that even woke her from sleep. Leslie had withdrawn from her husband (described as a nice guy that didn't know about her father) and couldn't even tolerate his effort to hold her hand. Leslie's childhood had been traumatic in other ways. For example, she had lived in several foster homes before being returned to her mother's home in late adolescence. As an adult, Leslie worked as a child welfare advocate, and this was the light in her life at the time of the consult. At work, she felt competent, and she enjoyed the forty-five-minute walk that she took at lunch.

The BHC acknowledged Leslie's strengths (e.g., a career focused on promoting child safety and health, a pattern of regular exercise, the ability to pull back when she needed to) and normalized the experience of intrusive images. The BHC explained that the patient's mind "… was trying to make sure she remembered.…" and that the best way to help one's mind when it is caught in a repetitive loop is to allow it to spin rather than to try to stop the thoughts and feelings. The BHC suggested she focus on the thoughts, feelings, and bodily sensations triggered by memories of the sexual abuse during the first five or ten minutes of her daily walk before turning on her CD player, as was her habit. Leslie agreed to consider this and to ask her husband to stop initiating touch with her for two weeks. She would explain to him that she needed to pull back to work on personal issues and that she wanted to be the only one to initiate any touching for the next two weeks. Leslie agreed to bring her husband to the planned follow-up consultation in two weeks, if he was willing and if it made sense to her for him to come.

At follow-up, Leslie's Mental Health score on the Duke had improved significantly, and her Physical Health score had also moved in the desired direction. Leslie reported that she had talked with her husband about her memories and the distress they caused her. His response was caring and supportive beyond what she could have imagined. While he was very angry with her father, he was kind and considerate to Leslie. She began to initiate touch with him after the talk, and she subsequently felt calm when he took her hand and comforted when he held her in bed. She had not focused on thoughts of the abuse during her walks, but reported that they were less troubling for her anyway. The BHC suggested writing in a journal as a possible strategy for becoming less sensitized to the content of intrusive thoughts and images. Leslie responded very positively to this suggestion. The BHC described sensate focus exercises to Leslie, and she planned to talk with her husband about these. She planned to see Dr. Mason for her prenatal check-up in two weeks. If she was not continuing to improve, she agreed to stop by to see the BHC while in the clinic for that visit. Leslie did not return for follow-up with the BHC. Feedback from Dr. Mason revealed that Leslie was continuing to improve and that weight gain was now occurring at a normal rate.

BHC Interventions for Patients with Symptoms of Depression and Traumatic Stress. The BHC identified Leslie's strengths and helped her redirect her control efforts from thoughts and feelings to her actions (walking) and interactions (talking with her husband). As indicated in Table 10.17, behavior change plans of this type are basic interventions, and the BHC may use a variety of patient education materials for support. At follow-up, the BHC planted the idea that intrusive thoughts and feelings might return in the future and suggested a strategy for Leslie to use if such did occur. With Leslie, the BHC also offered to work with her husband, and this offer may have felt helpful, even though it did not occur. Marital dissatisfaction is common among depressed women. In fact, it is the single factor that best predicts relapse of depression symptoms in women.

A variety of interventions are helpful to patients with fatigue, sleep problems, concentration problems, sadness, and anxiety, and the BHC's job is to match the intervention to the results of the functional analysis. Often, the BHC consulting with a patient with multiple symptoms of depression will use behavioral activation strategies. With more anxious patients, the BHC may lean toward interventions involving relaxation training and exposure. Most patients benefit from instruction in problem-solving, and many will agree to bring a family member to a consult when the BHC suggests this. Generic classes that aim to improve skills for reducing stress and improve quality of life can provide a means for more to intensive skill training for this group. (See Chapter 12 for a discussion

Table 10.17. Possible BHC interventions for patients with symptoms of depression and traumatic stress

1. Identify patient strengths (at present; at time of a past trauma) and activities or times of the day when the patient feels best.
2. Teach the patient to be present in the moment and to choose to engage in activities that promote desired affective states (e.g., feeling calm, content).
3. Direct the patient to focus on controlling events to external (e.g., going for a walk, calling a friend) rather than internal events (e.g., avoiding recall of traumatic experiences, suppressing depressing thoughts).
4. Use patient education materials to support behavior change (e.g., the Change Plan Worksheet on the compact disc in Appendix D).
5. Suggest planned exposure to avoided thoughts and feelings as an option (but don't require it).
6. Address specific symptoms that trouble patient, such as sleep, using patient education handouts (e.g., Beating Insomnia and/or Healthy Sleeping Tips on compact disc in Appendix D).
7. Offer to include members of the patient's family in the behavior change process.
8. Use behavioral activation strategies to help reverse patterns of lethargy and isolation.
9. Develop and place a relapse prevention plan in the medical chart. Recommend that the PCP support the patient in implementing the plan for at least six to twelve months after remission in symptoms.
10. Offer a drop-in class series supported by materials, such as *Living Life Well: New Strategies for Hard Times* (Robinson, 1996).
11. Suggest community resources (e.g., group programs based on leisure activities, exercise, or spirituality).

of generic classes.) We encourage BHCs to think about prevention opportunities and to encourage PCPs to refer patients to the BHC for relapse prevention planning. Books listed in Appendix C contain useful material for BHCs concerning intervention development for this large group of primary care patients.

PCP Teaching Points for Patients with Symptoms of Depression and Traumatic Stress. The BHC can improve diagnosis and treatment of patients with symptoms of depression and traumatic stress by encouraging PCPs to take a biopsychosocial approach and use behavioral interventions as the foundation for treatment, as suggested in Table 10.18. PCPs struggle with employing the DSM system for many reasons, including the reality that the rule-out process often requires more time than a PCP has

Table 10.18. PCP teaching points for patients with symptoms of depression and traumatic stress

1. Teach PCPs to educate patients in the biopsychosocial model of depression and traumatic stress and to employ the "watchful waiting" strategy.
2. Encourage PCPs to curb urges to diagnose "illness" and instead use available time to identify specific stressors and encourage use of coping resources.
3. Teach PCPs to identify symptoms of anxiety and depression that trouble the patient and/or interfere with functioning and to state these (rather than a diagnosis) as the reason(s) for referring to the BHC.
4. Teach PCPs to conduct efficient values assessments (e.g., if asking, "What is important to you in terms of being a wife?" and perhaps hearing, "Good communication."), and to help plan activities that are consistent with stated values (eg., taking a 20-minute talking-walk with husband every day).
5. Teach PCPs to use objective information to decide whether to start a medication (thus creating a baseline against which to measure treatment response).
6. Teach PCPs to refer improved patients to the BHC for development of a relapse prevention plan one month prior to the start of a taper from antidepressant medication.
7. Teach PCPs to develop and support relapse prevention plans, particularly for patients with recurrent problems with depression and anxiety.

for an entire visit. In an effort to provide psychiatric services, PCPs may resort to catch-all diagnoses, like "depression" and "anxiety." The busy PCP can make this type of diagnosis and start a treatment (usually pharmacological) in less than ten minutes. However, this very approach leads to many unnecessary medication starts and stops, as about half of all patients prescribed antidepressants stop the medicine within the first month. This is often because treatment does not match well with the problem. One of us (PR) participated in two large clinical trials where PCPs were asked to identify and refer patients with probable major depression who were willing to take an antidepressant. When the research assistant conducted follow-up structured psychiatric interviews with referred patients, only 50 percent met criteria for major depression. These findings suggest that half of the patients PCPs diagnose with major depression actually have subthreshold conditions that most likely would respond to brief behavioral interventions.

An alternative to this costly approach to diagnosis and treatment involves the BHC teaching PCPs to use a "watchful waiting" strategy for patients reporting less severe depression and anxiety symptoms. The PCP can refer these patients to the BHC for assessment and a targeted behavioral intervention to improve one or more specific troubling symptoms (e.g., poor sleep, flashbacks, fatigue, etc.). The patient can come for follow-up with the BHC (or PCP) within the next month for evaluation of progress. We both use the PHQ-9 (as a supplement to the Duke Health Profile) to assist PCPs with implementing the "watchful waiting" strategy (See Chapter 6 for more information on the PHQ-9). Patients who are not improving and/or are experiencing more difficulties with functioning at the one-month follow-up might then be candidates for a combination of medicine and behavioral intervention. This strategy is consistent with a biopsychosocial approach to treatment of depression, anxiety, and traumatic stress, where the basic treatment is behavioral and medication plays a specific, time limited role in controlling symptoms that are interfering with the more basic goal of behavior change.

Introducing the idea of "watchful waiting" provides an opportunity for the BHC to teach PCPs to practice the biopsychosocial model. (See Robinson, Wischman, & Del Vento, 1996, for patient education materials that support this.) BHCs may encourage PCPs to forgo efforts to make a definitive psychiatric diagnosis, and instead to identify target symptoms (e.g., fatigue, poor sleep, weight gain, chest pain, etc.) or skill deficits (e.g., stress-reduction, self-management of diseases, etc.) that will be further assessed and targeted by the BHC. The BHC should also develop a battery of specific outcome indicators (e.g., health related quality of life, PHQ-9 total score and impairment score) that will be used to plan and evaluate the effects of treatment.

PCPs need to encourage a holistic approach to care for these patients and to involve the BHC as an auxiliary provider. Many PCPs were trained in the biomedical model and view depression as an illness rather than the result of an habitual and ineffective way of responding to life challenges. The BHC can help PCPs practice the depression management skills listed in Table 10.17, including development of relapse prevention plans. A relapse prevention plan usually includes: (1) identification of a way the patient will assess his or her own functioning on an on-going basis (usually weekly), (2) a plan for maintaining gains made in a series of consultations visits (such as exercising thirty minutes daily, engaging in two social activities weekly, eating breakfast), and (3) a plan for accessing support (such as a visit with the PCP or BHC) if planned assessment indicates a drop in functioning on two consecutive weeks.

SUICIDAL IDEATION

Most people who commit suicide make a visit to a primary care clinic within months of dying, and often within days. Men with medical problems, particularly when they have no wife, and adolescents, particularly males who are using alcohol and have been rejected by a girlfriend, are probably among the most at risk for completed suicides among primary care patients. Jose's case example shows how patients frequently reveal thoughts of suicide to a PCP just prior to an attempt and the role the BHC can play in helping the patient and PCP, as well as the entire clinic.

Jose's Wife: He wants to kill himself

P.A. Avondale referred this forty-two-year-old, Hispanic man for a consultation concerning thoughts of suicide. Jose's wife brought him to the clinic requesting help after he told her that he wanted to die so badly that he thought he shouldn't even go into the kitchen because he might stab himself. Jose had seen P.A. Avondale one week prior, and he had received a prescription for a SSRI at that visit.

At the initial BHC assessment, Jose's Duke Scores suggested mild depression and concerns about his physical health (i.e., a score of fifty on the Perceived Health Scale). He explained that his thoughts of suicide had started about ten days prior when he was diagnosed with diabetes. As recommended, Jose was checking his blood sugar, making dietary changes, and attempting to exercise more. He cried as he explained that he was unable to keep thoughts of suicide out of his mind, and what was even more disturbing was that these thoughts were getting more and more frequent and compelling. He felt overwhelmed by worries about his ability to care for his wife and their children. He felt that he had failed his family by having failed to maintain good health. Jose explained that he had always worked in the fields and worried he would not be able to continue. Other stresses included the recent loss of his father who had suffered from numerous health problems. Jose loved music and found prayer helpful. He denied using alcohol or drugs.

The BHC explained to Jose that the more we try to stop ourselves from thinking of something (e.g., a red apple) or feeling something (e.g., fear or sadness about having a chronic disease), the more we tend to have the avoided thought or feeling. The BHC used an ACT technique by extending her arms to depict an imaginary time line going from birth (the left hand) to death (the right hand). She asked Jose to point to the place where he thought he was at that moment on the time line. He said he wasn't sure, but thought he might be close to death. She explained that being diagnosed with a chronic disease requires a person to be courageous and to look at that time line multiple times throughout the day. Further, she explained that it is by developing the courage to look at the time line four or five times a day (and feel the fear and sadness, etc.) that the person with a chronic disease is most able to make decisions that support health. Many people don't want to feel bad and don't look at the line. Then, they have trouble staying aware of the choices that would help them live longer with better health. The BHC also suggested the following metaphor to Jose (another ACT technique).

"Imagine that there is a pot of beans cooking on the stove, and the temperature is a little high. The beans start boiling and there's quite a bit of steam. Let's say you don't like steam, so you put a lid on the pot. What happens? Right, the steam builds up and soon you have a mess on the stove and you probably like that even less than the steam. Well, you could still put the lid back on, but then you'd probably soon have a bigger mess on the stove and perhaps a burned pan as well. If you really don't like steam though, you have to find a way to live with it so that you can leave the lid off (who knows— the heat could die down!). That's what I want you to try with your thoughts of suicide and your fears about not being able to take care of your family. Keep the lid off of your mind and let them bubble up. Notice when you start to put the lid on, try to take a slow deep breath and remember that painful thoughts, like steam, tend to come and go (unless you try to control it by putting the lid on)."

As a final ACT intervention, the BHC suggested that Jose take daily walks at a moderate pace with his wife and talk about his values concerning their relationship. Jose agreed to return for follow-up in one week and to call the clinic or the twenty-four-hour crisis line number should he become worried about acting on his thoughts of suicide.

At follow-up two weeks later, Jose's Duke Scores suggested a high level of health-related quality of life. He was walking with his wife almost daily, and his children were joining them on walks some of the time. His family enjoyed talking about their values, and they all wanted to help him look at his personal time line and make good choices. He was using the timeline metaphor at daily choice points related to his diabetes and the pot of beans metaphor to help him look at his uncomfortable thoughts and feelings. He proudly reported that he had taught these skills to his mother, who was also diabetic and who had originally encouraged him to "just not think" about his new diagnosis. At work, he was singing and talking with others and even felt comfortable eating his new food selections with his co-workers. He had accepted an invitation to dinner at a friend's house and brought food for himself, but was pleasantly surprised to find that the friend had anticipated his needs. He agreed to follow-up with his P.A. and to return for an additional BHC consultation if needed in the future.

Possible BHC Interventions with Suicidal Ideation. The consultation with Jose and his wife provides a good example of a patient overwhelmed by a new diagnosis of a chronic disease. While it is difficult to predict which patients might be so disturbed as to consider suicide as an alternative to living with a disease, the proportion of patients who become highly distressed is significant. Rarely does anyone in primary care see a patient who has made up his or her mind to complete suicide. Most patients who seek care are ambivalent about dying and troubled by problems for which they see no solution. Most often, thoughts of suicide function as a form of avoidance-based problem solving behavior. In a functional analysis of suicidal thoughts, the BHC can quickly come to understand when the thoughts started, what happens just before and after they occur, etc. Other questions can help establish level of risk (e.g., use of drugs and alcohol, availability of fire arms, etc.). Armed with this information, the BHC will often be able to help the suicidal patient formulate a plan to approach the problem that provoked the suicidal thoughts. In the case of Jose, the problem was fearing that he would fail to meet his responsibilities as a father and husband if he had diabetes. In a brief intervention, he came to see that it was not an either/or (either good health and good provider for family or bad health and inadequate provider) situation.

When unsure about safety issues, the BHC can shorten the return visit to as little as a day if need be. In addition, the BHC can coordinate the safety plan with the PCP and assume a more central role in care of the patient. If in need of hospitalization, some counties will be able to send a mental health professional to the clinic to assist with transportation, while others prefer that transportation be arranged through 9-1-1 services. The resources and methods for accessing these services vary from state to state and often from county to county within a state, and the BHC needs to be aware of back-up transportation options as well.

Consistent with possible interventions listed in Table 10.19, the BHC assessed the level of risk for Jose, focused on completing a functional analysis of the suicidal thoughts, developed a coping plan for suicidal thoughts and developed a behavior change plan consistent with remaining alive and successfully managing diabetes.

PCP Teaching Points Concerning Patients with Thoughts of Suicide. When a patient expresses suicidal ideation, the PCP must invariably slow down the patient flow to address the crisis. The BHC needs to let PCPs know of his or her ability to help with this type of situation so that the PCP's schedule is not overwhelmed. However, the BHC's schedule also

Table 10.19. BHC interventions for patients with thoughts of suicide

1. Assess level of risk and arrange transport to an inpatient facility if needed.
2. Conduct a functional analysis of the suicidal thoughts with particular emphasis on their emotional avoidance problem solving function (i.e., "What problems would you solve if you in fact killed yourself? How effective do you think suicide would be here as a way of solving these problems?").
3. Ask the patient what keeps him or her from acting on suicidal thoughts (this will often promote talk about what the patient values, e.g., children, religious convictions, belief in the ability to always find a solution) and rein-force this as a significant deterrent.
4. Address the problem(s) that the patient has been unable to solve and which he or she wants to avoid (through suicide) with skill-training and a specific plan.
5. Come down on the side of life in interactions and focus on behavior changes that implicitly affirm being alive.

needs to remains accessible, as it is easy to spend an entire morning or afternoon placing an acutely suicidal patient in the appropriate community program. Ensure the clinic has a strong triage plan for addressing emergencies, as this may sometimes help both PCP and BHC avoid being overwhelmed. (We discuss this at length in Chapter 13).

While many PCPs will be comfortable with using BHC services in suicidal emergencies, an occasional provider may think that a psychiatric opinion is needed. This may be problematic, as psychiatric services are usually difficult to access. If encountering this, to take the provider to lunch (after the emergency!) to explore his or her thinking and to provide assurance of one's ability to address the needs of a suicidal patient.

PCPs may also benefit from specific training on the issue of suicidal behavior, so that it is "demystified." The current cognitive and behavioral models of suicidal behavior provide a much more operable framework for addressing suicidal behavior, rather than treating it as a symptom of mental illness (see Chiles & Strosahl, 2005 for more information). Additional training may teach questions to help highlight patient's beliefs and values that are inconsistent with suicide or to reveal problem solving strategies that don't require killing oneself, as suggested in Table 10.20. The reading list in Appendix C includes our favorite resource book on suicidal behavior (Chiles & Strosahl, 2005), and we recommend in particular the chapter by Robinson (2005) concerning the relative risk status of patients who have lost loved ones to suicide, as this group is large relative to the number of patients who complete suicide and is a good target for preventive efforts.

DRUG AND ALCOHOL PROBLEMS

Drug and alcohol problems are generally under recognized and under treated in primary care settings. Patients with substance problems, particularly those with chronic problems, are among the least liked patients in primary care. While this is not surprising, it is regrettable because there are now a variety of effective, brief alcohol and drug abuse screening tools for primary care use. In addition, studies have consistently found that brief interventions delivered by primary care providers have a significant impact on subsequent alcohol and drug abuse patterns in primary care patients. While there is tremendous potential for helping

Table 10.20. PCP teaching points concerning patients with thoughts of suicide

1. Involve PCPs in reviewing and revising, if needed, the clinic triage plan for psychiatric emergencies.
2. Encourage PCPs to save their schedules by involving the BHC early in a visit with a suicidal patient.
3. Teach PCPs to use the BHC to assess risk level and develop appropriate plans.
4. Teach PCPs to recognize that most people do not want to die, but simply face problems that overwhelm them and that asking questions that shift the focus to these problems may be helpful (e.g., "What problem, if solved or even somewhat solved, would tip the balance toward your wanting to live?").
5. Teach PCPs that few patients attempt suicide while many have thoughts about it.
6. Teach PCPs to implement a problem solving, value based approach to suicidal behavior, rather than a "mental illness" approach.
7. Present information on the prevalence of survivors of suicide (meaning primary care patients who have lost a loved one to suicide) in primary care and explain their health risks (e.g., problems with intimacy, mood, and apprehension; under-achievement in relation to life goals).

patients in the initial stages of problematic use, the BHC is also likely to receive referrals for many patients whose lives were derailed by substance abuse long ago. These range from the young pregnant woman who is trying to stay free of methamphetamine while pregnant to the older marijuana-abusing man with multiple health and psychosocial problems. The case example of Ed demonstrates ways the BHC can help strengthen a substance dependence patient's commitment to health and active participation in health care.

Ed: I haven't had anything to drink in two weeks, and it's kind of hard

P.A. Jones referred this forty-two-year-old, Native American man for consultation to reduce or stop drug and alcohol abuse and to find stable housing. The patient had a long history of alcohol and drug abuse and had recently been released from jail. He had come to the clinic as a new patient, seeking treatment for a serious burn on his hand. The patient reported numerous chronic health conditions and his P.A. was attempting to obtain records and start medications as needed. The patient had been hit by a car several years ago, resulting in serious facial injuries and loss of vision in one eye.

At the initial consult, Ed's Duke Scores suggested some problems with physical health and social health, while mental health was a relative strength. When the BHC explored health issues, he explained that he had a plate and screws in his head and similar orthopedic hardware in his arm and shoulder. He had not used drugs or alcohol for two weeks, as he had been in jail. He wanted to continue to be straight and sober now that he was out and living temporarily with his brother. In the past, he had bene-fited from attending AA meetings in another city. He had no way to get to local AA meetings, but agreed that this would be helpful. Winter holidays were approaching, and he felt like he might relapse because his favorite recreational activity was partying, and he didn't know much about party-ing without using psychoactive substances to excess.

The BHC used the ACT Bull's Eye prescription pad (see Figure 10.3) with Ed, taught him an exercise to help him be mindful of urges to use, and provided him with resource information. As an additional ACT interven-tion, the BHC asked Ed about his values concerning love, and he said he wanted to be a playful person who was liked by his nieces and nephews and who could stay out of trouble. He was proud when he told the children tra-ditional Native American stories and taught them the traditional ways. In the past, he had been one of the best huckleberry pickers in his family. When asked to make an X on the bull's eye in terms of how close his activi-ties of the past week came to the bull's eye of being the playful uncle and teacher of tradition, Ed made a mark outside the target. The BHC helped him make a plan to bring his behavior closer to his values over the next week. Specifically, Ed planned to avoid drugs and alcohol and to tell a story every night to his brother's children.

The BHC told Ed about the WAVE metaphor (Marlatt, 2001), which is demonstrated in the following passage:

"Ed, I want you to think about the ocean shore and to imagine that you have become a surfer. A surfer has a board and watches the waves. In fact, a good surfer usually watches the ocean for fifteen minutes before going in. That is because surfers can't see currents under the surface that affect wave patterns; they just need to wait and watch for waves to emerge. Now, Ed, think for a moment about waves at the ocean. What's true about every wave? … Right, they start out there somewhere and they end at the shore. So, now tell me how waves differ? Right, some are small, some medium, some large. I want you to spend some time everyday thinking about urges as waves; notice the difference between one urge and another. Remember your board because it's what helps you watch or ride the surf. And, Ed, do you think a surfer would ever go out and start to swat the waves with his board? No, probably not, because he'd just get pulled under. A board is for riding the waves, watching the urges. Good luck, Ed, be a surfer."

The BHC also provided Ed with information about resources in the community, including a number for a sponsor who could possibly provide transportation to meetings, and other numbers concerning both dry and wet (i.e., alcohol permitted) housing. Finally, the BHC explained to Ed that the clinic was taking a team approach and that she would be a member of the team of people trying to help him get closer to the Bull's Eye.

Possible BHC Interventions with Patients with Drug and Alcohol Problems. Ed's case illustrates many of the possible interventions listed in Table 10.21 that a BHC can provide to patients with drug and alcohol problems. The BHC helped Ed develop a plan that increased his sense of purpose and meaning. Use of the behavioral prescription pad resulted in a written copy of the plan, which is very helpful to patients with concentration and forgetfulness problems, such as those withdrawing from drugs and alcohol. The

Table 10.21. BHC intervention possibilities for adult patients with drug and alcohol problems

1. Assess readiness for change and provide a brief intervention that matches the patient's level of readiness.
2. Provide the patient with a written copy of the plan that results from the visit.
3. Look for interventions that increase the patient's greater sense of meaning and social support base.
4. Maintain current information about resources (Alcoholics Anonymous, Narcotics Anonymous, and Moderation Management meeting schedules, housing resources, etc.).
5. Schedule follow-up with PCP and emphasize availability of same-day service from BHC.

metaphor gave Ed a tool to use in his attempts to cope with urges to drink. The BHC also provided a toll-free number that Ed could dial from a pay phone to find a sponsor, as well as numbers for emergency housing.

With patients just entering into risky drinking patterns, brief interventions can be very helpful. To improve detection of these patients, passive screening activities, such as exam room posters, may be helpful. Standardized screening tools such as those reviewed in Chapter 6 may also be effective.

PCP Teaching Points Concerning Patients with Drug and Alcohol Problems. While more and more PCPs are learning the basics of motivational interviewing and brief interventions, stigma may continue to be a barrier to successful intervention with patients with drug and alcohol problems. It is probably painful for many, if not most, PCPs to witness the long-term impact of excessive consumption of alcohol on the human being, as it is harmful to all organ systems. PCPs have committed themselves to improving health, and witnessing the destruction of the human body associated with use of unprescribed, unregulated, and sometimes illegally obtained substances can easily pull forth a sense of indignation and disgust. On more than one occasion, we have heard PCPs make statements, such as, "I've seen people treat their cockroaches better than you've been treating your body." While understandable, this line of intervention is usually not helpful. We recommend that the BHC talk with PCPs about the common problem of stigma and explore the impact it has on engaging in collaborative health care with the patient. We use the "thank your mind for that thought" technique from ACT to help PCPs provide more mindful care to these patients, most of whom differ from us only in the number and nature of traumas endured.

As suggested in Table 10.22, BHCs should also encourage PCPs to take a team approach with the BHC, particularly with patients with long histories of abuse and substantial health problems. More frequent follow-ups may improve outcomes with this group of patients, many of whom need a great deal of treatment, but in fact receive little. In addition, PCPs should be encouraged to prioritize the medical and psychological needs of the patient at each visit, being sure to focus only on the most important. This helps prevent feeling overwhelmed. The bottom line with this group of patients is to promote the sense that they are being accepted as human beings, while keeping the issue of making choices about drug/alcohol abuse on the table.

Table 10.22. PCP teaching points concerning adult patients with drug and alcohol problems

1.	Teach PCPs to assess readiness for change and to use brief interventions.
2.	Facilitate PCP discussion concerning stigma and teach PCPs the "Thank your mind for that thought" technique, so that they can be present with patients and make a strong effort to engage them in medical care.
3.	Encourage PCPs to prioritize care needs for patients with numerous health problems and to use the BHC to provide additional care.
4.	Encourage PCPs to access current referral information from the BHC (and make these easily available in wall files in common areas).
5.	Suggest that PCPs ask patients at the end of the visit, "How did this go for you? Did you get the care you needed?" (Greater satisfaction with care often leads to better engagement in care and better outcomes).

SERIOUS MENTAL ILLNESS

Increasingly, patients with serious mental illness are receiving treatment in primary care settings. This is due in part to the serious financial problems besieging Community Mental Health Centers (CMHC). As requirements for accessing CMHC services have become more complex and restrictive, more patients with serious mental illness have been driven out of the mental health system and into the primary care system. The integration of behavioral health services provides a platform for delivering one-stop services for these patients, who tend to underutilize all health care and to have elevated risk for physical as well as mental health problems. The case example of Elizabeth highlights how the BHC and PCP can take a team approach to helping a seriously mentally ill patient makes gains in both mental and physical health.

Elizabeth: I am hearing voices again and can't sleep

Dr. South referred this thirty-one-year-old, single mother of two for a consultation concerning sleep hygiene and medication adherence. Dr. South had cared for Elizabeth in the past, and she was now returning to the clinic after having lived in another area for several years. Elizabeth had a diagnosis of schizophrenia and a history of living with a man who behaved violently toward her. She had received care in the past from a local CMHC, but reported to Dr. South that they didn't want to see her there anymore and that she wanted him to prescribe her medication.

At the initial contact, Elizabeth's Duke Scores suggested poor Mental and Social Health Scores. She was very concerned about her difficulties with sleep and the extent to which voices distracted her from relaxing and from attending to her children. Elizabeth had recently separated from her violent partner and moved in with another family, who had meager resources, but were supportive of her and her children. They transported Elizabeth to her clinic visit, and they were helping with her children.

The BHC provided education about sleep hygiene practices (see Healthy Sleeping Tips handout on the compact disc in Appendix D), taught Elizabeth a visual metaphor from ACT for observing the voices that troubled her, and explored issues related to medication adherence. The BHC also introduced the possibility of Elizabeth seeing the BHC in a ping–pong pattern with Dr. South. Dr. South would attend to her physical health problems and prescribe her medication, while the BHC would help her to be a good mother and get along with her adoptive family. She agreed to follow-up with both Dr. South and the BHC in two weeks or earlier if her symptoms worsened or she was unable to take the medication as prescribed.

At follow-up, Elizabeth's Duke Scores suggested improvement in Mental Health, and she indicated success in taking the medication as prescribed. She had implemented the sleep hygiene plan, but continued to have problems relaxing at night when she was more aware of external noises as well as hearing voices. However, she reported the voices were a little less troubling to her when she used the observing technique. The BHC taught her the CALM Exercise (see handout on compact disc in Appendix D), and Dr. South increased her medication dosage. Elizabeth agreed to continue with her sleep hygiene practices and to practice the mindfulness and relaxation exercises in the morning and evening. She felt she was more attentive to her children, but wanted to talk about parenting issues at her next follow-up with the BHC.

Elizabeth came for monthly follow-ups over the following three years, alternating visits with Dr. South and the BHC. She attained stability and began to provide care for the children of the adults in whose home she was living. The BHC helped her learn specific skills related to parenting and addressing common behavioral problems exhibited by young children. Elizabeth resumed knitting and made several things to sell in a craft fair.

She took her medication consistently, and, when she began to put on weight, the BHC helped her develop a plan involving controlling portion size and taking daily walks. Elizabeth then lost twelve pounds over a six-month period.

BHC Intervention Possibilities for Adult Patients with Serious Mental Illness. Elizabeth's case demonstrates the essentials for successfully managing a patient with serious mental health problems. The PCP provided medication, and the BHC supported medication adherence, initiated development of a plan to improve quality of life, provided skill training as needed, and initiated a weight management program. The Primary Care Patient Values Plan (see in Appendix D) is an ACT tool that is useful in structuring a behavior change plan directed by values. It can be integrated into an electronic medical record and supported by multiple providers. The BHC also provided support to Elizabeth's children once or twice over the course of several years of care. BHCs may often become involved in assisting the parents or partners of patients with serious mental illness.

Table 10.23 summarizes the numerous interventions a BHC can provide to patients and PCPs to help improve both mental and physical health. Because many patients with serious mental illness may not be organized enough to describe their medical and psychological needs, it is important to create a welcoming protocol for such patients. Most primary care scheduling programs allow for creation of "patient alert messages," which can be used to support welcoming plans. Alert messages for patients with serious mental illness typically instruct the receptionist to call the BHC, PCP, or a specified nurse on the patient's care team immediately, so that the patient is not left waiting in an often noisy and sometimes confusing room full of strangers. These patients benefit from having a specific team of three or four providers that are familiar with and responsible for the care plan over time. This assures that someone who knows and understands them is always available in the clinic. A charge nurse is often a good team member, as she or he will probably be the person talking with the patient over the phone when an appointment is scheduled. The goal is to create a welcoming experience and the BHC may need to take the lead in creating a welcoming committee of providers for each patient with serious mental illness.

Table 10.23. BHC intervention possibilities for adult patients with serious mental illness

1.	Support medication adherence by carefully exploring and addressing barriers to use of medicine as prescribed.
2.	Develop a plan to improve health-related quality of life (e.g., use of the Primary Care Patient Values Plan) and provide skill training as needed for the patient to succeed in behavior change plans.
3.	Assist the patient's family members as necessary with problem-solving issues related to the patient's health. Refer them to community support groups, if available.
4.	Support development of a team of three or four providers for the seriously mentally ill patient, so that at least one informed provider will be available when the patient comes to the clinic.
5.	Create a welcoming protocol for patients who have frequent periods of instability and place it into the scheduling program alert system.
6.	Address health-risk behaviors, such as smoking and weight gain associated with medication adherence.

PCP Teaching Points Concerning Adult Patients with Serious Mental Illness. PCPs feel frustrated by barriers to obtaining psychiatric care for patients with psychosis. While some respond to this challenge with a commitment to learn more about psychiatric care issues, others recoil and try to avoid these patients. Therefore, it may be helpful for the BHC to address PCPs individually when pursuing the activities suggested in Table 10.24.

The BHC does need to be aware of community resources for psychiatric care and to network with local agencies and resources. When resources are scarce in the specialty sector, it is important for the BHC and PCPs to use them wisely. For example, the PCP may reserve requests for psychiatric assistance for new, unstable patients and agree to assume prescribing responsibility once the patient is stabilized. PCPs may also want to use precious psychiatric resources for telephone consultations at the time of need. The BHC can also be an advocate for educational resources that provide PCPs training for prescribing antipsychotics. While perhaps not interested enough to go to a weekend workshop, a significant number of PCPs might be willing to view a series of thirty-minute videos aimed at improving their prescribing skills.

Table 10.24. PCP teaching points concerning adult patients with serious mental illness

1. Address frustration with lack of psychiatric resources by learning about community resources and networking with psychiatric providers in an effort to make a plan that uses limited resources strategically.
2. Teach PCPs to better understand the function of various symptoms in psychosis, rather than to simply view symptoms as a sign of "mental illness".
3. Since PCPs vary in their interest in learning more about psychiatric care, support learning venues that are feasible and give providers a choice (e.g., a series of short videos about prescribing antipsychotic medications).
4. Help PCPs learn key strategies supporting patient adherence to medications (e.g., regular visits scheduled in a ping-pong fashion with the BHC, exploring barriers to adherence, devising cues for reminders, and reinforcing for adherence, etc.)

SUMMARY

1. While domestic violence often motivates patients to seek care, patients may present with vague pain complaints and even deny domestic violence when providers inquire about it. We recommend that providers find culturally sensitive ways to screen for violence and be prepared to develop safety plans and refer to community resources. The single most important goal beyond detection is having the patient leave the clinic with a feeling of having been understood and an intention to return.

2. BHCs need to teach patients who complain of pain a variety of skills, such as mindfulness, acceptance, pacing, relaxation, and comfort strategies. Additionally, these patients benefit from value-driven behavior change plans drawn from ACT and on-going support from a PCP. Development of a clinical pathway utilizing a Pain and Quality of Life class provides more opportunities for in depth skills training. Pathways also provide a structure that allows for systematic evaluation of pain treatment outcomes, where the focus is on improving functional status.

3. Hypertension, obesity, and diabetes are common in patients. The BHC can offer patients skill training to support implementation of a healthy lifestyle plan and can offer PCPs instruction in motivational interviewing.

4. Dizziness and chest pain are common complaints among primary care patients. Often, these complaints mask an underlying anxiety state such as panic or somatization. A BHC can complete a functional analysis and help the patient learn skills that address the troubling symptoms and reduce stressful life circumstances.

5. Many adult primary care patients are trying to learn to live with chronic conditions (such as diabetes), and they often struggle with avoidance patterns. The BHC can help newly diagnosed patients face their disease and partner with PCPs to offer group services for ongoing support and medical monitoring. Practice support tools may help the BHC take a systematic approach to newly diagnosed patients (See BHC Diabetes Screener on the compact disc in Appendix D).

6. Fatigue, sleep disturbance, and other symptoms of depression and traumatic stress are common in primary care. The BHC can use the functional analysis to identify and target the most troubling symptom for the patient. When improvements occur in the targeted symptoms, many other symptoms improve spontaneously as the patient develops self-efficacy. BHCs can offer a range of services to these patients, including behavior change support, evaluation of response to medication treatment, and relapse prevention training. The BHC can teach PCPs the biopsychosocial model and encourage a practice philosophy emphasizing behavioral interventions as the active ingredients necessary for long term change.

7. The BHC will see patients in primary care who are considering suicide and needs to be prepared to assess risk and respond appropriately. In addition, the clinic needs to have an emergency protocol in place so that a suicidal emergency does not disrupt the flow of patient care for either the PCP or the BHC. A new diagnosis of a chronic disease and any other number of other life problems can trigger a sense of hopelessness that results in health-care seeking.

8. While there are many primary care patients with alcohol and drug problems, they may be difficult to recognize until problems become more severe. Much can be gained from screening and brief intervention. The BHC also can help patients with more chronic problems by functioning as a "safety net," linking the patient with

existing community programs and using motivational interviewing and harm reduction strategies.

9. Many patients with serious mental illness seek care exclusively in the primary care setting. BHCs can support the PCPs who want to develop expertise in pharmacological treatment by organizing in-house trainings provided by a consultant. The BHC can also help with medication adherence, family support and education, connections to community resources, and assistance with reducing health risk behaviors.

11

EXAMPLES OF CONSULTATIONS WITH OLDER ADULTS

"I used to think getting old was about vanity—but actually it's about losing people you love."

—Joyce Carol Oates

The greatest challenges of aging well are those related to mastery of the art of losing. As we age, we lose friends, family members, some physical and mental abilities, economic earning power, and activities basic to independent functioning, such as driving. Unfortunately, our society does little to prepare its members for these experiences or to link them to activities that use the strengths of aging, such as wisdom and ample leisure time. Further, many health care reimbursement policies effectively work against the values of our senior citizens (such as remaining in their homes, maintaining contact with their friends, and being able to afford medications that help them preserve health). It's no wonder that as many as one in four adults experience mental health problems in old age.

In America, many older adults experience the double jeopardy of stigma against both aging and mental problems. It's as if the world is saying, "Yuk, old and losing all this stuff and feeling down about it ... better stay home and keep it to yourself." It is no surprise that few seek help for mental problems and that the few that do, go to their PCPs. Since the majority of older adults have been in their homes and communities for a long time (and plan to stay in them), they have established relationships with their PCPs and value their opinion on many issues.

A visit with the PCP is an important social event for many patients over seventy-five, and while PCPs know this, they experience a great deal of pressure to keep visit lengths down and completed encounters up. Many PCPs lack the time to stay current with evidence-based mental health treatments for older adults or to develop and support behavior modification programs to assist with lifestyle changes. The resulting "expertise gap," in combination with inadequate funding and time, often collude to prevent the delivery of high quality BH treatment to older adults.

However, research is generating evidence-based treatments for older adults, particularly for dementia and depression, and the PCBH model creates a platform for delivery of these services. The consultation based nature of PCBH services also gives us a golden opportunity to provide education to PCPs about the psychological aspects of aging. The addition of BHC services to the PC setting is an urgent matter when it comes to older primary care patients, as the U.S. population is growing older and living longer. Over seventy-five million baby boomers (born between 1946 and 1964) will begin reaching age sixty-five in 2011, and this will eventually lead to a doubling of the current population of seniors.

This chapter offers the reader an opportunity to shadow a BHC who is providing consultations to a variety of older adult patients. We provide templates for several classes specific to older adults and ideas for teaming with a nurse to improve care to older adults. We end the chapter with some ideas for delivering proactive, preventive behavioral health services to seniors. Appendix C offers a reading list for BHCs to use to further develop skills for providing care to adults in general, and the work of Molinari and colleagues (2003) is particularly useful for evaluating one's competencies for providing geriatric interventions. Appendix D offers a compact disc that includes patient handouts, most of which are useful with adults of any age (e.g., Diaphragmatic Breathing Tips, Managing Chronic Pain, and Healthy Sleeping Tips).

So let your imagination take over, as BHC work begins with a group of older adults. We invite the reader to learn by looking over our shoulders and into the eyes of patients—Janet, Andrew, Louise, Thelma, George, and Bob. As can be seen from a quick review of Table 11.1, it's a busy afternoon that starts with a Life Satisfaction Class for fifteen patients.

Table 11.1. An afternoon in the life of a BHC (providing care to older adults)

Chapter section	BHC # 1442	Referral reason
	1:00 (15 patients)	Life satisfaction class
Demoralization	2:15 Janet	Diabetes, vascular disease
Medical adherence	2:45 Andrew	Multiple medical problems
Stress (caregiving and other problems)	3:15 Louise	Shortness of breath, fatigue
Dementia	3:45 Thelma and George	Agitation
Loss and preparation for death	4:15 Bob	Lung cancer, bereavement

DEMORALIZATION

Multiple losses and setbacks in life, particularly those in the last few decades of life, may undermine one's confidence in meeting the challenges of life transition successfully. The rapidity with which these hardships appear, as well as their psychological scale, can be disheartening and result in a profound sense of demoralization. Many demoralized seniors visit the clinic with the hope that their PCP will help them recover their energy and zest for life. Often, the PCP offers a pat on the back, a few kind words and medication. Sometimes this is enough, and the patient leaves feeling encouraged and takes the medicine with some benefit. At other times, the PCP uses the available time to address medical concerns, as is often the case when laboratory findings suggest poor disease control. Demoralized patients may not see self-managing their disease as a top priority but will still respond to the PCP's concern with a shallow promise to do better. As is sometimes the case in primary care, the patient is presenting with one set of needs; the medical provider is delivering care to address a different set. This is a difficult situation at best, but the BHC may play a pivotal role in improving care to these patients. Janet's case demonstrates how the BHC can help reverse the cycle of demoralization associated health problems.

Janet: Yes, I'm doing okay with my diabetes

Dr. Reese referred this sixty-six-year-old married mother of four for a consultation concerning diabetes and atherosclerotic vascular disease.

Dr. Reese worried about lab results suggesting problematic control over the patient's diabetes, but noted that Janet insisted that she was "pretty much doing okay ..." with her diabetes. Dr. Reese knew that Janet had many psychosocial concerns and asked her to consult with the BHC about ways to manage stress as well as her diabetes.

Janet was tearful at her initial BHC consult, as she explained that her seventy-five-year-old husband had asthma and was in poor health. They both worried about two of their children, one of whom had lost her job and the other who had problems with alcohol. Their son was serving time in Montana for a driving under the influence conviction. She missed him terribly and asked if the BHC would write a letter to prison officials requesting that he be moved to a local facility. Janet indicated that she was testing her blood sugar on a regular basis, did not exercise, and found it hard to make dietary changes. She reported that she was taking all medications as prescribed including a SSRI that she had taken off and on for years. She agreed to take daily walks with her husband and to ask for his support in making dietary changes. Janet also agreed to initiate brief daily phone calls to her daughter who lived nearby. The BHC wrote the letter to prison officials during the visit and gave it to Janet to mail. She left with an agreement to follow-up with Dr. Reese and the BHC in one week.

Janet returned ten days later and reported that she and her husband were walking together for about ten minutes every day. She volunteered that she was checking her feet daily and that both she and her husband were eating better. She had talked with her daughter almost daily, and they were considering buying a treadmill together, as it happened that the daughter was now re-employed. She had sent the letter to the prison officials, and her son had sent her a Mother's Day card indicating that he might be transferred to a facility near her.

At the initial BHC consultation, Janet's Duke scores suggested a person with mental and physical health problems that interfered with her functioning. However, Janet's Perceived Health score of 100 suggested that she saw her physical health as good. This is an important score, as it is related to patient utilization of medical services, and Janet had a history of underutilizing services (i.e., not visiting her doctor when she needed to). This configuration is not uncommon among demoralized older adults with chronic conditions. They are simply unable to put the reality of their chronic disease burden on the table, given the extent to which the table is

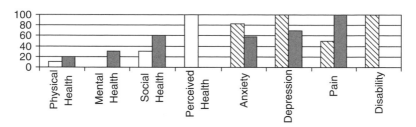

Figure 11.1. Janet's Duke Health Profile Scores at the Initial and Follow-up (shaded bars) Consultations (Scores range from 0 to 100. On Physical, Mental, Social, and Perceived Health Scales (white bars), higher Scores indicate better functioning. On Anxiety, Depression, Pain, and Disability Scales (striped bars), higher Scores indicate more severe symptoms).

crowded by other problems. Figure 11.1 is a graph of Janet's scores at her initial consult and again at her second follow-up consult. As can be seen, Physical, Mental, and Social Health scores improved, while symptoms of anxiety and depression decreased. Interestingly, her Perceived Health score dropped from 100 to 0 (suggesting that she felt she needed health care services) and her Disability score dropped from 100 to 0 (suggesting that she stopped seeing herself as disabled). This flip-flop may indicate that, after three visits with the BHC, Janet's motivation for using needed health care services improved.

Janet came for a second follow-up consultation with the BHC a month later and reported that she was now walking six or seven times per day for five to six minutes on the treadmill that she and her daughter purchased together. She was socializing more and enjoying outings with her daughter. She was eating more vegetables, and she was concerned about how high her morning blood sugars had been for the past few days. She had a visit scheduled with Dr. Reese later that day. The BHC showed Janet her change in scores on the Duke and stressed the importance of her working with Dr. Reese to maintain her gains. The BHC recommended that Dr. Reese support Janet's efforts to socialize more, use exercise to reduce stress, and ask for help when she needed it. Janet agreed to follow-up with the BHC if need be in the future.

BHC Intervention Possibilities for Demoralized Older Adult Patients with Chronic Disease. Patients like Janis often benefit from efforts to form a positive working relationship that allows them to become engaged in their care. In many ways, they feel that life has been unfair in giving them a chronic condition, which is often only one of many unhappy circumstances for which they didn't volunteer. Like most people, Janet wanted to improve her life and had her own set of priorities for doing so. At the top of her list was being a mother that could help her children, and the BHC accepted that goal and proceeded to help. The form that this took for Janet was the letter to a prison official, an act that demonstrated that the BHC was engaged with her and was interested in helping her achieve a desired social support outcome. As indicated in Table 11.2, using Duke Health Profile scores to plan and evaluate interventions is useful with patients like Janet. The Perceived Health score of 100 was a red flag, suggesting that Janet did not see herself as sick but rather as a person with psychological stresses that were detracting from her quality of life. The BHC also used motivational interviewing strategies to help her identify areas for behavior change to improve her diabetic control.

Many cognitive behavioral interventions are useful with older patients who are demoralized by multiple medical and life problems. Problem solving therapy (PST) (Harpole et al., 2005) offers an excellent methodology for older adults to use to effectively address various life events that trigger discouragement. PST appeals to older adults, who have solved many problems in their long lives. It is very useful in class formats, and we discuss its use in a health promotion class venue (the Life Satisfaction Class) in the

Table 11.2. BHC intervention possibilities for demoralized older adult patients with chronic disease

1. Engage the patient by addressing and validating their expectations (i.e., what the patient wants the BHC to address in the visit).
2. Use health-related quality of life scores in planning interventions.
3. Use motivational interviewing in regards to specific disease management skills, and target the one for which the patient reports the highest level of readiness.
4. Use intervention tactics that promote social interaction, effective personal problem solving, and healthy lifestyle behaviors (e.g., health promotion classes or group clinics).
5. When it is an issue, empathize with the patient's sense of loss in life and explore specific age-related changes that may act as barriers to behavior change (i.e., having less energy and endurance, visual or hearing impairments.

last section of this chapter. Robinson, Del Vento, and Wischman (1998) provide information on how to start a group clinic program for frail older adults, as well as detailed information on curriculum, and these are discussed briefly in Chapter 12.

PCP Teaching Points Concerning Demoralized Older Adult Patients with Chronic Disease. Probably at least one in twenty visits to a doctor is due to depressive symptoms, and most patients prefer talking treatments to medication treatment. Most PCPs know this, but at the same time are responsible for addressing other aspects of care. The time left after treating acute issues often doesn't allow them to address other issues. Table 11.3 provides suggestions for teaching PCPs how to work with demoralized older adults. Along with lab results, the Two-Minute Test on Proficiency in Self-Management helps the PCP accomplish a quick assessment of self-management efforts. This test, developed by Dr. Jennifer Gregg at the Veteran's Administration Hospital in Palo Alto, involves the PCP asking an open-ended question about the patient's success in managing his or her chronic condition and then (nonchalantly) timing the patient's response. Patients who cope well with chronic conditions tend to pursue self-management as one might pursue a hobby. These patients can easily talk in a focused manner for several minutes about their management efforts and discoveries. Patients who struggle with disease management usually provide a brief, vague response intended to reassure or placate the PCP and then change the subject, often in less than two minutes. When the patient doesn't make it to the two minute marker, the

Table 11.3. PCP teaching points concerning demoralized older adult patients with chronic disease

1. Encourage use of the Two-Minute Test on Proficiency in Self-Management to gauge the involvement of patients in their self-care.
2. Teach PCPs to ask the patient, "What is most important for us to talk about today?" rather than limiting discussion to medical issues.
3. Provide PCPs with information about problem solving therapy.
4. Provide PCPs with training on use of motivational interviewing strategies.
5. Encourage PCPs to consistently support patient development of a social support base. Consider having PCPs with a larger panel of aging patients shift the locus of care to a group medical appointment.

PCP's next question might be, "What do you most want to talk about in our visit today? What concerns you the most?" When a patient with a chronic disease is demoralized or depressed, this question invites them to discuss life stressors.

PCPs resonate to Problem Solving Therapy (PST), as it is consistent with much of their orientation as caregivers. They often describe themselves as problem solvers, therefore most will readily work to help the patient develop a plan to reduce stress, when time allows. Many will also be willing to recommend that the patient participate in interventions for reducing stress (such as attending a relaxation class, attending programs at the senior center, finding a volunteer job, restarting a hobby, consulting with the BHC, etc.). The BHC can also teach PCPs to explain that getting a handle on stress usually makes it easier for people to adapt to the realities of effective chronic disease management. Rather than trying to address everything in one visit, the PCP can invite the patient to return for a follow-up visit, where they can look at the patient's level of readiness for changing a variety of possible behaviors related to better disease management.

In all visits if possible, the PCP needs to help the patient rebuild (if necessary) and activate a competent social support network. Numerous studies have shown that competent social support is a very strong disease buffering attribute in the life of a senior. Towards this end, BHCs may partner with PCPs in building programs that help meet patients' social needs during delivery of medical care. Older PCPs tend to attract older patients, thus they may be ideal candidates for developing group care clinics for older frail patients. Older patients exposed to this visit model quickly use the group itself as a new social support base. Finally, we recommend that BHCs teach PCPs to be mindful of the patient's readiness to change before referring him or her to disease educators. Sometimes patients with low readiness will benefit from first seeing the BHC and then later seeing educators.

MEDICAL ADHERENCE

Only medicine that is taken can potentially help a patient. While this is obvious, many patients do not take prescribed medications for a variety of reasons. Most of the reasons or barriers can be addressed successfully by improving the patient–PCP relationship and the quality of their communication. To help PCPs develop relationships that promote adherence, the BHC may need to model techniques that bring patient beliefs about health and treatment to the forefront of patient interactions.

An often overlooked factor in medication under-use is that of the cost or affordability of medications. Older adults may take six or more medications every day, and psychotropic medications are among the most expensive. While many Medicare beneficiaries have a supplemental insurance program, up to one-third may pay out-of-pocket. In a survey of 660 older adults with chronic illnesses who reported under-using medication in the prior year because of cost, two thirds never told a PCP in advance that they planned to under-use medication because of the cost. Sixty-six percent reported that nobody asked them about their ability to pay for prescriptions and fifty-eight percent reported that they did not think PCPs could help them (Piette, Heisler, & Wagner, 2004). While conveying information about no-cost or low-cost drug programs is part of the solution, improved trust in the patient–PCP relationship may also impact the cost barrier (Piette, Heisler, Krein, & Kerr, 2005). Andrew's case provides an example of how BHC services can help address adherence problems.

Andrew: Sure, but I don't have the money for all those pills

Dr. James referred this seventy-five-year-old widow for a consultation concerning management of multiple medical problems and suspected difficulties with using medications as prescribed. Dr. James explained that Andrew often missed medical appointments and that he didn't take all of his medicines. He didn't see Andrew as experiencing problems with dementia as Andrew was an avid chess player and liked to talk about his success in competitive play in Internet-based games.

At the initial consultation, Andrew completed the Duke and teased the BHC about whether he looked "demented" or "nutty." His scores suggested generally positive mental and physical health and were probably realistic. He was not depressed, but his scores suggested some anxiety. When the BHC discussed Duke Scores with Andrew, he explained that he had lived a good life and was not afraid to die. He was not avoidant of his medical regimen for emotional reasons. He continued to enjoy contact with his adult children and daily chess games on the internet, but also welcomed the day when he would see his wife again, as she had "left to be with her maker" two years prior. The BHC explored Andrew's beliefs about his various health conditions and the treatments he was being asked to adhere to. He explained that he had made some dietary changes and walked a little every day. He was willing to take medicines to improve his quality of life, but lived on a fixed income. He took pride in supporting himself without any assistance from his children, and he didn't mind turning down the heat in his apartment or skipping a few pills in order to make his check last to the next month.

The BHC explained that there might be options that Dr. James could pursue to obtain needed medications at a cost saving, and Andrew agreed to have the BHC initiate that discussion. Dr. James was able to switch several medications to less expensive generic forms and to access a special program for one medication, given Andrew's income level. The BHC did not plan follow-up with Andrew, but did spend some time with Dr. James taking about the development of a Medication Adherence Form on which patients would be asked about potential barriers to adherence. Dr. James agreed to experiment with the form to see if it helped clarify adherence issues during general medical exams.

BHC Interventions for Older Adult Patients with Medical Adherence Problems. The consultation with Andrew highlights the importance of conducting a functional analysis concerning medication adherence when it is a reason for referral. Andrew's beliefs about using medications were not a barrier and, he had no difficulties remembering the medicine. The main issue was the cost of medicines that then triggered his value about being independent. On countless occasions, patients referred for being allegedly "noncompliant" turn out to be patients who have very good reasons for doing what they are doing. This disconnection between the viewpoint of the PCP and the world view of the patient is precisely what a BHC can bridge.

Table 11.4 lists possible BHC interventions with patients who have problems adhering to medical plans. Certainly, the BHC can develop a form that assures systematic assessment of risk factors for medication nonadherence. (See Robinson et al., 1996 for an example of a medication adherence plan). Once the BHC identifies problem areas via functional analysis, he or she can address them one at a time, as the BHC did

Table 11.4. BHC intervention possibilities for older adult patients who don't adhere

1. Complete a functional analysis of medication nonadherence, targeting belief systems, family influences, and external barriers such as cost, transportation, etc.
2. Build consultative interventions that address key barriers to adherence.
3. Develop a form for evaluating adherence (see Robinson, Wischman, & Del Vento, 1996 for an example).
4. Provide timely telephone follow-up when patient motivation is lacking or medication side effects are troubling.

with Andrew. When the risk level is high, timely follow-up is particularly important to the patient's successful adherence.

A patient's beliefs about his or her illness and the perceived value of medication in addressing uncomfortable symptoms are important components of a medication adherence assessment. If medication use makes sense to the patient in terms of his or her unique world view, then the BHC can go on to explore other beliefs pertinent to medication adherence, such as those suggested in Table 11.5. When a patient admits to beliefs that obstruct successful use of medications, the BHC may use Socratic questioning to help the patient address these potential barriers. For example, if the patient says his family would be disappointed if they knew he took

Table 11.5. Beliefs that conflict with medication adherence

1. These kinds of drugs are not the answer to problems in one's life.
2. These kinds of drugs are a crutch.
3. I would be the one to get severe side effects.
4. I should be able to get by without using these kinds of drugs.
5. I could get addicted.
6. My family would not want me to use these kinds of drugs.
7. I will not be able to work if I take these kinds of drugs.
8. These kinds of drugs are overused.
9. It is harmful to take too many different kinds of drugs.
10. These kinds of drugs should not be taken long-term.
11. Drugs that doctors prescribe for anxiety and depression are dangerous.

Note: The BHC might show the patient a list of these beliefs and ask the patient to indicate any of the statements that he or she believes, even a little.

Note: Reprinted by permission from Context Press from *Living Life Well: New Strategies for Hard Times* pills, the BHC can facilitate an exploration of how this would affect willingness to use a prescribed medicine.

The BHC needs to listen carefully to the patient's use of language concerning medication and to incorporate the patient's language into the planning process. For example, if a patient referred to her antidepressants as a vitamin for her nervous system, the BHC should use similar language in the remainder of the consultation. Potential barriers to use of medications are numerous and include lack of understanding of directions for taking the medicine, inability to pay for medicine, difficulties remembering to take medicine, avoidance of side effects, lack of support from loved ones, and inability to detect any beneficial benefits from taking medication. Table 11.6 provides a list of strategies for addressing these barriers.

As mentioned previously, timely follow-up is important with patients who have problems with adherence. Factors pertinent to planning the nature of follow-up include the patient's level of confidence in taking the

Table 11.6. Potential barriers to medication adherence and possible plans for resolving barriers

Potential barriers	Plan
Patient beliefs	Phrase patient use of medication in language consistent with patient beliefs (a vitamin for the nervous system); focus patient attention on detection of beneficial effects
Patient access	Patient can afford medicine; understands use and refill instructions
Patient tolerance	Give patient information about how to cope with side effects
Organization, memory	Link taking medication to daily routines (e.g., brushing teeth); suggest use of a medication organizer
Patient support	Plan for patient to report successful adherence to loved one or plan to give patient a telephone call in a timely manner
Patient confidence and collaboration	Check patient to see if patient is confident about taking medication and that he or she understands a specific strategy for evaluating medication impact

medicine, the probability and severity of negative side effects, and the availability of support to patient for adhering to the plan. Timely follow-up is critical when a patient's confidence is low, the probability and negativity of side effects are high, and the availability of interpersonal support is lacking. When this is the case, the BHC may want to give a call to the patient within a few days of the consult to support adherence or ask a nurse to provide this support to the patient.

PCP Teaching Points Concerning Older Adult Patients with Medical Adherence Problems. Andrew's case illustrates the unique role the BHC can play in educating PCPs about a functional analytic approach to the problem of nonadherence. The BHC suggested development of a medication adherence assessment, and the PCP agreed to pilot test the protocol in his general practice. Dr. James's involvement would likely result in a better product, and his participation in the project would increase his success in evaluating other patients and prepare him to influence other providers to improve their identification of at risk patients.

As suggested in Table 11.7, medical adherence is an area where BHCs can offer training to enhance PCP and nursing skills. The BHC can use the information in Tables 11.5 and 11.6 for workshop handouts. If some PCPs are surprised by the BHC interest in medical adherence (as he or she is not a prescriber), the BHC can explain that taking a pill is a behavior and that the tools of behavior analysis may be applied to help patients demonstrate that behavior consistently. In addition to PCPs, nurses have an important role to play in improving medical adherence, as they frequently are the staff members that perform telephone work. Meresman and colleagues (2003) describe a medication adherence protocol in which PC nurses

Table 11.7. PCP teaching points concerning older adult patients who don't adhere

---

1. Teach PCPs to ask about the patient's beliefs and barriers (e.g., cause of and cure for illness, acceptability of use of medications, barriers to use of medication).
2. Offer to develop a form for PCPs that systematically assesses risk for medication adherence failure.
3. Offer PCPs training on how to make a specific plan to support adherence (including needed follow-up).
4. Consider adapting evidence-based programs that involve nurses in improving medical adherence.

---

provided ten telephone calls to depressed patients over a four-month period. In the calls, nurses supported focused behavioral activation plans, provided education, monitored treatment response, and addressed barriers to medication adherence. Medication adherence rates were significantly higher in the group of patients that received the nursing intervention.

STRESSES RELATED TO CAREGIVING
(AND OTHER PROBLEMS)

One of the most common sources of stress for older adults is providing long term care to aging parents or to a life partner. Caregiver stress is receiving a great deal of attention from researchers interested in evaluating the impact of exposure to chronic, long-term stress. Many caregivers experience increased symptoms of depression and anxiety, and are themselves at greater risk for developing stress sensitive diseases. Educational programs, as well as BHC consultation services, are helpful to caregivers, particularly at the beginning of their experience of providing care when they can learn key skills for preventing burnout. During periods of more severe strain, caregivers will often benefit from a series of consultation visits with a BHC. Dr. Funk recognized the potential help the BHC could provide for her patient, Louise.

Louise: I can't breath, and I am so very tired

Dr. Funk referred this sixty-seven-year-old married mother of two for a consultation concerning shortness of breath and fatigue. Dr. Funk started the patient on a SSRI because she believed Alice was experiencing depression secondary to caregiver burn-out. Louise provided care to her eighty-seven-year-old mother and her eighty-nine-year-old former father-in-law. Her first husband had died many years prior, and she had agreed to care for his father, as her husband had been an only child.

At the initial consult, Louise reported that she began having episodes of shortness of breath four months earlier when her mother went through a period of critical illness. She explained that this medical crisis triggered many of the same feelings she had experienced when her father died the previous year. With her responsibilities to her mother and her father-in-law, she hadn't had time to grieve the loss of her father. She and her husband were retired, and while they'd hoped to travel together during retirement, she felt too guilty to leave the people that depended on her. She had two brothers that lived out of town, and they wanted to help but were often in disagreement with Louise about various issues related to their mother's care. She avoided asking them for help because she dreaded their criticism. She explained that her husband, who was a little domineering, provided ample suggestions to her about ways to improve her situation.

While Louise had a list of activities that she enjoyed, she was doing them infrequently or not at all. She enjoyed playing the violin and had been a music teacher for many years, but she rarely played. She enjoyed walking but had walked only once during the past week. She reported worrying during the walk about not being present for her mother and father-in-law. She liked to quilt and had a commitment to make quilts with others for the Make-A-Wish Foundation, but she had not gone to the weekly quilting group since her father died. She liked to travel, and she and her husband had a recreational vehicle, but they had yet to plan a trip.

Louise's Duke Scores suggested significant mental health problems. Perceived Health was a relative strength, which is usually not the case for a person with panic disorder. Her Depression score was 90. During the consult, the BHC provided an explanation of the connection between stress and somatic symptoms and taught Louise a breathing exercise to promote relaxation. In developing a behavior change plan, the BHC challenged her to change her behavior and see if the scores changed. Louise agreed to walk for thirty minutes daily with her husband; discuss the specifics of several camping trips for the coming summer; and notify her brothers of the dates that she and her husband wanted to travel over the coming summer. The BHC suggested that Louise might find herself wanting to take more time for creative activities and for socializing as she began to take better care of her mind and body.

When Louise returned for follow-up a month later, she reported that she had implemented the plan and was feeling much better. She had stopped the SSRI because it made her feel funny, but had taken a benzodiazepine "prn" on an infrequent basis, after that was suggested by Dr. Funk as an alternative. Louise and her husband had begun walking every evening together. When walking, they had visited with their neighbors and decided to join them as participants in a horseback riding club. They had gone on a day ride to a local winery, and she had met an interesting woman who also enjoyed quilting. Louise was reading a book, *Coming of Age with Aging Parents,* and was taking its advice about how to improve her relationships with her older brothers. In the second consult, the BHC provided Louise with a brief overview of the differences between aggressive, assertive and passive communications, and they practiced this in relation to her making requests for back up care to her brothers.

At follow-up, Louise's Duke Scores suggested improvement in physical, mental, and social health and a decline in severity of symptoms of anxiety, depression, and disability. She planned to maintain her behavior changes, to plan her vacations over the summer, and to make assertive requests to her brothers regarding their role as caregivers during her planned trips. Louise did return for one additional consult two months later, and she was maintaining her gains. She felt her life was much more balanced, and her relationships with her brothers and husband had improved.

BHC Intervention Possibilities for Older Adults with Caregiver Stress. Table 11.8 provides a list of possible interventions for caregiver stress. The top item is what the BHC used in the initial consultation with Louise, namely, an explanation of the connection between stress and somatic symptoms. For many patients, this is "news" and it immediately results in a sense of relief. The relief often comes in the form of, "You mean this is just my reaction to stress and I'm not crazy?" The BHC also taught Louise skills to man-

Table 11.8. BHC intervention possibilities for older adults with caregiver stress

1. Explain the relationship between symptoms and stress response.
2. Teach skills that have an immediate impact on symptoms of stress (e.g., diaphragmatic breathing on shortness of breath).
3. Support development of a daily schedule that involves specific self-care behaviors (e.g., stretching, listening to music, longer baths, walking, drawing, or other creative activities, etc.).
4. Encourage development of relationship(s) with adults who do not need care.
5. Provide education about delayed grieving and help schedule "grieving" sessions if needed.
6. Provide targeted skill training (e.g., interpersonal assertion, mindfulness, etc.).
7. Start a Healthy Aging program.

age her troublesome stress related symptoms (i.e., fatigue and shortness of breath improved with daily exercise and use of relaxation strategies). The BHC provided training in assertiveness skills to help her begin setting appropriate limits on the demands of others, while making clear requests concerning her immediate needs as a caregiver.

For the stressed older adult, targeted skill training, particularly regarding any physiological manifestation of stress, increases the patient's sense of control or ability to respond in a way that makes a difference. Patients often have skill deficits that increase their vulnerability to the on-going stress of caregiving, such as being unable to say no or to take a mindful or accepting perspective in response to annoying behaviors exhibited by the person for whom they provide care. It is not unusual for older adult caregivers to also be grieving the loss of a loved one, as was the case for Louise. BHCs need to support healthy grieving by providing emotional validation and education about the grief process. Two helpful interventions are scheduling contact with adults who do not need care and scheduling a pleasurable activity such as walking or some type of craft or hobby (gardening, fishing, playing a musical instrument, etc.).

Older adults experience numerous stressors other than caregiving, including problems with adult children and spouses, problems with housing, and financial strain. The BHC can offer more intensive assistance with coping skills by offering programs such as the Healthy Aging program, which involves collaboration between a BHC, a nurse, and an older adult volunteer. In most primary care settings, it is relatively easy to identify older patients who are high utilizers of care because of psychosocial issues such as caregiver stress. For example, the BHC can use billing data to identify patients over sixty who are in the top 10 percent of utilization and then have PCPs identify patients at risk for caregiver stress. The nurse can then invite patients to participate in the Healthy Aging program, which offers patients a series of four weekly five to ten minute phone calls from nurses (see Table 11.9 for topics) and an invitation to attend a weekly Mind–Body Tea at the clinic, which can be co-led by the BHC and a volunteer. Table 11.10 provides an explanation of Tea activities (See Kabat-Zinn, 1994, for information on the meditation exercises). Of course, this approach also encourages PCPs to consistently involve the BHC in the care of older adults who are beginning to use medical care more but with less benefit.

Table 11.9. Healthy Aging nurse telephone topics

Week	Telephone call topics
One	Give examples of challenges to aging well, provide instruction in diaphragmatic breathing and suggest the use of such to support an accepting perspective on stress.
Two	Evaluate adequacy of social support, plan ways to improve quality and/or frequency of social interactions.
Three	Evaluate level of physical activity, plan ways to increase quality and quantity of physical exercise.
Four	Evaluate extent to which patient is able to provide valued services and/or to engage in creative activities, plan ways to increase quality and quantity.

Table 11.10. Healthy Aging mind–body tea class activities

Provider	Item	Activities
Volunteer	Tea	Prepare tea, facilitate discussion about resources for seniors in the community, record new resource information in the class resource book
BHC	Skill development	Rotating series of exercises to assist with development of mindfulness and generation of feelings of well being and to improve results of problem solving activities (e.g., Bending Tree, Meditative Walking, Yogic Breathing, Mountain Meditation, Lake Meditation)
BHC	Discussion	Experience of participants in applying mindfulness and problem solving skills to on-going psychosocial problems

PCP Teaching Points Concerning Older Adult Patients with Caregiver Stress. The upcoming population shift makes it particularly important for BHCs to team with PCPs in advocating for primary and secondary prevention services for caregivers. The magnitude of stress experienced by this group can have a very negative impact on health. In many ways, caregivers are health care provider extenders, and we need to prepare them to

Table 11.11. PCP teaching points concerning older adult patients with caregiver stress

1. Encourage PCPs to advocate for primary and secondary prevention programs for caregivers.
2. Suggest that PCPs refer caregivers to the BHC for development of a self-care plan.
3. Invite PCPs to partner with BHCs in designing and delivering Caregiver Hardiness Workshops and Healthy Aging programs.

succeed in their role. Programs such as the Healthy Aging program provide caregivers with an opportunity to access social support, to share ideas about resources in their community, and to learn skills commonly needed by those working in caregiver roles. If the PCP and BHC are successful in recruiting a nurse and volunteer to help in implementing the program, the demands on their time may be significantly reduced and the quality of care for patients will be improved. The Mind Body Tea also provides a resource for training PCPs and nurses in interventions typically provided by the BHC. See Table 11.11 for a list of teaching points for PCPs.

DEMENTIA

By definition, dementia is an acquired syndrome of decline in memory and at least one other cognitive domain (such as language, visuospatial, or executive function) of sufficient magnitude to interfere with functioning in social or occupational roles in an alert person. While dementia may be caused by any number of diseases, the two most common causes are Alzheimer disease and cerebrovascular ischemia (vascular dementia). Risk factors for dementia include age, having a first-degree relative with a history of Alzheimer, and cardiovascular risk factors such as hypertension. Current estimates suggest that 3 to 11 percent of persons older than sixty-five and 25 to 47 percent of those older than eighty-five have dementia (Cooper, Bickel, & Schaufele, 1996).

The human costs associated with dementia are substantial. For the patient, there is the frustration of loss of independence and the complications related to managing co-morbid diseases that require the ability to plan, remember and execute important self-care tasks. For the patient's family, there is the burden of caregiving, the loss of a period of retirement where recreation and rest were expected to be plentiful, and the challenge of negotiating a complex network of medical, respite, assisted living, and nursing home care.

Mild to moderately severe dementia is under-detected and consequently under-treated in primary care. Physicians diagnose around half of the patients with mild to moderate symptoms of dementia (Cooper et al., 1996). Improved detection, as mentioned in Chapter 6, would allow patients to receive treatment at earlier stages, which is the goal. The case example of Thelma and George illustrates the range of beneficial interventions that a BHC may offer to patients with dementia and their families.

Thelma and George:
It was not supposed to be this way

Dr. Davis referred George and Thelma for a consultation concerning coping with Thelma's symptoms of dementia, particularly episodes of agitation. Dr. Davis had provided PC services to both George and Thelma for many years, and he had diagnosed Thelma's dementia about eighteen months prior to the referral. George had read extensively about dementia and become an active participant in a support group for patients with dementia and their caregivers. He was a retired minister and was active in his community. He took Thelma with him to almost all of his activities, feeling that it was best for her to remain socially active.

At the initial consultation, Thelma had difficulty responding to the Duke questions. She made efforts to be socially appropriate but was confused about the role of the BHC and the reason for the consultation. George gave a patient and caring explanation to Thelma, and she appeared to relax. The BHC complimented George on his ability to calm Thelma with his soft voice and focused attention. George explained that Thelma often became agitated just prior to their leaving home. She often commented on his clothing and suggested that he was dressing up for someone. Sometimes, she cried and insisted that he tell her who was taking her place. He noticed that explaining patiently about where they were going and where they would sit—painting a picture of what was to come—alleviated some of her agitation. The BHC suggested that he take photographs of the facilities where he and Thelma went on a weekly basis and place the photographs on a large calendar. He could then refer to planned outings in advance, and she could refer to the picture for an image. He also agreed to request her assistance in selecting his clothes, which she had done for many years and had stopped only months before.

George called Dr. Davis a week later to report that Thelma was more relaxed and that he thought they could avoid use of additional medication at the present time. When Thelma and George came for a check-in with the BHC a few months later, George photographed the BHC with Dr. Davis, explaining that he wanted to add this to their calendar. George consulted with Dr. Davis and the BHC without Thelma present several times over the following year, and they helped him develop behavioral approaches to various problem behaviors and eventually to negotiate her placement in a nursing home. Perhaps the most painful experience for George and Thelma was when she was assaulted in the nursing home and her finger was sprained by the thief who took her wedding ring. George looked to Dr. Davis and the BHC for support insisting, "It wasn't supposed to be this way."

BHC Intervention Possibilities for Older Adult Patients with Dementia. For George, the BHC and Dr. Davis provided ideas for handling problem behaviors and support in making painful transitions. For Thelma, the BHC–PCP team offered behavioral treatment that helped her manage her confusion with less medication and boosted her ability to engage in usual activities and, ultimately, to remain at home for the longest possible time. Behavior modification programs are often helpful in preventing and/or lessening agitation in patients with dementia. For Thelma, George's selection of his own clothes provoked fears of losing him. This could be easily avoided, and the use of a calendar with photographs appeared to strengthen Thelma's visuospatial processing.

Table 11.12 suggests additional interventions that BHCs may provide to older adults with symptoms of dementia. Worthy of mention is the usefulness of behavior modification to promote independence and reduce problems other than agitation, such as incontinence. With support from the PC team, including BHC services on an intermittent basis, families can often significantly delay the relocation of patients into nursing homes. This is particularly important as placement in a nursing home often leads to a significant loss in functioning for the patient and can trigger anticipatory grieving in family members. While Thelma had difficulties in responding to health-related quality of life questions, many patients with

Table 11.12. BHC intervention possibilities for older adult patients with dementia

1. Provide caregiver support and education to prolong the period before nursing home placement is required.
2. Complete a functional analysis of behavioral dysfunction (i.e., identify causes, such as pain or environmental triggers, that can be avoided or minimized).
3. Develop behavior modification programs (e.g., scheduled toileting and prompted voiding to reduce urinary incontinence).
4. Teach caregivers to provide graded assistance, skills practice, and positive reinforcement to enhance the patient's functional independence.
5. Assess health-related quality of life of the patient and use it to inform pharmacological treatment by the PCP.

mild to moderate dementia will be able to respond. This information will be useful to the PCP in selecting appropriate medications, particularly in regards to treatment of both depression and anxiety, which are not uncommon among patients in the early stages of dementia.

PCP Teaching Points for Older Adult Patients with Dementia. Though a great deal of research is in progress in the area of PC management of dementia, there is consensus about the recommended teaching points offered in Table 11.13 (Doody et al., 2001). This is an area for the BHC to monitor and to discuss on an on-going basis with his or her PCP colleagues. It is important that the BHC attempt to share information on the patient's health-related quality of life with the PCP and encourage him or her to use this rather than caregiver reports. Caregivers tend to underestimate the quality of life for the patient, which is possibly related to the impact of the burden that the caregiver is experiencing.

LOSS AND PREPARATION FOR DEATH

While healthy patients and those with mild chronic illnesses want services that support prevention and cure, those with serious, progressive, disabling illnesses look to their PCPs for a different array of services. Medicine offers no cure and little in the way of rehabilitation for conditions that are most likely to lead to the end of life (such as cancer, stroke, heart disease, and dementia). As medical technology continues to improve, a sizable and growing group of patients will spend a significant

Table 11.13. PCP teaching points for older adult patients with dementia

1. Cholinesterase inhibitors benefit patients with Alzheimer's disease, although the average benefit appears small.
2. Vitamin E likely delays the time to clinical worsening.
3. Antipsychotic medications are effective for agitation or psychosis in patients with dementia when environmental manipulation fails.
4. Antidepressants are effective in depressed patients with dementia.
5. BHC services are useful to patients with dementia and their families (including development of behavior modification programs, assessment of health-related quality of life, and support to family members, particularly during transition periods).

portion of their lives coping with these terminal conditions. Our health care system is not prepared to deliver care to this group, as it continues to operate on the outdated assumption that most people die from unintentional injury, infections, and myocardial infarction (Lynn, 2001). Emergency resuscitation is available to most patients almost anywhere or anytime. However, continuity and comprehensiveness of care for patients who have little chance of recovery and their families is lacking.

The integration of BH services into PC can empower efforts to better meet the needs of those approaching the end of life. The needs of this group go well beyond conventional medical care and instead include anticipatory planning for medical crises, advance directives, and ways to involve family members in the transition between life and death. The BHC and PCP can help the dying patient to retain dignity and control, and help the family to bear the stress of providing care at the end of life and enduring the loss of a loved one. Bob's case example highlights how Dr. Myers and the BHC worked together as a team to allow Bob to retain dignity and control during his transition.

Bob: I'm dying and my wife already passed away

Dr. Myers referred this sixty-seven-year-old man for a consultation concerning coping with lung cancer and bereavement. Bob was new to the clinic, having recently moved from another state to live with an adult child that received care from Dr. Myers. Medical records confirmed the patient's self report of poor health, including terminal cancer, diabetes, hypertension, and vascular disease. In the initial visit, Bob told Dr. Myers that his lung cancer was terminal and that he had moved to his son's home to die. He wanted Dr. Myers's support in arranging palliative care. Dr. Myers referred Bob for a same-day visit with the BHC with a request for an evaluation of his depression and bereavement symptoms.

At the initial consultation, Bob's Duke scores suggested poor physical and mental health, and his depression severity was high. When the BHC reviewed his scores with him, he explained that his wife of forty years had died six weeks earlier and that he wanted to join her. He denied suicidal ideation and stated that he would be patient and await his time. In fact, he had plans of taking a trip soon to see several grandchildren that lived in a different city. Bob talked at length about his wife and the goodness she had brought to his life for over forty-five years. The BHC asked Bob about his plans for care at the end of his life and his concerns about preparing for death. He said that he did not want any curative treatment, that he wanted to be comfortable, and that he wanted to leave something for his grandchildren that would help them remember him and his dear wife.

The BHC helped Bob develop a plan concerning leaving a legacy for his family, particularly his grandchildren. He had a wooden jewelry box that his wife had given him forty years earlier for an anniversary. He kept treasures from his life in the box, and he had brought it with him in his recent move. Bob agreed to write a note about every treasure in the box, so that his loved ones would understand their meaning to him. He also agreed to complete a Durable Power of Attorney for Health Care form and to talk with his son about arrangements for his funeral.

Bob returned a week later stating that he had followed the plan and had taken the trip to see his other beautiful grandchildren. His Duke scores suggested mild improvements. He was dressed impeccably, and he explained that every minute seemed to count. He was pleased with the hospice service staff and with Dr. Myers's care. At that visit, he worked with the BHC to develop another plan concerning his death. He agreed to ask his son to record him making a statement about each holiday that his family celebrated. In the statement, he planned to explain traditions that he and his wife had carried forward over the years and that he hoped others in his family would also observe at holidays. He would ask his son to make copies of the tape for his children and grandchildren and to mail the tapes to them after his death. Bob died ten days later.

BHC Interventions for Preparing Older Adult Patients for Death. The BHC helped Dr. Davis better understand Bob's symptoms of grief and depression as they might affect his end of life directives. Bob's preference to use as little medication as possible, just enough to comfort him, was relayed to the PCP. The BHC also helped Bob plan for his death and his care at the end of life. Bob planned his legacy and died with dignity.

As suggested in Table 11.14, the BHC may often be asked to provide input to the PCP concerning the role that bereavement and/or depression may be playing in the decisions of terminal patients who have recently lost a spouse or life partner. Conjugal bereavement is frequently associated with symptoms of depression and/or posttraumatic distress. As many as a third of widows and widowers meet criteria for a major depressive episode one month after the death of a spouse and a larger group probably suffers subthreshold depressive symptoms (Reynolds et al., 1999). Conjugal bereavement is a risk factor for suicide in later life, particularly for men. Negative changes in physical health and an increased mortality rate also accompany widowhood, particularly in men.

In conjunction with evaluating depressed and bereaved older adults, the BHC can partner with the PCP in planning and delivering useful interventions. With more severely depressed widows, a combined intervention involving, for example nortriptyline and interpersonal support, may have a stronger impact and enhance retention of patients in treatment more than single modality interventions (Reynolds et al., 1999). Warning signs of more severe depression in the bereaved older person probably include

Table 11.14. BHC interventions for preparing older adult patients for death

1. When the older adult that is preparing for death has lost a loved one in recent years, assist the PCP and patient with sorting out symptoms of depression versus bereavement.
2. Support healthier forms of reminiscing.
3. Define and/or teach nonmedication comfort strategies.
4. Help the patient and family members plan for use of resources (financial, emotional, and practical).
5. Provide transition coaching services (to assist with changes in levels of care).
6. Encourage completion of documents that support planning for care in the event that the patient loses the ability to make decisions (e.g., advanced directives).
7. Encourage completion of planning activities related to death (will, funeral home arrangements, and preparation of materials for loved ones).

isolation and a lack of responsiveness to usually pleasurable events. In our example, Bob displayed neither of these. In fact, he was seeking contact with loved ones and enjoyed their presence immensely. In regards to BHC interventions, we recommend that the BHC use those that are more specific to grief and suggest Dorothy Becvar's book as a resource (Becvar, 2001; see Appendix C). She suggests that grief is a fundamental and necessary emotion that provides a cleansing function, and this definition seems to be helpful to most bereaved patients.

Older people in general spend a considerable amount of time reminiscing, and BHC interventions may focus on structuring the reminiscing. Recent research findings suggest that different forms of reminiscing are linked to differing levels of life satisfaction. Specifically, reminiscences that foster conversation and prepare for death are linked to higher life satisfaction, while reminiscences that revive old problems and compensate for low cognitive stimulation (i.e., boredom) are associated with lower life satisfaction and greater psychiatric distress (Cappeliez, O'Rourke, & Chaudhury, 2005). Reminiscence directed toward maintaining a connection with a departed person also predicted psychiatric distress in this study. The BHC can promote patient satisfaction with life by supporting engagement in adaptive uses of reminiscence.

On occasion, the BHC may be asked to help patients and family members with the design of comfort activities. Dying patients may benefit from interventions that help them create images of peace and comfort. They may also choose to prepare a selection of reading and/or music selections that they find comforting. Family members may benefit from interventions such as providing gentle touch or singing or reading to the dying family member.

The BHC may also be the PC team member who helps patients and family members plan for use of their health care resources at the end of life. For most patients, there is no specific point that marks a dramatic transition from cure to care. While hospice programs are typically reserved for patients that will die within six months, many would benefit from care typical of hospice providers for at least a year prior to death. The BHC may be one of the providers in the newly emerging integrated health care system that helps to fill this gap in planning for use of financial, emotional, and practical services. It is difficult for patients and family members to navigate the complexities of changes in care, and the BHC in some PC settings may be a leader in developing programs that help patients during these difficult moments. While this is of course the humane thing to do, it will probably also save economic resources. For example, use of "transition coaches" (who provided assistance with planning for changes in care) for recently hospitalized patients resulted in a reduction in rehospitalization costs among a cohort of patients with terminal disease (Coleman et al., 2004).

Finally, the BHC can help patients prepare for a time when their capacities for memory, judgment, reasoning, planning, and decision-making decline. This will require learning the specific legal requirements in each state for advanced directives and for procedures related to guardianship. Unfortunately, patients are more likely to plan for their death (e.g., preparation of a will, arrangement with a funeral home) than for care at the end of life (Pinquart & Sorensen, 2002). The BHC can partner with PCPs in designing programs that educate dying patients and their families about the planning strategies summarized in Table 11.15.

PCP Teaching Points Concerning Preparing Older Adult Patients for Death. The BHC can be of great assistance in reducing confusion, suffering, and unnecessary spending of medical dollars at the end of life by helping PCPs increase the percentage of their patients who execute advanced directives. Since most patients do not currently have an advanced directive, this tops the list of teaching points for PCPs in Table 11.16. The Patient Self-Determination Act of 1991 initiated the requirement that anyone entering a health care facility, such as a hospital or nursing home, be asked if he or she has an advance directive, but the Act requirements did not extend to out patient settings such as PC clinics. We recommend that the BHC find a provider champion that supports the idea of asking all patients, new and continuing (particularly those over the age of 50), if they

Table 11.15. Advanced directives

Strategy	Definition
Instruction types	Express the patient's desires and instructions as to what life-prolonging medical procedures the patient would accept if he or she is unable to make or convey such decisions at the time
Proxy directives	Patient gives an agent, person or persons, or institution the power or authority to act in his or her behalf

Table 11.16. PCP teaching points concerning preparing older adult patients for death

1.   Teach PCPs to encourage patients and family members to actively plan the direction of care, transitions, and wishes at end of life.
2.   Encourage PCPs to suggest completion of an advanced directive at new patient visits, particularly for patients over fifty years of age (with BHC assistance as needed).
3.   Let PCPs know that you are available to process their loss of a patient.

would like to complete an advanced directive. Posters and buttons for physicians and nurses can be used to generate a sustained focus over the course of a year, so that completion of advanced directives becomes a part of routine care. This will save many patients and their families from confusion, disagreement, and distress and could prevent guardianship hearings. Finally, we recommend that the BHC approach the PCP to talk about the death of a patient with whom the BHC has been involved and to let providers know in general that he or she is available to discuss issues related to the death of any PC patient.

PREPARING TO CARE FOR MORE OLDER ADULTS IN PRIMARY CARE

In the next few decades, the current population of older PC patients will double. BHCs can be leaders in helping PC prepare for this shift in the population. The question is, "How do we provide services to a large group of older PC patients who want to use our services to help them live vital lives until they die?" Many older patients will need assistance from PC in order to learn skills for experiencing loss and making new connections.

One way a BHC can help is to start health promotion classes. In the late 1980s, one of us (PR) participated in a study designed to evaluate delivery of six health promotion classes to older PC patients (on topics such as hearing, vision, exercise, diet, etc.). The health promotion class targeting improvement of behavioral health was modeled after Gallagher's Life Satisfaction Class (see Thompson, Gallagher, & Breckenridge, 1987 for general information about psychotherapeutic treatments for depressed older adults). Not surprisingly, this class was selected as the favorite of the series by patients. It was a six-session class that offered practical cognitive behavioral strategies for solving the challenges of aging well. The health maintenance organization sponsoring the study agreed to on-going delivery of a four session version of the class after the end of the study because the PCPs insisted on having this resource for their patients. The PCPs explained to the administrators, "Life satisfaction is what all of our patients want." Classes are an excellent format for meeting the behavioral health needs of older patients because participation in a class links patients with the same kind of problem together in one space. Also, to attend a class is itself a social activity and thus defeats the tendency toward withdrawal and isolation.

In addition to classes and group care clinics (which we discuss further in the next chapter), the BHC can be an advocate for other program changes, perhaps the best of which is forming a clinic committee whose mission is to develop services that promote healthy aging. Increasingly, materials are available to support such efforts. The National Council on Aging (NOC) offers tool kits to use in promoting healthy physical activity, management of depression and diabetes, and good nutrition (see NOC ordering information in reading list in Appendix C). However, these evidence-based self-management programs will have little impact if no "champions" appear at the clinic level to promote their implementation.

Nurses are essential members of a Healthy Aging Committee, as they offer a great deal in the way of clinical management services. Nurse–BHC partnerships have great capacity for relieving the burden on PCPs and increasing the value of services to older adults. A Healthy Aging Committee may also create links between PC clinics and community resources. While many older adults find ways to stay involved in their communities, as many as a quarter voice a need for greater involvement with others. In some communities, committee members may need to advocate for development of resources that prevent older people from becoming isolated, depressed, and more vulnerable to disease. Both local and state governments stand to gain from programs that reduce seniors' health care costs by preventing depression and improving fitness, and grant funding may be available for the clinic (and BHCs may help write the grant applications). Finally, the BHC, as a member of the Healthy Aging Committee, also needs to be alert to the possibility of involving older adults as volunteers to meet social service needs and overcome the workforce shortages that are common in PC clinics. In these ways, BHCs can be leaders that bring clinics closer to a future where the circle of life and death meet in the context of community-based health care.

SUMMARY

1. Americans are growing older and living longer, and the current population of seniors will soon double. The BHC needs to evaluate his or her preparedness for delivering evidence-based geriatric services to this group and plan continuing education efforts accordingly.

2. Many referrals of older adults will come with the request that the BHC help them self-manage chronic diseases, because as many as four out of five older adults have a chronic disease.

3. Medical adherence is also an issue, as older adults face many barriers to successfully participating in their care. Cost, along with personal views of illness and treatment may be barriers. A good functional analysis of adherence problems can lead to clear plans for improvement.

4. Caregiving is a common role for the older adult, one that is replete with daily stressors and carries both psychological and health risks. BHCs can help patients maintain independent functioning and family members manage their stress. These services are best delivered early in the caregiver role and in groups where social support and sharing of resources occur spontaneously.

5. Many patients with mild to moderate symptoms of dementia are managed in PC, and BHCs can improve care to this group by supporting early detection efforts, developing behavior modification programs, and assisting patients with planning and negotiating changes in levels of care.

6. BHCs can both develop and support clinic efforts to prepare patients for death with dignity, and family members for negotiating the pain of loss.

7. BHCs can advocate for a clinic-based Healthy Aging Committee, whose role is to create a structure for planning and implementing various programs for the growing number of seniors over the next two decades.

12

MORE THAN ONE PATIENT AT A TIME: GROUP VISITS IN PRIMARY CARE

"Coming together is a beginning. Keeping together is progress. Working together is success."

—Henry Ford

The BHC has many patient care opportunities in PC, and some are best realized by seeing patients in a group context. When using groups, their basic structure should be guided by the PCBH mission goals of improving patient access and PCP learning opportunities. Possible group visit formats in PC include classes, group medical visits, family visits, couple visits, and visits with patients and their caregivers together. Although many of these same formats are used in specialty MH, their structure and application is quite different in the PC setting. In this chapter, we provide ideas for developing PC-friendly formats for all types of group visits. We also suggest ways to integrate group visits into clinical pathways. Clinical pathway development offers excellent opportunities for integrating BHC services seamlessly into care for a targeted group of patients.

ADAPTING GROUP VISITS FOR PRIMARY CARE

Most MH providers are familiar with the concept of group visits and have experience providing services to families and couples as well. A variety of types of group visits, such as support groups, therapy groups, and psychoeducational classes, play important roles in the delivery of special-ity MH services. In PC, though, offering group visits to patients unrelated to each other is a relatively new phenomenon. It is developing partly in response to the needs of a changing health care population where people are living longer and with more chronic conditions and partly in response to the increasing availability of BHC services.

The basic rationale for group visits in traditional MH settings and PC settings is similar—providing more efficient and powerful services. In groups of unrelated persons, more patients can be provided with more support and more information using less provider time. Visits with family members and couples can also make a more powerful and appropriate intervention than an individual visit, whether in a PC or MH setting. However, this is often where the similarity stops. Beyond these basics, the goals, format, processes, size, and leaders for group services are often quite different in PC compared to traditional MH groups. While the group visit approach (for patients unrelated to each other) in PC may be new ground for both BHC and PCP, a BHC with group experience from MH settings will have few problems making adaptations. Providers in PC may need some coaxing to try group visits in clinics where there is no history of such. However, the benefits of group services quickly become apparent to all once begun.

What to Change and Why

Many BHCs who enter PC attempt to apply the same group visit strate-gies they used in MH, only to find that something gets lost in translation. The typical group or class format used in MH often seems inadequate when conducted in PC. For example, MH groups usually start on a spec-ified date and last a certain number of weeks (usually six to eighteen weeks), and the therapist often uses a manual to guide the content of classes (e.g., Barlow et al., 1992; Craske & Barlow, 2000; Craske, Barlow, & Meadows, 2000; Lewinsohn, 1984). Therapists lead groups with the expectation that clients who complete them will be ready for termination, or at least a level of care that requires less frequent contact, by the end. However, evaluation of the effects of these types of group services when offered to medical patients has produced mixed results. For example, the use of traditional support groups for patients with diabetes improved patients' subjective sense of well-being, but did not result in desired changes to important diabetes outcomes (Gilden, Hendryx, Clar, Casia, & Singh, 1992; Maxwell, Hunt, & Bush, 1992). Additionally, attendance at traditional groups is often low, which hurts the BHC more than a MHP because of the greater productivity expectations on the former. To improve the potency and reach of PC groups, one needs to create a format that is unique and that differs significantly from formats employed in specialty MH.

Why doesn't the structure and format of traditional MH groups work as well in PC? How does one decide what adaptations to make? The following section attempts to answer these questions. The reality is that there are as many options for group models as there are primary care clinics. Each clinic needs to find a format that works for its providers, patients, and staff. Suggestions in this chapter are geared toward ensuring that whatever format is used it is consistent with two important aspects of the PCBH mission: maximizing patient access and improving PCP learning opportunities. Consider these as guideposts against which to measure the success of group adaptations in primary care. In hopes of providing readers with a sampling of the wide variety of possible group formats, we provide descriptions of groups used in our own clinics. Later in this section, ideas are also provided for adjusting visits with couples and families so they are consistent with the PCBH model. In case the reader desires to use manual-based psychoeducational treatments in a primary care group format, we also provide suggestions for adapting their curricula. Table 12.1 helps the reader put all of this together with a list of group visit guidelines for BHCs and their colleagues. While not all of the guidelines will apply to every group service, a review of items in this table can help ensure the most PC-friendly group format.

Patient Access. There are many more patients in PC than in specialty MH that can benefit from group visits, so every effort must be made to create group services that can accommodate a large number of participants (e.g., fifteen instead of five). However, PC patients in comparison with MH patients may be even less consistent in attendance and prone to dropping out. If inconsistent attendance happens in a typical sequential MH class the patient may have to drop out because each week builds on

Table 12.1. Guidelines for BHCs to use in creating group services for primary care

1. Ensure the minimum number of participants per hour of a group exceeds by at least one the number that would be seen per hour individually by each provider involved (usually 3 per hour for a BHC and 4 or 5 per hour for a PCP).
2. Increase attendance and provider efficiency by involving PCPs and suggesting patients use the group in place of individual visits with the PCP.
3. Minimize economic barriers to attendance by offering group visits at a rate that is significantly lower than that of individual visits.
4. Transform sequential curricula into a series of stand-alone offerings that can be delivered flexibly (rather than each week building on the one before).
5. Make group services available at the time of need (i.e., allow patients to start at any visit, attend a single visit or a series, and return at times of need) to capture patients during "teachable moments."
6. Build group cohesion activities into every group visit so that patients feel welcomed and connected to the group whether they are first-time attendees, regulars, or returning after a period of nonparticipation.
7. Develop relapse plans (or healthy lifestyle plans, diabetes management plans, etc.) during group visits, request that PCPs support these plans, and encourage patients to return to the group for making updates to plans.
8. Maximize opportunities to teach PCPs by creating groups aligned with their interests and using formats that involve their presence and direct participation.
9. Improve population penetration rates by embedding the group in a clinical pathway so that PCPs refer consistently to the group.
10. Make patient education handouts for groups that PCPs can also use in individual visits with patients.
11. Allow both PCP and patient self-referral to group services.
12. Avoid strict membership rules for the group or requiring lengthy screenings for new patients wishing to join a group.
13. If PCPs are not involved, use measurements or assessments (e.g., goal attainment self-ratings, quality of life ratings) in group visit chart notes so the PCP knows how the patient is progressing.
14. Consider forming classes that are PCP-specific (e.g., only patients from Dr. Brown's panel are invited) to encourage PCP participation and enhance PCP–patient relations.
15. Train a substitute for the BHC so groups can maintain a predictable, ongoing schedule unaffected by BHC absence.
16. Keep use of forms in groups to a minimum and assure that they serve an important purpose (such as facilitating communication between the patient and PCP and/or supporting patient efforts toward improved self-management).

17. Adapt group visits with couples and families by orienting patients to the educational (rather than therapeutic) nature of the visit, and establishing feasible educational goals for the visit.
18. If using a manual-based curriculum, condense content as needed so that the maximum number of contacts required for exposure to the full curriculum is no more than seven. Repeat the curriculum continuously and allow patients to drop in and out over time.

---

skills taught or experiences shared in previous week(s). Similarly, patient access usually stops after the first week or two because starting later means crucial information has been missed. Patients who drop out early may not ever get exposed to class curricula because classes are offered sporadically (and sometimes just once). Transferring the tradition of sequential classes into PC will severely limit the number of patients who access the group service and will have a negative impact on provider (PCP and BHC) productivity measures. It is not a format that is consistent with the PCBH mission.

Productivity standards are important for group encounters in PC because of the tremendous demand for individual encounters. In MH, groups may survive despite low attendance week after week because the MHP typically sees one patient per hour. A MH group lasting two hours may thus be justified as long as at least two or three clients attend. Obviously one would hope to have more than two or three clients attend, but from the standpoint of productivity nothing is lost if only two or three people attend. In PC, where a BHC might see four to six patients in two hours, one has a harder time continuing a group with low attendance. This is especially true for PC group visits that involve a PCP. Given the usual expectation for PCPs to see three to four patients per hour, a two-hour group would need a minimum of six to eight patients to justify the PCPs time (in simple productivity terms). If a BHC and PCP work together to deliver a two-hour group service the group size necessary might be as high as fourteen from a productivity standpoint (though one can argue that the long-term cost-savings of group visits potentially offsets the immediate, direct revenue lost).

So, how can BHCs offer groups or classes in PC in ways that maximize their use by patients? For starters, one must create inviting economic contingencies. As mentioned in Chapter 4, the Health and Behavior Codes series includes a code for classes or group services, 96153. The reimbursement rate suggested by Medicare for classes is $5.00 per fifteen minutes, while suggested rates for individual services are around $25.00 per fifteen minutes. This suggests that classes cost 80% less than services delivered in an individual format. This type of pricing will encourage patient access. While MH groups typically cost less than individual services, the percentage used for discounting in primary care may need to be even greater in order to bring in the large number of patients who can benefit.

The ideas of Advanced Access, which promote immediate access to care, can also help maximize group attendance. The ideal is a primary care group that is immediately accessible, available on an ongoing basis, and, when possible, supported by a clinical pathway. One of us (PR) offered a class simply called the Good Life Class in a PC clinic for years that met the first two of these criteria. PCPs could refer patients, or patients could self-refer. The group program included six classes offered on an ongoing basis, and patients could start participation during any of the six classes. It was a generic class, applicable to patients with a variety of problems. The following example of Ezra illustrates how open and immediate access to a group such as this can operate in PC. Ezra, a PC patient waiting in a pharmacy line, heard a medical assistant announce over the clinic public announcement system that the Good Life Class would be starting in five minutes in room 107. After picking up his prescription, he rushed into room 107 explaining, "I hope I am not too late. I was in the pharmacy line and I heard about the class. I think this is what I need help with—making my life good. May I stay?" In contrast to a structured ten- or sixteen-week class with closed membership after the first week or two and strict exclusion criteria, an open access policy assures that patients will not need to wait when desiring help. Placing announcements of group services around the clinic can help ensure that patients know of the offering and that PCPs are reminded to refer patients.

Groups in PC are even more accessible when their design allows for patients to participate sporadically (or consistently) for as long as desired. While MH groups tend to be time-limited (often returning patients to PC at the group's conclusion), PC groups need to serve patients perpetually. The longitudinal care design of PC demands this. Even patients who attend MH group treatment sometimes need more help later in PC (especially if the patient dropped out, failed to benefit or benefited minimally). Formats such as that of the Good Life Class allow patients to continue participation indefinitely and encourage completers to drop-in for support of relapse prevention plans as needed. The example of Sandra demonstrates how these features can work in PC. Sandra, a patient with a history of chronic depression, had participated in various specialty MH treatments including psychopharmacology regimens and manual-based cognitive behavioral group therapy. These somehow never seemed adequate for her, though. Sandra began the Good Life Class and continued through four 6-session, repeated series of the class. With each repetition of the series she strengthened her skill base and her connection to the class. She then declared herself improved and offered to serve as a volunteer in the class (distributing handouts, etc.).

Of course, one must think through strategies for building cohesion in groups where there is variation in membership from one meeting to the next. Group cohesion supports retention of patients in group services. We have found that having a welcoming routine, such as asking participants to introduce themselves by first name and to describe something (e.g., something that made them smile earlier that day, or that got them to class that day, etc.) helps veteran and new participants feel a part of the same group experience. A heavier, but potentially more powerful, option is to have members give their first name and a description of one strategy they have used to help with the problem/condition that brought them to the class. As an alternative to self-introductions, groups might start by having each member talk to the person beside him or her for two to three minutes and then introduce each other to the group (this is easier for some members than introducing themselves and helps develop relationships between members from the outset). Also important at the beginning of these classes is to provide a brief summary of the previous class and allow a brief check-in for returning participants to report results of homework activities.

Some classes in PC may be generic (i.e., not problem- or condition-specific). These classes have content that is easily applied and relevant to the growing group of patients who are learning to live with chronic diseases. Other classes may be more narrow in focus (i.e., diabetes- or depression-specific). Condition-specific classes offer instruction in self-management skills specific to the condition of concern.

Whether generic or problem-specific, groups should be as open as possible and avoid lengthy screening requirements for new patients who wish to join. One of us (JR) was recently expressing the mixture of amusement and frustration he felt when trying to help a patient access a trauma group offered by a nearby MH clinic. This was a free ten-week group and sounded like an excellent opportunity for JR's patient, who was uninsured. The patient was a non-English speaking refugee who had been severely traumatized during conflict in Azerbaijan years ago and was severely depressed and suicidal. Unfortunately, the following were the requirements for joining the group: trauma from a crime (war-related trauma was specifically excluded) or motor-vehicle accident or natural disaster; meets DSM criteria for PTSD (established via a required evaluation); no suicidal ideation; no substance abuse; English-speaking; no significant psychiatric co-morbidity. Not surprisingly, JR was told that the group was being delayed because they were having difficulty finding people to join. Rigid or extensive rules regarding group membership do not usually work well in MH and they certainly will not work well in PC.

Linking patients to group services through clinical pathways may also improve patient access. A clinical pathway identifies a target population and stipulates care processes related to that population. The point is to make certain aspects of a care plan routine, so that they are seamlessly and automatically integrated into care. An example of a simple clinical pathway program that links patients to group services might target obese children. The pathway could outline screening processes for obesity and state that any overweight children between the ages of six and ten and their families must be referred to a class that is co-taught by a dietician and a BHC. Patients would be dropped into an ongoing class that provides them with information about a healthy lifestyle and about behavioral technology needed to pursue lifestyle change over time. Embedding a group service in a pathway improves the consistency of referrals and naturally leads to opportunities for educating PCPs about BHC interventions.

PCP Training Opportunities. Group services offer many opportunities to pursue the PCBH mission of influencing PCP practice. Prospects for training range from minimal to extensive depending on the group model used, but this is ideal in that PCPs vary in their interests and their level of interest in any specific area. One PCP might be very interested in behavioral treatments for mood problems while another has a strong interest in behavioral treatments related to diabetes care. Similarly, some PCPs will enjoy being "on stage" in a group and will want to provide didactics, while others may simply prefer to join a group for a few minutes at the end.

A good strategy is to develop a variety of group services for a variety of problems and find innovative ways to get PCPs involved. For example, if the BHC is seeing a family for the third and final visit, the PCP might be invited to join the last five minutes to witness the family's commitment to using a specific problem-solving technique. In ongoing, generic life skills classes, BHCs may invite PCPs to sit in on a class (or part of it) offered at the end of the clinic day, if the PCP lacks the time or interest to attend on a regular basis. Even a brief showing can bolster patients' perceptions of the class and of PCP–BHC collaboration, and provides the PCP a sense of the group's benefit. Other group visit models (discussed later in this chapter) involve PCP participation during the entire visit, thus providing immense opportunities for training (and cross-training). BHCs can also influence PCPs by creating patient education handouts for group visits that are brief and practical. Many PCPs are eager to employ such tools in individual visits.

Adaptations for Family and Couple Visits

Modified formats for family visits are used in the PCBH model, and might include couples, a parent and child, two parents with multiple children, or multiple couples and families. Adjustments that allow for delivery of these services in the PCBH model include orienting patients to the educational (rather than therapeutic) nature of the visit, establishing feasible educational goals for the visit, and suggesting measures for evaluating goal attainment.

Of course, the goals for group visits with people related to each other need to be tailored to the specific referral issues. Goal(s) may be for a single consult or a series of consults, and examples include teaching a couple to apply the Caring Days procedure (Jacobson & Margolin, 1979) or reviewing a list of communication strategies to help the family improve relationships between an adolescent child and his or her parents. Handouts that support work toward the goal can be helpful (e.g., a handout summarizing common barriers to parent-adolescent communication, or describing the Caring Days procedure). Other examples of adapted interventions could include teaching a spouse to help her husband use the squeeze technique for premature ejaculation, educating family members about how to support a patient with diabetes, or helping a family in conflict increase the frequency of praise or positive collective experiences.

While one cannot hope to meet all the needs of all couples and families in PC group visits, more can certainly be accomplished than would normally be accomplished during a visit with the PCP. Quite often, families and couples can be taught skills by a BHC that they can use with future problems and PCPs can gain ideas about how to better interact with families in crisis. A BHC can help facilitate a referral to specialty services, if needed and possible, but should also offer educational interventions while patients await the specialty care. After the specialty care ends the BHC might also need to provide occasional support to patients as they continue to strive to apply skills learned.

Adapting Psychoeducational Materials for Primary Care Classes

As in specialty MH, psychoeducational group visits may be helpful to patients, and these, along with family and couple visits, are often easiest for the new BHC to integrate into practice. These simply require a space (large enough for a group of ten to twenty patients), a curriculum, a referral method, a plan for communicating with the PCP, and an enthusiastic BHC. Surveying PCPs to select the one or two populations that they perceive as most in need of a class is a good place to start. Needs will vary from clinic to clinic, but common groups of concern include obese patients and patients with chronic conditions. We offer specific examples below of psychoeducational formats that can be used with the all-too-common problem of obesity.

There are a variety of books and programs available to inspire development of group services for obese patients, but we mention two for illustration purposes. The Bienestar Health Program is a curriculum that offers a diabetes risk-factor prevention workbook designed for use with fourth grade Mexican–American children (Trevino et al., 1998). In research evaluating the effect of this program in a school environment (which is similar to PC in terms of constraints on how much care can be provided), the primary goals were to decrease two established risk factors for diabetes, namely overweight and dietary fats. Preliminary results suggested that the Bienestar Health Program significantly decreased dietary fat, increased fruit and vegetable servings, and increased diabetes health knowledge. Given that the workbook is provided in both Spanish and English and has wonderful illustrations, it is useful with parents with limited literacy in English and Spanish.

One of us (PR) is using this curriculum in a PC class in combination with behavioral parent training. To accomplish this, two to three chapters are covered in a single class instead of one (thus reducing the number of contacts required to get through the entire curriculum). Additionally, a skill-training component was added to enhance parenting skills related to lifestyle issues (in an effort to increase patient interest in the group). The behavioral skills training component includes modules that link to the lifestyle change curriculum. For example, the BHC invites parents and children to identify their values concerning health, along with the current discrepancies between their valued directions and their daily activities. Early in the class series, the BHC introduces the concept of modeling and helps the parents make behavioral plans to model specific healthy lifestyle behaviors. In later classes, parents learn to use positive reinforcement and differential reinforcement of other behaviors to shape healthy lifestyle behaviors in their children and to reduce or eliminate the use of high caloric, low nutrition foods as reinforcers.

For adult patients who are overweight or obese, the *LEARN Workbook* (Brownell, 2004) is a useful psychoeducational resource that JR uses in his clinic. Again, the highlights of two or three chapters can be combined into a single class (meaning the finer points of chapters will be sacrificed to capture the main points). Group members might select specific chapters as a focus for any given class. Members might vote, for example, to discuss chapters 1 to 3 or 9 to 10, based upon the interests of those present for that class. Obviously the BHC must have a thorough familiarity with the workbook in order to be this flexible, and must be prepared to talk on any of the chapters for each class. If this is not feasible, the option of having members select the topic can be omitted. Though participants are encouraged to purchase and follow the workbook, it is not necessary that they purchase it or read it prior to class. If possible, maintaining a collection of several copies of the workbook that can be loaned to participants during the group (not to be taken home) is helpful.

Table 12.2 provides an example of a class agenda using the LEARN curriculum adapted to fit the needs of PC. With flexible membership policies and no end dates, new members can be present on any given week (or veteran members can return after a long absence), while other attendees might have been present for several consecutive weeks or even months. Thus, each group includes material for newcomers and for returning members. For the former, a brief overview of the group and an introduction to basic concepts of weight management is covered. The latter group is indulged by a discussion of their progress toward goals. Both benefit from the forty-five-minute didactic topic, which is sure to reveal new information even to those who have heard it before. If all of the patients are from a particular PCP's panel, the PCP is always invited to stop in during the last fifteen minutes, even if just for a minute, to praise the participants for attending and show support for their efforts.

Remembering the Details

The less exciting, and sometimes deterring, aspect of conducting groups is getting them organized. Fortunately, if a group is successful it will often

Table 12.2. Agenda example for a primary care psychoeducational class

Weight management class: Wednesdays, 2:00–3:30 (leader: _____)

Time	Activity
2:00–2:20	• Introductions of leader(s) • Review of group visit structure and rules • Welcome routine (members talk with and then introduce neighbor) • Review of progress toward goals (for returning members)
2:20–2:30	• The basics of weight management (discussed each week, covers the concepts of calorie balance and lifestyle change)
2:30–3:15	• Specific didactic topic (differs each week; combines content from 2 or 3 LEARN chapters; members might choose topic)
3:15–3:30	• Individual goal-setting and wrap-up (including visit from PCP, if possible)

continue long enough that it becomes routine, but start-up is always a challenge. If a BHA is available, he or she can provide much of the organizational assistance, but if there is no BHA the BHC can ask the clinic manager to assign a staff person to help. Some clinics do have patient care coordinators whose job is to help precisely with activities such as groups.

One important start-up task is to locate and train a substitute to fill-in when the BHC is out of the clinic. This allows groups to be held on a predictable schedule (e.g., the third Tuesday of every month at 5:30), so members can develop a routine for attending and PCPs can develop a routine of referring patients. When a class is first beginning, or if attendance is waning, efforts to recruit participants may need to be stepped up. This can involve placing brochures and/or flyers around the clinic, sending announcements to select patients, reminding PCPs to refer, and even making phone calls to potential members. If a group is developed specifically for one PCP's panel that PCP will often offer to make some calls to patients as well. Blocking one's schedule for the group and locating and reserving space for the group is obviously also a must. If a clinic is tight on space, consider holding groups after regular clinic hours in the waiting area. Attendance is often better for evening groups than for daytime groups.

A final recommendation is to simplify forms used in PC groups and make sure that they are practical and necessary. The two forms that are perhaps most important are a homework planning form and a form for conveying plans to the PCP. The former might be more extensive, walking patients through the process of establishing a self-management goal, while the latter might be a simple one or two line summary of the goal(s). The summary can be placed in the chart (or dictated to the electronic medical record) by the BHC after the group.

PRIMARY CARE GROUP MODELS AND EXAMPLES

Assuming an understanding of the rationale for different models of group care in PC, we can now introduce some specific models in detail. Increasingly integrated clinics, acceptability of clinical pathways in the PC setting, and the growing pressure to adopt a different model of care for chronic conditions have all resulted in interest in innovative group visit models. Three well-known models designed for use in PC are the

Cooperative Health Care Clinic (CHCC), the Drop-In Group Medical Appointment (DIGMA), and the cluster visit. These models originated mostly in Kaiser-Permanente medical centers, and while their use has spread, the number of facilities currently using group visits (of any sort) is not known. Efforts to compare these types of PC group visit approaches with usual care suggest that the group visit approaches are superior on a number of indices (Beck et al., 1997; Sadur et al., 1999; Scott, Conner, Venohr, Gade, McKenzie et al., 2004). However, there are no randomized, controlled studies comparing one group model to another, and no controlled studies at all of group versus usual care approaches for some common problems (e.g., depression).

Because there is little empirical basis for choosing one group model over another for a given clinical condition, the BHC and his or her colleagues need simply to consider the clinic's resources and preferences when designing group visits. Most clinics seem to use some combination of the CHCC, DIGMA, or cluster visit models, making adjustments to meet their unique needs. It would probably be quite difficult to find two clinics using the exact same group care model in exactly the same way. We provide below a brief summary of each of these three common models, and then introduce versions that are or have been useful in our own work as BHCs. Additionally, we recommend visiting the website of the Robert Wood Johnson Foundation's Improving Chronic Illness Care (ICIC) project, www.improvingchroniccare.org. It is probably the most comprehensive source of information on the topic of group visits, and includes a helpful starter kit for those seeking practical advice.

The Cooperative Health Care Clinic (CHCC)

Credit for the CHCC model usually goes to Dr. John Scott, an internal medicine physician who wanted a more effective, sensitive, and cost-effective way of caring for his sizeable geriatric panel. The model he developed is detailed in Scott et al. (2004) and Beck et al. (1997). In the CHCC model, groups do not typically involve a psychologist or BHC. Instead, they are run by a PCP and nurse. Behavioral health and/or other specialists are invited to attend depending on the topic of planned discussion (if this was used in a clinic with a BHC the role of the BHC could likely be enhanced significantly). Patients are usually invited to participate if they utilize medical services frequently for one or more chronic conditions. Groups meet every month for ninety minutes and follow a consistent format:

- Warm-up (fifteen minutes; involved organized approaches using reminiscence therapy techniques at the beginning then became spontaneous over time)
- Education (thirty minutes; focused on a specific topic decided upon by the PCP or patients, and sometimes delivered by other members of the healthcare team)
- Caregiving (twenty minutes; nurse takes blood pressure and makes sure labs, immunizations, etc., are up to date; PCP attends to minor concerns and refills medications; participants not talking to the nurse or PCP simply socialize)
- Question and Answer (fifteen minutes; questions on any topic are taken)
- Planning (ten minutes; scheduling the next month's meeting and planning an educational topic)
- Individual Visits (PCP meets individually with patients as needed for five to ten minutes each)

Both Beck et al. (1997) and Scott et al. (2004) found significant advantages of the CHCC model compared to usual care. In the former, group participants had fewer emergency room visits, fewer visits to subspecialists, and a lower rate of repeat hospital admissions. They made more visits and calls to nurses than control group patients and fewer calls to physicians. In addition, group participants had greater overall satisfaction with care, and PCPs reported higher levels of satisfaction with the groups than with individual care. The cost of care per member per month was $14.79 less for the group participants. Results of the Scott et al. study were similar except that the cost savings amounted to $41.80.

The Drop In Group Medical Appointment (DIGMA)

The DIGMA approach is credited to Ed Noffsinger, PhD, a clinical psychologist who worked for Kaiser Permanente in California. It differs from the CHCC approach in a few ways. First, DIGMA groups are usually co-led by a PCP and behavioral provider (rather than a nurse) and meet weekly for ninety minutes. A medical assistant takes vitals and performs other functions (e.g., doing a foot check for a patient with diabetes) and a scheduler calls potential patients each week (identified by the PCP) to invite them to the group. DIGMA groups are open only to patients on the panel of the PCP leading the group, but in another point of departure from the CHCC model they are not limited to any particular subpopulation. In other words, attendees may be any age and come with any type of health problem (usually chronic problems). Recommended (and typical) attendance is ten to sixteen patients and three to six family members. Another difference from the CHCC model is that the group consists of different patients every week. Each patient accesses the group on a "drop-in" basis, usually after being told about it during an earlier visit with the PCP or when calling in for an appointment. The goal of DIGMA groups is to address the many commonalities patients have regarding their health, to provide enhanced patient education, and to allow the PCP to see many more patients than would be possible in individual visits.

The behavioral health professional in the DIGMA model introduces the group, manages group dynamics, addresses emotional and psychosocial issues, provides behavioral health evaluations and interventions, responds to any psychiatric emergencies, and helps keep the DIGMA running smoothly and on time. He or she runs the group alone when the PCP leaves for a brief individual visit with a patient. This might be necessary if a particularly confidential issue needs addressed or if equipment from another part of the clinic is needed. In general, DIGMA groups are designed to target patients whose significant psychosocial needs drive a lot of their care, so the presence of a BH provider is important.

Outcome evaluations of the DIGMA model, though less rigorous than those done for the other two types of approaches, have shown improved access to physicians, increased patient satisfaction and PCP job satisfaction, and reduced organizational costs (Noffsinger, 1999).

Cluster Visit Model

In the third group approach, called "cluster visits" (Sadur et al., 1999), groups are focused on patients with a particular condition. In the original Sadur et al. study, patients with diabetes were used in an approach titled the Diabetes Cooperative Care Clinic (DCCC). The study authors formed a multidisciplinary DCCC team consisting of a diabetes nurse educator (the team leader), dietitian, pharmacist, "behaviorist" (a psychologist), and two physicians with specialist expertise in diabetes. The team essentially took over diabetes care for the patients for six months, without direct involvement of any patient's actual PCP. Willing patients met monthly for two hours, during which a didactic topic was covered (the patients chose the topics they wanted covered), referrals were made as needed, and as needed basic diabetes education was provided (e.g., meter education for self-monitoring of blood glucose). The physicians did not meet routinely with individual patients during the groups, but were indirectly involved in monitoring and managing care via regular meetings with the nurse educator. They also examined patients during the group if necessary.

The behaviorist and dietitian met individually with patients on a referral basis. The behaviorist saw thirteen of the ninety-seven patients in the study group, for a total of one to four visits (the length of the visits was not specified in the paper) but also helped with other aspects of managing the group, such as helping transition patients back to their original PCPs at study's end. (Probably he also delivered some of the didactics, though this was not specified in the paper.) The pharmacist reviewed medication profiles and educated patients as needed, and a medical assistant collected vitals and helped with clerical needs. Groups were moderately sized, with ten to eighteen in attendance at a given meeting.

The results of the Sadur et al. (1999) study were encouraging, showing significant advantages to those enrolled in the DCCC intervention compared to patients provided usual primary care (with their usual PCPs). Specifically, group patients showed improved glycemic control, greater self-efficacy, and higher satisfaction with care, as well as reduced healthcare utilization after the six-month group ended.

Home-Grown Approaches

As mentioned earlier, there are as many varieties of group approaches as there are clinics. Even the developers of these three well-known approaches acknowledge that clinics that use their approaches do so in a distinctive, individualized fashion. Thus, having provided the reader with an understanding of how and why groups are different in primary care and of the most commonly referred to approaches, we now offer descriptions of the models we know best—our own! Some of these derive directly from the models just described, while others deviate. Our hope is that in providing a diverse array of approaches readers will begin to get a sense for what might work in their own clinics.

The Hybrid: One Model for Many Conditions. A hybrid model developed at JR's clinic contains features of the CHCC and DIGMA models and has been used with depression, diabetes, and attention deficit hyperactivity disorder (ADHD). In this model, group visits are 90 to 120 minutes in length, and the BHC and PCP provide the service together. A third staff member, often an office assistant, oversees the logistics of the group (e.g., scheduling patients, providing them with reminder calls, reserving space for the visit, blocking providers' schedules, etc.), and for some groups a nurse or medical assistant takes vitals. Each group serves a specific PCP's patients, so on any given day there may be different groups with the same topic but with patients from different panels. For example, depression group visits might occur on Mondays for Dr. Chau's patients and Dr. Monahan's patients and on Thursdays for Dr. Ricking's patients. In the same week there may be group visits for other chronic problems, such as a Tuesday ADHD group for Dr. Heisey's patients and a Friday diabetes group for patients of Dr. Walsh. For most problems, an intensive scrics of visits (e.g., once a week for four weeks) allows for focused skill instruction, which can then be supported by a less intensive maintenance schedule (e.g., once a month or a quarter). The intensive visits are repeated annually or at some other regularly occurring interval. The groups run indefinitely on this schedule, continuously adding new patients while losing others.

The content of hybrid group visits usually includes a brief welcome by the PCP, followed by an interactive didactic talk by the BHC, and ending with an open-ended question-and-answer session facilitated by the BHC. During the question-and-answer session, the PCP huddles briefly, away from the rest of the group, with patients who need medication refills or alterations. These individual huddles are a crucial component because they allow patients to attend the group in place of a normal individual visit. However, they are kept brief and limited in content to the problem that is the focus for the group visit. For example, patients do not receive treatment for a sinus infection during a depression group visit.

During the didactic portion, the BHC usually teaches a self-management strategy, and the topic varies from visit to visit. For example, ADHD group visit topics might include effective use of Time-Out, development of reward plans, and/or ways to improve basic organizational and study skills. Depression group visits might include talks on behavioral activation, problem solving, and assertiveness. Different topics are discussed at every group visit. A good rule of thumb for didactics is to limit them to the basic information a patient might normally get during an individual BHC visit. If research and trips to the library are needed to put together the didactic portion, the talk is likely to become unnecessarily detailed and cumbersome.

Clearly, in this model, the BHC does the bulk of the work during the visit, but the presence of the PCP is equally vital. By attending the entire visit, the PCP not only learns behavioral techniques but also sends the message to patients that these techniques are valid and important. We have noticed that many providers begin to talk with patients about behavioral strategies once they have been introduced to them in the class, and patients often bring such topics up during subsequent PCP visits. Additionally, by spending an entire 1.5 or 2 hours in the group with patients, the PCP gets to know each patient better and vice-versa. In our clinic, both patients and providers greatly appreciate the relationship-building qualities of the group visit.

For providers, one of the most attractive features of the group visit is the ability to use the group for problem-solving. Unlike the individual visit with the PCP, there is time to explore issues in greater detail. Group members provide support and ideas for coping, which are often different from those offered by the PCP and BHC. One of the PCPs in our clinic described her pleasant surprise at this aspect of the group visit after the conclusion of one of the first ADHD groups. She had been apprehensive about the idea of brief individual medication visits with patients during the group, fearing this would put her behind in her schedule. She anticipated that patients would bring up complex psychosocial issues rather than staying with basic medication management issues. In the first huddle, her worst fear was validated when a patient's mother asked for advice on a difficult situation at the patient's school. However, before the PCP even began to answer, the mother stopped her and said, "You know, maybe I should just bring this up for discussion in the group. I'll bet someone else has had a similar problem." The PCP happily agreed and quickly realized that the group could provide more support and ideas on this issue than she.

For the BHC as well these group visits can be a boon. Patients who might otherwise never have been referred have the opportunity to become familiar with the BHC and with typical BHC interventions during the group visit. At our clinic, attendance ranges from five to twenty patients per group, thus ensuring a healthy patient count even at the low end of the range. At times, patients in these groups initiate an individual consult with the BHC to resolve a particularly difficult problem, thus circumventing the need for a referral from the PCP. The robust patient count provided by group visits is also very appealing to PCPs. Most PCPs need to see at least three patients per hour, and PCPs sometimes feel pressured to meet this goal, given the complexity of many of these patients. With attendance ranging from five to twenty, group visits are providing PCPs with higher productivity figures yet with little labor intensity. As this example shows, group visits often allow BHCs and PCPs to "work smarter, rather than harder."

The Generic Approach: The Living Life Well Class. For a clinic with a low ratio of BHC hours to PCP patients, a generic class might be used to address the needs of many if not most referred patients. One of us (PR) once worked in a PC clinic that included over a dozen PCPs and a single BHC who had only eight hours per week of clinic time. To implement the PCBH model in this context, a generic class was used with a format capable of accepting almost any PC patient at any time. Program content included chapters from the book, *Living Life Well: New Strategies for Hard Times* (Robinson, 1996), which are supported by a treatment manual for BHCs and PCPs (Robinson et al., 1996). The content for every class was based on one of the seven chapters, and the series repeated and thus provided ongoing group services. Table 12.3 provides a description of the class content. Many of the adaptations suggested in Table 12.1 were made in this group program.

The curriculum in *Living Life Well: New Strategies for Hard Times* is based on that used in one of the first studies to evaluate the impact of using brief cognitive behavioral interventions in combination with psychopharmacological treatments with depressed PC patients. Results suggested that use of the curriculum described in the book (in a series of

Table 12.3. A generic PCBH class: the Living Life Well class

Class/chapter	Topic	Critical concepts
One	Hoping/planning/doing	• Ongoing self-assessment is important. • Suffering is a biopsychosocial experience. • Hopefulness will improve. • Complete a behavior change form.
Two	Building acceptance and making value-based choices	• Psychological acceptance helps a person stop avoiding uncomfortable thoughts, feelings, etc. and start choosing a course of committed action. • People feel most vital when their behavior reflects what is most important to them.
Three	Appreciating your mind and body	• Practice improves skills for being aware of the mind–body. • People can create sensations of well-being by working with the mind–body. • Psychological neoteny improves health.
Four	Solving problems	• There are four necessary elements for personal change. • Self-efficacy is the belief that one can cope effectively. • Solutions do not always relate directly to problems. • Always evaluate results of problem solving efforts.
Five	Responding to interpersonal conflict	• The only way to avoid conflict is to avoid people. • One can learn to stay in touch with one's body–mind during conflict … and choose actions.

Continued

Table 12.3.—*Cont'd*

Class/chapter	Topic	Critical concepts
Six	Expressing yourself	• "Driven doing" is an avoidance strategy that takes a lot of energy and gives little back. • Acceptance is a form of validation. • "Not doing" allows time for personal assertion and creative expression, which restore health.
Seven	Continuing to live life well, planning your lifestyle	• What concepts from class are useful now? How? • Develop a plan for staying in touch with the mind–body. • Anticipate and plan for stressful times. • Associate with people you trust. • Know your values and live them.

four to six visits, not seven) with a BHC was associated with better clinical outcomes for patients and greater PCP satisfaction than usual primary care (Katon et al., 1996). When implemented individually with PC patients, over 90 percent attended at least four visits and rated the program very positively.

A Community for Aging Well: The Group Care Clinic. This program developed at an HMO in Seattle (Group Health Cooperative) in a clinic that served a large number of older patients with multiple medical problems and limited social support. A PCP and his nurse came to the BHC (PR) and asked for collaboration in developing a program similar in form and content to the CHCC developed in Denver (see the above and Beck et al., 1997). Unlike the Denver group, the Seattle group service expanded the provider team to include a BHC and a clinical pharmacist. The Group Health dissemination model was called the "Group Care Clinic." The nurse played the central role in coordinating care to patients assigned to the Group Care Clinic, while the BHC facilitated group visits (which included a "Behavioral Health Hour"), and the physician and clinical pharmacist provided brief updates and answered questions (Robinson, Del Vento, & Wischman, 1998).

In starting the program, the nurse sent invitations to twenty-four patients and nineteen of twenty-four (79 percent) agreed to participate. They ranged in age from seventy-one to eighty-nine and included seven males and twelve females. A chart review of the initial group of participants suggested that 70 percent had seen multiple specialty physicians in the past year, 50 percent had depression or dysthymia noted in their medical chart problem list, and 30 percent had no advance physician directive concerning end-of-life issues recorded in the medical chart. In preparation for the first class, the nurse prepared individualized packets of health care materials for each patient, which were called Patient Medical Diaries. The team defined the objectives for the Group Care Clinic, which are listed in Table 12.4.

The inclusion of a BHC probably improved the CHCC model experience in Seattle in several ways. First, the time commitment was less extensive for the PCP, and he was able to pull out patients as needed for in-room exams after the nurse completed vitals in the group setting during the initial fifteen or twenty minutes of the class. BHC attention to group process factors probably supported development of group cohesion and retention of patients (as no one dropped out over a four-year period). For example, the group agreed to have partners with whom they checked-in once between groups and again at the beginning of each group meeting; to celebrate birthdays together; to have tea as a part of

Table 12.4. Objectives of the group care clinic

1. Provide phone and clinic visits needed to address the care needs of chronically ill, older patients.
2. Make interventions in the group care context to prevent escalations in health problems that would result in delivery of more intensive services.
3. Build cohesion among group participants and facilitate actions among members to improve quality of daily life.
4. Teach specific skills for coping with medical and behavioral health challenges confronting patients.
5. Enlist patients as partners in updating medical diaries and determining Group Care Clinic norms.
6. Increase provider satisfaction in working with complex patients for whom there are no predictable protocols for resolving illness.

every class, and to have presentations by group members. All of these activities combined to increase patients' sense of identification with the group as a community.

The typical group meeting agenda included time for partner check-ins, self-assessment and vitals, updates to medical diaries and charts, a brief talk by the PCP (and/or clinical pharmacist), a time to pose questions to the PCP, tea and a presentation by a patient (often on a hobby or special interest), a behavioral health presentation by the BHC, and updates from the nurse. At least every other month, the class invited a guest speaker, such as a hearing specialist or physical therapist. The presence of the BHC probably also helped adjust the curriculum to different phases of the group's life, which in the Seattle project spanned four years. When the group lost its first member, the BHC encouraged group members to develop norms for observing the death of a member, as well as a process to guide the addition of new members. Group Care Clinic outcomes suggested that the program met its objectives. We encourage BHCs in clinics with a large number of older patients to seriously consider a group approach. The behavioral health curriculum used in the Seattle program is available to help with this (see Robinson et al., 1998).

A Class at the Heart of a Pathway: The Pain and Quality of Life Program. A group visit model that is currently proving useful in PR's clinic is embedded in a clinical pathway program for patients with chronic pain. The program is called the "Pain and Quality of Life" Program. Patient involvement in the pathway begins when the PCP asks a patient to sign an agreement concerning participation. This agreement defines roles and responsibilities for the patient, PCP, and BHC. After signing the agreement, the patient comes for an individual consultation with the BHC for further orientation, including an introduction to the monthly class. The PC nurse works with PCPs in preparing prescriptions for distribution at the end of the monthly class, and patients must attend the class to receive their prescription. At the beginning of each class, the BHC helps patients complete a measure of health-related quality of life and then provides instruction in various strategies for pursuing behavior changes consistent with patient values. At the conclusion of the class, the BHC charts patient scores and briefly summarizes patient behavior change plans, so that the PCP is able to support these in medical visits.

When a patient fails to come to the class (and did not call to make a plan prior to missing the class) or violates any other term of the agreement, he or she enters a Three Strikes program, which spans a two-month period and requires the patient to come for two individual monthly consultation visits with the BHC in addition to the group visit. The purpose of these visits is to address barriers to meeting the terms of the agreement. Violation of any term of the agreement during the two-month period in the Three Strikes program constitutes a strike (e.g., missing an appointment with their PCP or failing to show for a requested urine screen). Patients who are able to stay under three strikes during the two-month term in the Three Strikes program return to the usual program, but PCPs stop narcotic pain medications for those who do not.

The Pain and Quality of Life Program is popular with PCPs and patients. Nurses and PCPs feel that their interactions with patients are improving, and they often remark that they have relatively few conflicts with patients about medications on the telephone or in clinic visits. PCPs like having health-related quality of life scores to use in assessing their treatment plan and making updates. They also like learning about behavioral strategies used in the class. The BHC is using the Bull's Eye technique (Fortrin, Robinson, & Walsh, in preparation; Ludgren & Robinson, in preparation) to support ongoing value-driven behavior change efforts for patients in the class, and PCPs are learning this technique in professional detailing sessions with the BHC (see Chapter 10 for example of using the Bull's Eye Prescription pad). The approach is an example of a pathway program that spans the entire range of care opportunities in the PC setting, as it also addresses identification of patients who are at risk for development of chronic pain and specifies interventions to increase their hardiness. Similar approaches to behavior change are used for both prevention and intervention, which makes it easier for PCPs to learn and reinforce the approaches.

Patients like the Pain and Quality of Life Class program because of its holistic approach and its effort to address their needs for convenient, prompt service. The program serves a wide range of patients, some of whom are not taking pain medications and come solely to learn behavioral strategies. While some patients stop using pain medications as they learn effective behavioral strategies for living well with pain, others appreciate the one-stop shopping feature of the program and often find that the addition of behavioral strategies improves their ability to live meaningful lives.

SUGGESTIONS FOR STARTING GROUP SERVICES

The plan that a BHC makes for starting group services needs to reflect the needs of the clinic and its resources. Small clinics may differ from large clinics in both areas. We recommend that the BHC partner with PCPs in forging a start that generates enthusiasm for group services and build from there. Primary care clinics are structured historically to support delivery of individual services, so addressing the logistics of providing group services will require effort and support from a broad base. Additionally, PCPs, like BHCs, have habits and routines that help them to survive the frenetic atmosphere of the clinic, and they can be understandably wary of altering those to try something for which operational support is undeveloped. Many also have fears that are ultimately unfounded. The following list is typical, and so that the BHC can be prepared to answer concerns we include more realistic responses in parentheses:

- "I'm too busy to start a group!" (The truth is that groups allow PCPs to work smarter rather than harder, and most of the legwork is done by others.)
- "I'm not comfortable delivering medical care in a group." (Some PCPs have social anxiety that makes groups difficult, while others have concerns about confidentiality and yet others are simply anxious about breaking habits they have honed over the years in individual visits. Ultimately, groups are not for everyone, but try to discern the exact reason for the discomfort and discuss it. Many will find they like groups better than individual visits once they begin.)
- "I still need individual appointments with my patients." (True, but many high-utilizing, high-need patients can be captured in a group, which will ultimately save time. Studies of the CHCC and Cluster models suggest they help avert emergency care, as well, meaning individual visits may be less complicated.)
- "I'm concerned about confidentiality." (Some groups ask patients to sign special confidentiality waivers. Others simply review strict confidentiality rules with the group. Very rarely do patients express concern about this.)
- "What if I attract more patients because they want the group?" (This actually could happen. However, if most or all PCPs are doing groups,

this is less likely. If it is a major concern, suggest a small-scale pilot to test the PCP's fears.)

The first step to implementing group visits may be to provide a presentation on group visits (and models for group medical visits in particular) at a provider meeting. This will help the BHC find an interested provider (there will always be at least one daring soul!). A successful group experience with that provider will often break down resistance from other providers. Another strategy for starting group services in clinics that track care for patients with chronic conditions (e.g., diabetes) is to review patient outcomes with each doctor and to suggest group visits as a strategy for improving care. If Dr. Smith's patients are having trouble maintaining healthy LDL cholesterol levels, she may be interested in partnering with the BHC to deliver a group visit that focuses on behavior change strategies for improving cholesterol. Rarely will all PCPs in a clinic agree to start group visits. However, with persistence the number of PCPs who recognize and support group visits will likely grow over time.

SUMMARY

1. Traditional MH groups and classes are not used in PC. However, traditional formats may be adapted to better fit the PC environment. There are two central reasons for doing groups—access enhancement and improved opportunities to influence PCPs.

2. Seeing more than one patient at a time in primary care can mean using group medical visits, adapted psychoeducational classes, family visits, or conjoint couple visits.

3. An adjusted approach is also needed for couple and family visits in the PCBH model. Still, a great deal may be accomplished when the BHC frames the consultation as an opportunity to discover and implement an educational intervention to improve the day-to-day functioning of the couple or family.

4. Psychoeducational classes offer the BHC an opportunity to provide more in-depth skill training for PC patients. However, to fit the PC setting, sequenced programs must be transformed into stand-alone offerings and rules for membership in the group must be minimal.

5. The three best known group medical visit models for use in primary care are the Cooperative Health Care Clinic (CHCC), Drop-In Group

Medical Appointment (DIGMA), and Cluster visit models. However, there is no clear empirical support for using one over another and most clinics use their own "spin-off" version of one of these.

6. The Group Care Clinic approach is an example of a CHCC spin-off that involves a BHC. It can be quite useful in PC clinics that serve large numbers of older adults. This approach allows the BHC, PCP, and nurse (and in some settings a clinical pharmacist) to become members of an ongoing health care community that exists to help patients maintain health, manage disease, and die with dignity.

7. The Hybrid CHCC/DIGMA model can be applied to a variety of chronic conditions and places didactics from the BHC at the fore. In this model, groups are co-led by the BHC and PCP. Both PCPs and patients give very positive feedback about this model.

8. The Pain and Quality of Life program is an example of a pathway that incorporates a class. PCPs will welcome BHCs that help them provide a structure such as this to address the high impact of patients with chronic pain, particularly those that become dependent on narcotic medication. This program puts functioning at the top of the list and supports the creation of a meaningful relationship between PCPs and some of their least satisfied patients.

9. As exciting as the highly integrated group services described in this chapter may sound, they are often hard to sell initially and can prove to be logistical challenges. Scheduling the personnel to participate, advertising, and/or recruiting for the group, procuring space and resources, and other requirements can stymie even the most eager of BHCs. However, once they become routine they typically run more smoothly, and in the meantime other adaptations such as those involved with couple, family, and psychoeducational classes can be made quickly and with few barriers. Once begun, group visits typically win proponents.

PART VI

UNCHARTED TERRITORY

Margaret Chase Smith suggested that "When people keep telling you that you can't do a thing, you kind of like to try it," and this captures the pioneering spirit that keeps the PCBH model alive and growing. As with any new field, BHCs will discover (and address) numerous obstacles (and self-conscious moments), and there's no way to anticipate and prepare for all of them. In Chapter 13, we share with readers what we have learned from our puzzled and embarrassing moments thus far. Befuddled moments in BHC practice have led us to search out a meaningful response for the all-too-common problems of dependence and abuse of prescription drugs; develop strategies for hanging in there with providers that lean toward the biomedical perspective, and formulate a structure for responding to various psychiatric emergencies. In Chapter 14, we provide case examples as a way of introducing the more common ethical issues encountered by new BHCs. Chapter 15, the final chapter, provides guidance for evaluating the PCBH model and BHC services. This is an important section, and one that the BHC will want to read to prepare for successful exploration of unfamiliar territory.

13

CHALLENGING MOMENTS

"Not failure, but low aim, is sin."
— Mary Frances Berry at the College of Wooster (OH)
commencement, 1987

Reflecting on our time in specialty MH, we both can recall many diffi-cult situations. Every MH provider has gone to bed worried about a possibly suicidal patient, felt frustrated with patients who demand a lot of time but never seem to improve, or struggled through a conflict with a col-league. Indeed, every job comes with its own stresses, and BHC work is no different. However, the BHC who has worked in specialty MH will face some very different challenges in PC. In some cases problems occur that are unique to the PC setting, while in other cases the PC work will require a different approach to a problem that might also be encountered in MH.

In this chapter we provide ideas for handling some of the most com-mon problems in each of these categories. We start with a discussion of prescription drug abuse, which is an ubiquitous, corrosive, and—without exaggeration—enormous problem in PC (especially community health care). Quite a bit of space is devoted to this topic because of the signifi-cance of the problem and because most new BHCs will lack (but need) a thorough understanding of the issues involved. Next will be an introduc-tion to the "biomedical" provider, i.e., those PCPs who show little interest in the psychosocial component of patient care and can be difficult for a BHC to engage. We devote significant space to this topic as well, because every clinic will have at least one biomedical provider and it can prove frustrating for a BHC. Following that section will be shorter sections discussing tips for handling psychiatric emergencies in the busy PC setting, managing patients who don't improve, helping PCPs who want a diagnostic workup on a patient, and responding to patients who ask for more than the BHC can or should provide.

We certainly don't have all of the answers for these problems, and indeed we often still struggle with them in our own clinics. What this chapter hopefully can offer readers is at least an improved awareness and understanding of challenges they will face, along with some suggestions for confronting them. Sometimes these suggestions will help and sometimes they won't, but to paraphrase the advice from Mary Frances Berry that introduced this chapter, trying nothing will be worse than trying something.

PRESCRIPTION MEDICATION MISUSE AND DEPENDENCE

The typical BHC is not a prescriber and as such he or she usually (before working in PC) has probably only been on the periphery of decisions about medications. He or she might have called a patient's physician to voice concern about potential medication abuse, or referred the occasional patient to drug treatment. However, once in the PC setting, the BHC will become intimately and frequently involved in managing patients who abuse medications. This can easily become the most challenging of a BHC's challenging moments.

A typical problem scenario is that of Terri, a forty-year-old female patient at the clinic of one of the authors. For several years Terri complained of chronic back pain and was managed with narcotic analgesics, among other medicines. She also complained of depression and anxiety and was prescribed several antidepressants for this. Terri maintained a relationship with her PCP whom she trusted, and she generally followed-up well with appointments. Because of this relationship the PCP was willing to continue narcotic medications for pain relief, even though Terri's functioning was not improving. She spent a great deal of time in bed and had not been employed regularly for several years and generally had a great deal of stress in her life. Additionally, she continued to complain frequently of pain, despite the narcotic analgesics.

The PCP felt somewhat guilty about Terri's lack of improvement and was sympathetic to her pain complaints. If the PCP broached the topic of stopping her narcotic medications, Terri expressed great resistance and insisted that she would be even worse off without them. The PCP certainly did not want to cause more stress in Terri's life. Additionally, the PCP of course had limited time for clinic visits, and had other of Terri's health issues to address during the visits. Thus, the PCP got into the habit of simply refilling the narcotics rather than struggling over discontinuing them. On several occasions Terri called to insist on an urgent, same-day visit with her PCP because her medication had been lost or stolen or because she needed an early refill (prescriptions were generally written for one month at a time). Staff and the PCP were disinclined to allow a same-day visit for this, but Terri would plead and be very insistent over the phone. Eventually, not wanting to spend more time in conflict, the PCP would often agree to let Terri come in (squeezing her in between scheduled patients, thereby cramping time with those patients). Despite being highly suspicious of the need for an early refill, the PCP on the first occasion opted to refill them rather than tussle further over the issue. However, on subsequent instances, the PCP refused the early refill, which resulted in loud and tearful protest by Terri toward the PCP, her medical assistant, and other staff (often in front of other patients in the waiting area).

Over time Terri did begin to improve as her PCP helped her to accomplish some functional goals that improved her self-efficacy. However, after a few years Terri's PCP left the practice and Terri had to follow-up with other PCPs who did not know her. This was stressful for Terri, who expressed to the BHC her concern that they would not refill her narcotics. Indeed, lacking the relationship Terri had with her previous PCP, the subsequent PCPs she saw usually revisited the idea of discontinuing the narcotics. This always resulted in fervent protest from Terri, as well as more frequent clinic visits during which she displayed rather dramatic pain behavior that staff viewed as manipulative. Although Terri's narcotics were generally refilled each month, the frequency of conflicts with staff rose sharply, and her functioning deteriorated again.

The case of Terri exemplifies a number of reasons that many PCPs loathe prescribing medications that can be habit-forming. Terri was likely abusing the medications. She was using them sometimes in greater quantities than prescribed (e.g., when she requested early refills), and on more than one occasion claimed they had been last or stolen. Special accommodations needed to be made when she complained of acute pain or needed an early refill, and staff often struggled with Terri on other occasions about this as well. The PCP did not feel good about continuing the prescriptions, yet found it very difficult to stop them. And, despite all of this commotion, the medications had no apparent positive effect on Terri's functioning. In fact, her functioning deteriorated when there was a change in PCPs and less consistent support of her efforts to change behavior.

Cases such as Terri's are unfortunately all too common in PC. They can exact a great deal of strain on the system and inject conflict into the patient–provider relationship. They also provoke suspicion of other patients who use similar medications, even though these patients may be using them legitimately and therapeutically. A certain amount of distrust often develops among PCPs toward patients requesting habit-forming medications. After all, physicians, like anyone else, do not enjoy being duped.

A BHC can offer a great deal to the management of patients such as Terri who abuse prescription medications in PC. In this section, we review characteristics of the most commonly abused medications and discuss strategies a BHC can suggest to combat this problem. The reader should note that, while abuse of some prescription medications is a significant public health concern and a disruptive phenomenon in PC clinics, most experts agree that the majority of patients prescribed these medications use them appropriately and safely. Many patients benefit from the same medications that others abuse, and PC staff need to resist the temptation to label all patients that seek these medications as "drug-seeking."

Narcotics, Depressants, and Stimulants ... Oh, My!

Three classes of medications comprise the list that many PCPs prefer to avoid prescribing. These include narcotic analgesics (a.k.a. opioids), central nervous system (CNS) depressants (including barbiturates and benzodiazepines) and psychostimulants. Table 13.1 displays the generic and brand names of the most commonly encountered medications in each of these categories, along with the most common clinical uses and consequences of each. This table is adapted from one available at the website of the National Institute on Drug Abuse (NIDA, 2005), which is a good

Table 13.1. Common prescription drugs with abuse potential

Opioids	CNS depressants	Stimulants
Oxycodone (Percodan, Percocet, Oxycontin)	BARBITURATES	Dextroamphetamine (Dexedrine, Adderall) Methylphenidate (Ritalin, Concerta)
Propoxyphene (Darvon)	Mephobarbital (Mebaral)	Sibutramine hydrochloride monohydrate (Meridia)
Hydrocodone (Lortab, Vicodin)	Pentobarbital sodium (Nembutal)	
Hydromorphone (Dilaudid)		
Meperidine (Demerol)	BENZODIAZEPINES	
Diphenoxylate (Lomotil)	Diazepam (Valium)	
Codeine	Chlordiazepoxide hydrochloride (Librium)	
Fentanyl		
Methadone (Dolophine)	Alprazolam (Xanax)	
Morphine (Roxanol)	Triazolam (Halcion)	
Morphine sulfate, Controlled release (MS Contin)	Estazolam (ProSom)	
	Clonazepam (Klonopin)	
	Flurazepam (Dalmane)	
	Lorazepam (Ativan)	
	Temazepam (Restoril)	
Generally prescribed for:	Generally prescribed for:	Generally prescribed for:
Postsurgical pain relief	Anxiety	Narcolepsy
Management of acute or chronic pain	Tension	Attention-deficit hyperactivity disorder (ADHD)
Relief of coughs and diarrhea	Panic attacks	
	Acute stress reactions	Depression that does not respond to other treatment
	Sleep disorders	
	Anesthesia (at high doses)	Short-term treatment of obesity
		Asthma
Effects of long-term use	Effects of long-term use	Effects of long-term use

Continued

Table 13.1.—*Cont'd*

Opioids	CNS depressants	Stimulants
Potential for tolerance, withdrawal, abuse and/or dependence	Potential for tolerance, withdrawal, abuse and/or dependence	Potential for abuse and dependence
Possible negative effects	Possible negative effects	Possible negative effects
Severe respiratory depression or death following a large single dose	Seizures following a rebound in brain activity after reducing or discontinuing use	Dangerously high body temperatures or an irregular heartbeat after taking high doses; Cardiovascular failure or lethal seizures; For some stimulants, hostility or feelings of paranoia after taking high doses repeatedly over a short period of time
Should not be used with	Should not be used with	Should not be used with
Other substances that cause CNS depression, including: Alcohol Antihistamines Barbiturates Benzodiazepines General anesthetics	Other substances that cause CNS depression, including: Alcohol Prescription opioids Some over-the-counter cold and allergy meds	Over-the-counter cold medicines containing decongestants; Antidepressants, unless supervised by a physician; Some asthma medications

source of information on this topic, as well as from a thorough review article by Weaver, Jarvis, and Schnoll (1999).

As suggested earlier, concerns about the use of these medicines are many and varied. First, concern exists about iatrogenic effects and public health issues. Physicians often worry about the potential for "addiction" (i.e., "substance dependence" in DSM-IV terminology) with these medicines. A patient who develops dependence on a medication has developed a new health problem in addition to whatever the medicine was being prescribed for, thus violating the physician's important medical ethic of "doing no harm." Additionally, in this scenario more work is created for an already busy health care system, as it must manage the newly created substance dependent patient. Prescribers also worry about "misuse" of these medicines, as for example when a patient uses the medicine for recreational rather than for medical purposes. Some patients "divert" their medicines to others for this exact purpose, meaning they sell them on the street or give them away for recreational/nonmedical use by others.

Diversion and misuse raise concerns among physicians about criminal liability and licensing matters, in addition to the public health concerns. Some high-profile criminal charges have been made against physicians following Oxycontin overdose deaths, including at least one conviction (Meier, 2002; Mishra, 2001), which of course fuels physician anxiety. The Drug Enforcement Administration (DEA) also worries prescribers with threats of investigative or punitive actions outside of those threatened by the criminal court system. Surveys of physicians suggest that fear of DEA investigation is one of the most frequently cited deterrents to opioid prescribing (Clark & Sees, 1993; Olsen & Daumit, 2004).

In the background of all of these concerns is the reality that most PCPs have very little foundation and support regarding the treatment of conditions for which habit-forming medications are prescribed. Olsen and Daumit (2004), in a helpful summary of the problems surrounding opioid prescribing, explain that much of the frustration physicians feel when treating patients with chronic nonmalignant pain stems from a lack of knowledge about how to handle these patients. Such a situation can be very frustrating for a person who genuinely desires to help. Olsen and Daumit (2004) note that medical school and residency curricula and continuing medical education regarding chronic pain are "sorely lacking" (p. 142). They further note that PCPs often have little specialty back-up to guide them and as a result are often left to conjecture about treatment options. No clear guidelines exist to help providers make treatment decisions, and medical boards vary from state to state in their opioid prescribing philosophies. Although Olsen and Daumit (2004) focus on opioid prescribing, the picture is much the same for the CNS depressants and the psychostimulants. It is a messy situation, indeed.

On top of all this, serious questions remain regarding the effectiveness of these medications. Find virtually any PC clinic and you will also find a multitude of patients on chronic narcotic, benzodiazepine, or stimulant regimens without any clear improvement in functioning. Many studies have suggested that improvement in long-term social and occupational functioning for chronic noncancer pain patients remains elusive even when pain is controlled (Portenoy & Foley, 1986; Savage, 1996), and surveys of physicians support that impression (Turk, 1996). Prescribing narcotic medications for use "as needed" for pain flare-ups might even worsen a chronic pain syndrome because the pleasant effects of the medication become a reward for the increased pain behavior (Fordyce, 1976). Psychostimulants are also a concern for PCPs. Although the effectiveness of stimulants for children with attention deficit hyperactivity disorder (ADHD) is well established, their effectiveness with adults is less clear. To date, just twelve randomized, controlled studies have been conducted on the treatment of ADHD in adults, even including unpublished conference presentations (Wilens, 2003). As noted by Dodson (2005), these studies have shown variable results and none have looked at long-term outcome (i.e., longer than six months). As a result, many providers feel comfortable prescribing stimulants for children but not for adults. The use of benzodiazepines for anxiety is also controversial. Clearly, they may play a role in managing acute anxiety, as in the case of a person who is profoundly distressed in response to a recent stressor, but they have not been shown to be effective long-term treatments for anxiety disorders. Nonetheless, patients are commonly kept on benzodiazepines for long periods by providers who feel they have no other options.

The Extent of Abuse and Misuse Problems

Physicians have good reason to be concerned about abuse/dependence, misuse, and diversion issues. According to the NIDA (2005), prescription drug abuse/misuse has risen sharply in recent years. They cite increases of 181 percent, 132 percent, 90 percent, and 165 percent in the nonmedical use of opioids, tranquilizers, sedatives, and stimulants, respectively, during the 1990s. Overall, approximately 2 percent of the population reports nonmedical use, which is a disconcerting but not staggering percentage. However, this figure includes a particularly pronounced increase among twelve- to seventeen-year-olds and eighteen- to twenty-five-year-olds, which is more unsettling.

Medication misuse and dependence problems appear to be more common among certain medical patient groups than among the general population, though data can be difficult to come by and interpret. For example, depending on the criteria used to define abuse and on the population sampled, reported rates of prescription opioid abuse in pain clinics range from 0 to 90 percent (Chabal, Miklavz, Jacobson, Mariano, & Chaney, 1997; Portenoy & Foley, 1986; Zenz, Strumpf, & Tryba, 1992). Studies of PC patients, though limited in number, have been more consistent. Two recent studies of PC clinic patients (Chelminski et al., 2005; Reid et al., 2002) found a high prevalence of opioid abuse. The first found a rate of 32 percent and the second 24 percent or 31 percent (depending on the clinic sampled). Given that the authors of the latter study (Reid et al., 2002) relied on a chart review to obtain their estimates, they acknowledge that the study likely underestimates the true extent of the problem. The exact prevalence of the problem might be difficult to ascertain, but these studies at least suggest that a person working in PC will have very frequent contact with persons abusing opioids.

CNS depressant abuse/dependence is probably also much more common than most medical providers would guess. Diazepam and temazepam are considered the most commonly abused of the class, but others are often abused as well (Fraser, 1998; Garretty, Wolff, Hay, & Raistrick, 1997). Depressant misuse may occur orally or intravenously, the latter leading to concerns of human immunodeficiency virus (HIV) infection from dirty needles or other consequences beyond those inherent in abusing the medicine. Benzodiazepines are often misused to prolong or enhance the effects of opiates, and thus they are very commonly misused among persons using heroin and methadone (Garretty et al., 1997). Similarly, concerns about opioid medication abuse and benzodiazepine abuse often go hand-in-hand (Hermos, Young, Gagnon, & Fiore, 2004). One of us (JR) learned about this the hard way, after several patients presented to his clinic requesting benzodiazepines to help them withdraw from opioids. These patients, who interestingly came to the clinic within a week or two of each other, claimed a long history of opioid abuse that they now purportedly wanted to stop. Each displayed a great deal of distress and pleaded with his or her PCP to prescribe a benzodiazepine to help cope with withdrawal symptoms. The PCP, though somewhat perplexed by this request, decided to give the prescription in the hopes that he was supporting a valid attempt to recover from opioid dependence. Ultimately, as each patient avoided meeting with the BHC (JR), failed to show for follow-up PCP appointments, and resisted referrals to free specialty drug abuse treatment, we realized the patients had likely been seeking benzodiazepines for nonmedical use. We (JR and the PCP) both felt naïve and exploited but vowed to use the experience to improve our handling of similar requests in the future.

Stimulants are most commonly used to treat attention deficit hyperactivity disorder (ADHD), a condition known to place one at an elevated risk for substance abuse. In addition to concerns that persons with ADHD might misuse prescribed stimulant medications, there are concerns that introducing stimulant use might increase the risk of abuse of other substances, especially cocaine or methamphetamine. However, most researchers and clinicians now agree that the risk of substance abuse is greater if ADHD is left untreated (Faraone & Wilens, 2003). In addition, the risk of stimulant and cocaine abuse in persons with ADHD may be no greater than in those without ADHD (Pliszka, Carlson, & Swanson, 1999). Nonetheless, as noted earlier, misuse of stimulants among the general population has risen in recent years, particularly among young people, and it is a valid public health concern. Misuse typically involves use of diverted stimulants to create a pleasing effect (not obtained by oral administration but possible by snorting the medicine) and to enhance performance on tasks (such as on exams or projects) (Dodson, 2005).

While all PCPs are familiar with problems associated with opioid/CNS depressant/stimulant abuse, prescribing practices actually seem to vary widely. Some PCPs refuse to prescribe certain of the medicines while others prescribe them liberally. (Of note, there is medico-legal pressure to prescribe in at least some cases. Olsen and Daumit (2004) remind us of a recent action in which a PCP was successfully sued for *not* prescribing opioids for an older patient with chronic pain.) Some PCPs prescribe these medicines for short-term use but refuse long-term prescriptions, while others have few qualms about long-term use, provided the patient appears to be using the medicine appropriately. In many cases, patients come to a PCP already on opioids/stimulants/CNS depressants that another PCP has been providing long term, which can pose a particularly difficult dilemma for the new PCP. Some PCPs in this situation will continue the prescription, while others will insist the patient wean off. This variation in prescribing practices is really a symptom of the greater underlying problems discussed previously; i.e., that clear guidelines for prescribing these medications generally do not exist, that training regarding their use is often inadequate, that concern exists about abuse and misuse issues, and that perceptions of the efficacy of the medications vary greatly from one PCP to the next.

Upon entering a PC clinic, the novice BHC may be surprised how frequently these medications are utilized, given the aforementioned concerns. The bottom line is that many PCPs, time-strapped and sympathetic to the pleadings of patients, often feel compelled to begin these medicines, especially for patients who have "failed" other treatment approaches. Similarly, they often avoid weaning patients off the medications, thinking the patient will escalate demands, show inappropriate aggressive behavior, and/or use services more frequently.

Any review of this topic would not be complete without also mentioning the pervasive influence of the pharmaceutical companies. Consumers are inundated with pharmaceutical advertisements in the popular media (including television, the internet, e-mail and land mail), and pharmaceutical representatives are a frequent presence in PC clinics, taking any opportunity possible to sell PCPs on the benefits of their products. An example of the influence of these companies is Oxycontin, as described by Olsen and Daumit (2004). They note that Purdue Pharma, the manufacturer of Oxycontin, used marketing tactics that were so aggressive they were written about by the lay press. However, the tactics worked. Oxycontin burst out of the gates with dramatic success upon its release and became one of the fastest selling drugs on the market. This may be one of the more publicized examples of the influence of pharmaceutical companies, but it is a phenomenon repeated daily with numerous other medications in PC clinics around the country.

Available data suggest that direct-to-consumer (i.e., patient consumer) advertising is likely to increase the request rates for the drug category and drug brands, as well as the likelihood that those drugs will be prescribed by physicians (Parker & Pettijohn, 2003). While the majority of physicians in the Parker and Pettijohn study were either neutral or did not feel that accepting some types of gifts from pharmaceutical companies affected their ethical behaviors, more and more clinics and medical schools are creating policies that place limits on pharmaceutical company activities. In fact, recent recommendations now include (1) establishing a system to enforce and monitor vendor policies and measure their effectiveness and (2) monitoring and regulating use of continuing medical education funding (much of which comes from pharmaceutical companies) (Zarowitz, Muma, Coggan, Davis, & Barkely, 2001).

The relevance of all of this, for our purposes, is simply to explain that PCPs face real quandaries when it comes to prescribing opioids, stimulants, and CNS depressants. They almost always worry about abuse and misuse and efficacy issues, yet they are pressured from many sides to prescribe regardless. All of this can lead to unpleasant patient encounters and a good deal of stress on the system. Given this backdrop, a BHC in any clinic will need to consider ways he or she can support the PCP in managing patients using and/or requesting these medicines.

Strategies and Solutions

Make Your Presence Felt. Fortunately, there are many ways a BHC can help. At the most basic level, the simple presence of a BHC on the PC team is helpful. The BHC can strengthen the behavioral component of care for the underlying condition (chronic pain, anxiety, etc.), perhaps decreasing the need for medication. Additionally, most PCPs will feel more comfortable discontinuing a medication if they are able to offer a viable clinical alternative, such as behavioral techniques. The BHC can also alleviate some of the load on the PCP when a patient is being weaned from a medicine. He or she can be available to field phone calls (instead of the PCP) from patients in distress, and may schedule frequent visits with patients who are weaning. This availability of the BHC is often reassuring to patients, especially when patients know the BHC is working closely with the PCP.

Develop Medication Agreements. Beyond assisting with direct clinical care, the BHC may also help a clinic implement systemic changes in the management of these patients. One of the simplest yet most appreciated (by clinic staff) changes involves use of a medication agreement (American Academy of Pain Medicine, 2005; Fishman & Kreis, 2002; Jacobson & Mann, 2004). Traditionally these have been called medication "contracts," but medico-legal experts recommend that they be called "agreements" instead (Doleys & Rickman, 2003). (Agreements are allowed more flexibility legally, which may benefit patient and/or provider in the event of hostile legal action.) The use of medication agreements is actually fairly common in PC, but typically they are only used sporadically (after problems have arisen with a patient) and only for narcotic analgesics. A great number of problems can be avoided by helping staff to utilize an agreement routinely and for all classes of medicines with abuse potential.

There exists no universally accepted medication agreement, but most simply stipulate conditions under which the PCP will be willing to prescribe. For example, it might state that refills will not be given for lost or stolen medications, and that the patient is expected to obtain the medicine only from his or her PCP. An agreement might have a fairly lengthy list of such mandates. Both the patient and PCP sign the agreement (though in practice the BHC, nurse, or medical assistant can help by reviewing the agreement in detail with the patient after the PCP has completed dosing information), and it is then placed in a visible location in the patient's chart, such as on top of the medication list. Ideally, the patient will also be given a copy of the agreement, and it will be reviewed during each follow-up visit. Content recommendations for opioid agreements are also outlined in an article by Jacobson and Mann (2004).

There is no clear evidence that medication agreements affect the probability of misuse or abuse of prescription drugs, but medical assistants and PCPs (and sometimes patients) appreciate them. A clear agreement can improve physician and patient comfort level with the treatment plan, evoke a sense of partnership between them, decrease communication problems, protect patients from harm, and possibly afford legal protection to both parties (Doleys & Rickman, 2003; Fishman & Kreis, 2002; Jacobson & Mann, 2004). Medical assistants and nurses who frequently field patient requests for refills like agreements because they do not have to interrupt the PCP to make a decision regarding whether to grant the refill request. A quick review of the medication agreement can spare staff and patient the time and energy of an otherwise likely conflict. Of course, an agreement is only helpful if it is adhered to, so staff must be encouraged to stick firmly and consistently to its terms.

The BHC may also help the clinic develop a PCP–patient agreement that stipulates terms of treatment beyond use of medications. One of us (JR) is involved in an organization-wide effort to make continued use of habit-forming medications contingent on improvements in functioning. The goal is to develop a medication agreement in which PCP and patient agree on functional goals, meaning that if progress toward those goals is not improving on the medications, the prescriptions may be stopped. The other of us (PR) is using an agreement that requires attendance at a psychoeducational class and participation in more intensive levels of care as needed. This type of agreement is most often useful when a clinic develops a pathway program for the problem of concern, such as chronic pain or ADHD or anxiety. (See Chapter 12 for discussion of a program that uses this expanded medication agreement, the Pain and Quality of Life program.)

Suggest and Implement Screeners. Another helpful systemic change involves the routine use of risk screeners. These are brief self-report measures used to identify patients at risk of abusing medications. A risk screener may be given to a patient when the issue of using a medication with abuse potential is first discussed. An example of such is the Screening and Opioid Assessment for Patients with Pain (SOAPP) (Butler, Budman, Fernandez, & Jamison, 2004). It is a fourteen-item screener developed for use with patients with chronic pain and is consistent with the requirements for a PC screener. If used as part of a pathway program in which patients are routinely referred to the BHC, this screener can be completed during an initial visit with the BHC. No screener is sensitive enough to detect all patients at risk of medication abuse, but they likely provide medico-legal support to prescribers and communicate to patients that the clinic takes the issue seriously.

Random urinalysis is another tool that clinics employ to ferret out patients who are abusing or misusing prescription medications. A urinalysis is not generally a test that BHC's order, but it might be helpful to suggest use of such by a PCP in certain situations. Some PCPs insist on a urinalysis from every patient started on a medication with abuse potential. If the patient tests positive for an illicit substance the PCP might decide not to begin the prescription, given that a history of substance abuse is a risk factor for prescription drug abuse and misuse. Other PCPs conduct random urinalyses on patients, which serves the dual purpose of checking for illicit drug use and also making certain the prescribed medications are being taken. Regarding the latter, if a patient prescribed narcotics for the previous several weeks shows no evidence of them in his or her urine, he or she presumably is misusing the medicine (e.g., giving it to a friend, selling it, or even stockpiling it for a suicide attempt or for future needs). In such cases, the PCP might decide to discontinue the prescription or refer the case to an oversight committee (see discussion later in this section for a definition). Random urinalysis typically means testing patients during clinic visits at irregular intervals, although some clinics (usually specialty pain or substance abuse clinics) call patients randomly to come into the clinic for testing. A small percentage of PCPs will conduct a urinalysis at every visit for patients on medications with abuse potential, but this can be quite costly and labor intensive. A more reasonable strategy might be to do this only for patients suspected of, or at higher risk of, prescription abuse.

Develop Pathway Programs and Groups. Yet another strategy for minimizing prescription drug abuse/misuse involves the use of group visits, discussed in Chapter 12. In addition to helping patients with chronic pain, group visits may be useful for patients with anxiety, insomnia, ADHD, or other problems for which the opioids/stimulants/CNS depressants are prescribed. The primary goals of the group approach are to make more comprehensive behavioral assistance and support feasible, while monitoring medication use more closely. If a PCP attends the group, as is done in some group models, his or her knowledge of behavioral strategies will also improve, which may shape how the PCP discusses and delivers future care. Some clinics make refills of narcotic medications contingent on attending monthly chronic pain group visits. Although we know of no clinics using this model for other problems, such as making benzodiazepine refills contingent on attending monthly anxiety group visits, this certainly seems feasible.

Along the lines of a pathway approach, consider creating a registry of patients having the problem of concern. A registry is simply a database for tracking care of patients with a chronic condition. The clinic of one of us (JR) recently completed a pilot study of a registry for patients with chronic pain, and results showed a significant spike in the number of these patients completing a medication agreement and seeing the BHC. The clinic is now in the process of implementing this consistently and for a much larger number of patients. A registry can be developed that tracks any aspect of care that is of concern to the clinic for the problem being monitored. In the case of chronic pain, it might track:

- Date the most current medication agreement was made
- Date of the last urine drug screen (and results)
- Date of any violations of the medication agreement
- Referral history for external services such as physical therapy or a pain clinic
- Studies obtained (e.g., X-Ray or MRI)
- Date of education (from the PCP or BHC) in behavioral pain management strategies
- Current medications
- Attendance at the clinic's chronic pain group
- Use of emergency services since the last PC visit
- Current pain intensity
- Date of last functional assessment (using a self-monitoring form or via PCP questioning)
- Date and results of risk screener
- Date of nurse visit for basic strengthening and stretching recommendations
- Any other items of interest

Each time a patient with chronic pain has a clinic visit, the PCP can check the registry to see which of these routine care components a patient needs.

Develop an Oversight Committee. A time-intensive but useful strategy that can be tried is to form an oversight committee that makes recommendations regarding discontinuing medications in individual cases. An oversight committee can also be used to make treatment recommendations on difficult cases or to review cases where serious problems arise. The Anchorage Neighborhood Health Centers (ANHC) in Alaska uses an oversight committee that includes two PCPs at all times, with the responsibility rotating among PCPs. The BHC would also be a member of the committee and other personnel to consider include a clinic nurse, a pharmacist, a medical assistant, the clinic manager, and the clinic's patient advocate. A PCP or, in some cases a BHC, can review the medical record in detail prior to the committee meeting and provide a brief summary. After discussing a case, the committee might vote on whether to continue medications and generate a note for the medical record and a letter to the patient. This model could easily be adapted for CNS depressant and/or stimulant oversight, and clinic policies may require that if a patient violates a medication agreement more than once his or her case will automatically be reviewed for a recommendation regarding medication continuation. Taking cases to the committee relieves the PCP from having to make such decisions under pressure and may help avoid deterioration in the patient–provider relationship that undermines needed care. Some PCPs might balk at the idea of an external review of their case, but most will probably favor it (Brock, personal communication, 2005).

The downside of a committee approach is that it takes time away from patient care, and patient–PCP medication agreements can clearly address the conditions under which the PCP may, by clinic policy, stop prescribing (e.g., presence of heroin, methamphetamine, or cocaine in a urinalysis, or receiving "Three Strikes" in the Pain and Quality of Life Class as discussed in Chapter 12). Use of a clear and enforced agreement should at least help decrease the number of cases sent to an oversight committee, though a committee still might be desired for cases that are less clear, e.g., for patients who repeatedly screen positive for cannabis use.

THE "BIOMEDICAL" PROVIDER

When George Engel introduced the "biopsychosocial" model in 1977 (Engel, 1977), it was hailed as a revolutionary idea that would change medicine. Whereas the prevailing "biomedical" model of earlier times emphasized linear, cause-and-effect thinking and a singular focus on disease, the biopsychosocial model introduced the notion that psychosocial factors are also important for medicine to study. Engel (1977) believed medicine would never fully understand and treat medical problems by focusing solely on biology, because such factors as culture, family, community, environment, personality, and emotions also influence health significantly.

Within a fairly short time the medical community became familiar with the biopsychosocial concept and began teaching it in medical schools (Novack, Volk, Drossman, Lipkin, 1993). However, despite this change, studies suggest the biomedical model continues to influence physician communication styles and to exert a negative impact on patient outcomes (Barry, Stevenson, Britten, Barber, & Bradley, 2001). For purposes of discussion, we refer to these PCPs as biomedical providers. The BHC may have fewer opportunities to influence biomedical providers because they may be less likely to refer patients. Further, they may be less interested in BHC recommendations. Biomedical providers may seem to favor psychiatric consultation over a BHC consultation and may be reluctant to screen patients for behavioral problems. Their chart notes may show scant mention of the patient's psychosocial history, which they often rely on a nurse or other staff person to obtain. Nonetheless, the presence of behavioral issues is so widespread in PC that no one can avoid them completely and all PCPs feel the weight of them, regardless of orientation or interest. In addition, many providers in this group probably do include some psychological and social aspects of care in their work and are amenable to influence if the right strategies are used.

The good news is that there are many ways for a BHC to engage the biomedical provider, and once a successful relationship has been established it can produce a bountiful harvest of referrals. Many of these providers show increased interest in attending to behavioral issues once they obtain some understanding of how to do so, while others will engage the BHC more once they learn it can take some work off of their shoulders or once patients show benefit from it. In this section, we review strategies for improving collaboration with biomedically oriented PCPs. These strategies include the use of group visits, development of a personal relationship with the PCP, making BHC referrals a routine part of care for certain conditions, and implementation of routine screenings to increase the likelihood of identifying behavioral problems.

Promote Group Visits

Group visits, discussed in detail in Chapter 12, provide one of the best means for connecting with a biomedical provider. Regardless of the model used, group visits entail much collaboration between a BHC and a PCP, which can help grow the relationship. Simply organizing and planning a group allows for personal interaction between the BHC and the PCP that might not have gone on otherwise. Beyond this, group visits give a PCP the opportunity to learn about what a BHC can offer. If present during the group visit, as occurs in some models, the PCP can see how positively patients respond to psychosocial interventions and how much they appreciate the attention to that part of their health. Group visits may also demystify the work of the BHC, and the PCP may discover psychosocial interventions he or she can use during subsequent patient visits.

We have noticed that even biomedical providers begin to talk with patients about behavioral strategies once they learn about them in classes. Sometimes they cannot avoid such discussions because patients bring them up during subsequent PCP visits! For example, shortly after starting depression group visits in his clinic, a BHC colleague of ours noticed the attendees bringing copies of Feeling Good (Burns, 1980) (the text recommended by the BHC during the group) to individual appointments with their PCP. The patients wanted to tell the PCP about their progress with the book and discuss their impressions of it.

Groups can be especially attractive to biomedical providers because they can be used to work out a patient's personal problems that otherwise might be raised in individual PCP visits. Group members, with facilitation from the BHC, can do a wonderful job of problem solving for each other, thus sparing the PCP the need to wrestle with this during a busy individual visit. The BHC struggling to obtain referrals from a biomedical provider may also find group visits to be a boon, as patients who might otherwise never have been referred have the opportunity to get familiar with the BHC during the group. At our clinics, attendance ranges from five to twenty-five patients per group, thus providing many patients exposure to the BHC. In addition, patients in groups may often initiate an individual visit with the BHC outside of the group and then provide positive feedback to the PCP concerning the visit.

Despite the many benefits of group visits, finding a willing biomedical provider to conduct one with can be a challenge. Though we discussed typical sources of resistance to group visits earlier, a few additional reservations are commonly heard from biomedical providers. Some may be reluctant to venture into psychosocial territory with which they are unfamiliar or uncomfortable. Others may have social anxiety in groups. Ironically, we have also heard concerns that a successful group would make the PCP a magnet for other patients with similar problems (e.g., a successful depression group might lead to more patients with depression seeking out that PCP for care). Whatever the source(s) of resistance, even a biomedically oriented PCP will often warm to group visits after trying one, so finding a way to get a foot in the door is crucial. Review Chapter 12 for ideas on how to accomplish this.

Be Personable

Politician Ralph Wright wrote a book titled *All Politics Is Personal*, and the title certainly describes the situation in most work settings, including PC. Many PCPs carry negative stereotypes of MH providers and have a limited understanding of the potential benefits of a BHC service, particularly if their orientation is biomedical. Stereotypes typically break down with personal contact, so the BHC needs to pursue this directly. Not long after starting work in the PC arena, one of us (JR) was problem solving with the other (PR) about how to elicit more referrals from a particular PCP colleague. After listening to the various strategies JR had tried to remedy the problem, PR asked, "Have you tried taking her to lunch?" This idea that a personal approach might boost referrals more than the technical approaches discussed in this text seemed simplistic and overly optimistic. Yet, it worked. During a brief but enjoyable lunch with the PCP, in which a number of personal commonalities were discovered, they discussed the idea of starting group visits. This led to a marked improvement in the working relationship, and a jump in the number of patient referrals followed.

Be sure to take advantage of opportunities to improve personal relations with all PCP colleagues. Keeping a central office location can greatly facilitate personal, as well as professional, interactions. Coming out of the office as much as possible when not seeing patients is also important. Attendance at clinic gatherings, such as farewell parties for departing co-workers and potluck lunches or informal lunch meetings, may also provide opportunities to talk about topics other than work. If invited to a gathering outside of normal work hours, make every effort to attend and socialize. One of us tries to host a gathering of co-workers each year (ideally scheduled around a significant date, such as the anniversary of the establishment of the BHC service in the clinic). In short, one should remember that the existence of a BHC service relies on referrals from PCP colleagues. In specialty MH one can usually work in relative isolation, but in PC settings (especially those with many biomedical PCPs) an effort to develop personal relationships with PCP co-workers can prove essential.

Develop Reminders and Registries to Increase Referrals

Primary care clinics are increasingly using computerized reminder systems and patient registries to guide the care of chronic conditions. These systems help to increase the use of evidence-based interventions and promote comprehensive care (Bodenheimer, Wagner & Grumbach, 2002a,b). As such, they are potentially effective vehicles for increasing BHC referrals from a biomedical provider. Consider the reminder system feature of electronic medical records. In clinics that use electronic medical records rather than paper records, patient information is entered into a computer by the PCP during the patient visit. This replaces the old process of scribbling notes on paper during a visit and then dictating a chart note afterward. Each exam room comes equipped with a computer and the clinician simply constructs the electronic chart note as the visit progresses. As information gets typed in, the computer will often prompt the PCP to take a certain action, and these prompts can sometimes be modified to suit clinic or health care system preferences and policies. The system can sometimes be modified so that if a PCP enters a diagnosis of depression a reminder pops up recommending a referral to the BHC for development of a mood improvement plan. Of course, the electronic medical record can offer similar reminders for a host of circumstances, such as referring patients with a BMI over 25, patients with tension headaches, etc. The simple presence of a reminder does not guarantee a referral will be made, but it at least brings the idea onto the radar screen of the biomedical provider.

Similarly, many clinics use computer registries to track care for patients with chronic conditions, especially diabetes, and providers are often graded on how their patients are performing on various indices. Registries, whether integrated into an electronic medical record or not, offer an excellent opportunity for increasing work with a biomedical provider. If a BHC referral is included in the registry's list of routine care components, it can greatly improve the likelihood of a referral from a biomedical provider.

Improve Screening for Behavioral Problems

For any PC provider, detection of behavioral problems can be difficult, and it may be even more difficult for the biomedical provider. In Chapter 6, we provided extensive information about screening tools and strategies. For the present purposes, suffice it to say screening can enhance opportunities to engage the biomedically oriented PCP. If, for example, a PCP in the clinic sees a lot of children but rarely refers to the BHC, then implementation of routine screening for psychosocial dysfunction in children may help spotlight patients in need of the BHC's help. Regardless of a provider's orientation, he or she most assuredly will want to help a patient once a problem is identified.

HANDLING PSYCHIATRIC EMERGENCIES

In PC, as in specialty MH, patients sometimes present with emergencies. This typically involves concerns about suicide, harm to other(s), or a gross inability to function due to psychiatric problems. One might assume these problems present more frequently in PC settings because of the greater volume of patients seen, though we could find no recent data on this in the United States. In Australia, available estimates suggest that general practitioners manage between 75 and 90 percent of patients with serious mental illness in the community (Working Party Concerning General Practice, 1995). We both have more psychiatric emergencies in our current roles as BHCs than we did as MH providers.

Emergencies are inherently stressful, but in PC they can result in additional stress if there is conflict between the BHC and clinic staff. Staff might expect the BHC to help with all such patients, while the BHC might be strapped for time with his or her own scheduled patients. Also, in the busy PC setting there is the possibility that a patient with a psychiatric emergency will not be adequately assessed for risk and may be unnecessarily directed to 9-1-1 or to a nearby emergency room. When this happens, the patient puts additional pressure on an already busy emergency system and may end up with a hefty bill. Unnecessarily incurred expense will add to the patient stress, especially for uninsured patients. Thus, the wise BHC will look for ways, such as the following, to help plan for psychiatric emergencies in the clinic.

Improve the Clinic's Triage System

The BHC can improve a clinic's ability to respond to psychiatric emergencies by assuring that the system for triaging this type of patient is adequate. Triage occurs when patients call or come to the clinic requesting a same-day appointment. Typically, in both PC and outpatient MH, a triage worker (usually a registered nurse in PC) will field the call or sit down with the patient and, in some cases, direct the patient to the nearest emergency room or call the police in an effort to address a high-risk emergency.

Triage workers in the clinic are trained to use an algorithm that suggests specific actions based on how patients answer specific questions. For example, if a patient calls to request an urgent visit for depression the triage worker might ask, "Have you been thinking of harming yourself?" If the answer is "no," the recommendation would likely be to schedule a routine visit with the PCP as soon as feasible, but if the answer is "yes," the triage worker might be guided to a follow-up question such as, "Do you have a specific plan to harm yourself?" This process continues until a specific action recommendation is reached. Unfortunately, differences exist between clinics in the algorithms used, and some are better than others. Some will recommend an ER visit merely for the presence of suicidal ideation, while others guide the triage worker through a more detailed assessment of risk before reaching an action recommendation. Less detailed algorithms may protect clinics better from liability actions because more patients are directed to emergency care. However, they may also produce problems for patients and the health care system because of unnecessary emergency service utilization.

With this background in mind, one strategy for improving triage is to improve the clinic's algorithm. The goal of such an effort should be to develop questions that assess psychiatric risk as thoroughly as possible, while keeping within the comfort and skill level of the triage staff. Because there are no universally accepted algorithms, and because every staff is different, the end-product will be different from one clinic to the next. Work closely with the triage nurse on this issue to develop a process that provides a good fit.

A prudent strategy is to accompany algorithm redesign with training to improve staff comfort and skill with psychiatric risk assessment. Staff will greatly appreciate an in-house training from the BHC on this topic, and this should further improve their ability to distinguish true emergencies. Such training is well within the intended role of a BHC, i.e., to elevate the system's ability to respond to behavioral issues. The more confident staff feel in their ability to manage psychiatric emergencies on their own, the less conflict will come from over-reliance on the BHC.

Develop a Team-Based Therapeutic Relationship with the Most Troubled Patients

Over time, most BHCs develop relationships with some patients that are similar in some ways to the patient–PCP relationship. Repeated contacts over time, for the same or various problems, build trust in the patient–BHC relationship and help the BHC to learn how to work most effectively with a given patient. In some cases, this relationship helps to create alternatives to unnecessary emergency services. For example, Gloria is a fifty-three-year-old uninsured and unemployed female patient at the clinic of one of the authors. For several years Gloria has been followed for problems related to severe anxiety and mood swings, as well as fibromyalgia, obesity, and chronic dermatological problems. In response to these problems, Gloria leads a very isolated existence with minimal social support. When she began coming to the clinic, she expressed a great deal of distress and used services frequently, including visits with the BHC. However, as she developed basic coping strategies and discovered the right medication mix, her visits became less frequent, less intense, and of shorter duration. Her functioning gradually improved as well, as she began experimenting with various work and social opportunities.

Occasionally, though, Gloria relapses and experiences intense anxiety and depression. When this happens, she often calls the PC clinic in distress, expressing suicidal ideation and feelings of hopelessness. Initially when this happened the triage nurse would direct Gloria to the emergency room, and Gloria went on several occasions. The emergency room had little to offer her, though, and never hospitalized her. Afterward, she would report that going there left her more frustrated and more financially strained from the added medical bills. Hence, on subsequent occasions when Gloria felt distressed and called the clinic she would ask to speak with the BHC. Together, they discovered after a few such calls that a fifteen- or twenty-minute phone conversation offered Gloria the support and guidance she needed to begin to relax and re-establish a healthy focus, and she never felt the need to use the emergency room after these calls. Although the BHC wasn't always available to talk with her immediately, over time the promise of a return call was sufficient to stabilize Gloria until the BHC had more time to talk.

Although this type of extended contact with Gloria might seem incongruous with the consultant approach, one must keep in mind that the mission of the PCBH model is to improve the overall functioning of the PC system as well as to improve the care delivered there for behavioral issues. By initiating this team-based therapeutic relationship with Gloria, her rate of episodes of distress gradually decreased and the triage nurse and PCP (and emergency room providers) gained needed time to focus on other medical needs. Further, these brief phone calls (which only occurred every couple of months and became less frequent over time) were usually easily accommodated into the BHC schedule.

Other patients with chronic mental problems that predispose them to psychiatric emergencies are handled in similar ways to Gloria in both of our clinics. This procedure has only evolved over time as we, as BHCs, have developed relationships with the most chronically troubled patients in the clinic. However, the approach suggested in the example of Gloria is best reserved for the most difficult and time-intensive of the clinic's patients.

Let Clinical Judgment Guide Routine Risk Assessments

Our discussion of handling emergencies would not be complete without also mentioning routine risk assessment. In MH clinics, questions regarding suicidal ideation are a part of most initial evaluations. In the specialty MH arena, clinicians conduct thorough patient histories that gather information about many areas of the patient's past and present functioning, whether directly related to the presenting problem or not. However, as a BHC with brief visits focused on functional assessment, questions about suicidal or homicidal ideation need not be routinely asked. Such questions are likely not relevant for a patient being seen for obesity or smoking cessation or a host of other commonly encountered problems. Instead of routinely asking about risk, the BHC can save these questions for consults in which safety concerns are an issue. Of course, if indicators of risk are present, they must be adequately assess regardless of the initial referral reason.

MISCELLANEOUS CHALLENGES

There are other challenges that the BHC will face in PC, but we include only three more in this chapter. We chose these three because they have been particularly difficult for us. Since we measure outcomes at all visits, we know in black-and-white when patients fail to improve, and after a reasonable number of consults and interventions, we have to decide what to do. Additionally, we both scratch our heads when a biomedical provider asks us about a patient's diagnosis, and we want desperately to engage him or her by meeting the expectation of a diagnosis. Last but not least are the challenges related to special requests from patients and PCPs.

When a Patient Doesn't Improve

The PCBH model described in this text is, by definition, consultative. A basic goal of the BHC visit is to develop a well-rounded treatment plan that includes a behavioral component the PCP can follow. Ideally the BHC has limited, if any, follow-up with many patients. This consultative model represents the ideal, but ideals often clash with reality and this is certainly true of BHC work. Try as one may to adhere to a purely consultative model, there will inevitably be patients who require (or simply desire) more than the typical care. Ask any PCP and he or she will easily be able to recite names of at least several patients who are regulars at the clinic. When one of the authors (JR) began working in a new clinic, a PCP colleague told him she had been meeting weekly for the previous six months with a patient who was chronically suicidal. This may be an extreme example, but PC clinics quite commonly have patients who are frequent users of care. Such patients are referred to as "high-utilizers," and they often push the BHC to step outside of a purely consultative role. These patients might require more frequent and/or more sustained support in making changes, might need follow-up as motivation to change waxes and wanes, and might have more frequent crises or more severe needs.

In such cases, the BHC needs to keep in mind that an important BHC function is to lighten the load on PCPs when possible. One way to accomplish this is to share visits with the PCP using the ping-pong strategy described earlier in the book. If a high-utilizer patient can be satisfied by meeting every other visit with the BHC instead of the PCP, this helps the entire clinic (and possibly the patient as well). Thus, a BHC might begin to develop his or her own list of high utilizer patients, but this can be consistent with the goals of a BHC service. These planned visits with the PCP and BHC should be scheduled in advance each month as guaranteed space for the patient. Often times this strategy will cut down on unscheduled appointments because the patient knows he or she will soon be able to talk with the providers.

One important clarification to make is that although some patients will be seen more frequently, the scope and goal of each visit remains the same. The goal is to improve functioning, and the methods involve teaching skills and establishing self-management plans. The BHC practice of assessing outcomes at all contacts allows for assessment of impact of BHC interventions, and results should be shared with the patient and PCP each time. Note any small improvement on any functioning scale and support the patient's identification of strategies for maintaining this. When there is no improvement, attempt to assist the patient with identifying what he or she is doing to maintain current functioning levels and encourage the continuation of these activities.

When scores suggest that the patient is declining, consulting with the patient and the PCP together to form a plan may be helpful. The plan may involve assertively pursuing more intensive services outside the clinic (when such are available and accessible) or increasing the frequency of the ping-pong visits with the PCP and BHC. Sometimes, despite one's best efforts, patients simply do not improve, and the best that can be done is to mitigate the effect they have on clinic operations in general.

"What's This Patient's Diagnosis?"

One of the essential skills to learn for day-to-day BHC work is that of conducting a functional assessment (See Chapter 7). Functional assessment allows the clinician to focus on the presenting problem behavior, determine the antecedent and contingent factors that maintain it, and then develop an individualized plan for changing the behavior. This approach works well for PC because it allows for a brief and focused visit that produces a set of pragmatic recommendations. Unfortunately, most MH providers are trained in a diagnostic approach to assessment rather than a functional approach, and this is simply not practical for PC settings. In a diagnostic approach, extensive history-gathering may be accompanied by testing or symptom checklists, all geared toward establishing a DSM-based diagnosis. The assumption is that once a diagnosis is established, a treatment program specific to that diagnosis (e.g., a manualized therapy approach or pharmacotherapy regimen) will be implemented.

Primary care providers are usually trained in specialty MH settings during residency, and thus they are also trained to use the diagnostic approach. This might make sense to them during a residency rotation, but it is difficult to transfer to the real world of PC. As a result, a frequent lamentation of PCPs is the lack of time they have to establish a patient's diagnosis. In many cases, they will ask the BHC to see a patient in order to "clarify the diagnosis." This can be stressful for the BHC, who also has limited time for assessment (though probably more than the PCP). Additionally, the BHC may want to accommodate the PCP, particularly a biomedical PCP, in an effort to further develop their relationship.

We recommend that the BHC answer this type of question honestly, explaining that making rule-out diagnoses is not consistent with the PCBH model but that use of functional assessments and brief assessments support development of interventions that improve patient functioning. In chart notes, the BHC may state an impression about diagnoses and may certainly discuss such with the PCP. However, the BHC needs to use the occasion of "What's the diagnosis?" to also teach the powerful skills associated with functional analysis. If a PCP seeks help with the diagnosis for purposes of starting a medicine (e.g., deciding whether to use an antidepressant or a mood-stabilizer), use of one of the self-report measures described in Chapter 6 may help.

"Can You Ask my Doctor about This?"

Patients understand that BHCs work closely with PCPs, and they will often ask the BHC to intervene on their behalf for certain problems. Requests may range from "Can you ask my doctor to prescribe X?" to "Would you ask my doctor to support my disability application?" and others. When patients ask for a request to be passed along, the BHC might explain that patients often get the best results from making direct requests to the PCP. We both usually agree to forward a question or concern in the chart note, along with any recommendations based upon our consultation. And, clearly, if an urgent issue is involved we do go directly to the PCP. However, it is best to avoid becoming a go-between and to instead try to strengthen the patient–PCP relationship by addressing barriers to communication.

Special Evaluations

There are some issues that the BHC should not be involved with. One is evaluations for lawyers or the Court. The limited amount of time for visits precludes doing the type of comprehensive assessments these entities need. One would not like to find him or herself in court, defending a diagnosis made during a 20- or 30-minute visit.

However, many BHCs complete forms for short-term disability. We expect that BHCs will vary in their handling of this issue. One of us does disability evaluations, and the other is still considering it. A positive for completing disability forms is that it can facilitate needed medical/psychiatric care or other support that might improve the patient's functioning. Also, as a provider who is familiar with the patient, a BHC's recommendations will possibly be more accurate than those of an evaluator who has never met the patient before. A negative is that the BHC–patient relationship can be hurt if the BHC does not make the disability recommendations desired by the patient. In addition, completion of the forms takes time away from other important tasks, and there is a risk of being inundated with requests for form completion. One strategy is to agree to complete forms only for patients who, in the BHC's opinion, clearly warrant disability. Others can be told they need to pursue disability through the usual means provided by the relevant State office. One practice we both avoid is conducting Social Security disability evaluations. These are simply too lengthly to accommodate in the PCBH model.

When a Patient Is Aggressive with Staff

Unfortunately, some patients lack skills for working productively with nurses, PCPs, and support staff when they are frustrated. Patients with low tolerance for frustration may make demands, speak loudly, use inappropriate language, and even make threats while in public areas of the clinic. These patients may call frequently and make rude remarks to nurses when their requests are not met. The clinic's triage system needs to include protocols for addressing these patients.

An example of a well-developed plan comes from Dr. Julie Rickard at the Columbia Valley Clinic in Wenatche, Washington (2005, personal communication). She and her colleagues have a plan that covers most every possibility for this challenging group of patients. The BHC role includes teaching patients specific skills for relating, as well as adopting a warning letter to individual patient needs. Their letters often include the requirement that patients participate in a series of consults with the BHC to build skills for working with strong emotions while in the clinic, and PCPs, after receiving BHC training, often can provide on-going support to the patient for using these. The BHC periodically trains PCPs as a group in how to help these patients. Of course, the best response may be to call 9-1-1 if a patient refuses to calm down or becomes physically threatening.

SUMMARY

1. The BHC will confront many new issues in PC. One of these is the abuse and misuse of prescription drugs. Given that this is a frequent problem, the BHC should learn about relevant issues and work on solutions that are feasible in the clinic. Potentially helpful can be medication agreements, screening to identify patients at risk for medication abuse, the use of registries and group visits, and development of an oversight committee.

2. Some PCPs have a bent toward the biomedical perspective and can be more challenging to get referrals from. Use of routine screening for behavioral issues, development of personal relationships with the PCP, and setting up reminder systems and pathways can help improve collaboration with these PCPs.

3. In PC, the BHC will probably encounter more psychiatric emergencies than he or she did in an outpatient psychotherapy practice. Prepare for these by improving the clinic triage system, developing team-based therapeutic relationships with the most troubled patients, and training staff to respond effectively to crises. Routine assessment of risk is not a part of the PCBH model.

4. Other challenges such as PCPs wanting a diagnosis, patients wanting requests passed along to a PCP, and pressure to do court-ordered evaluations and disability forms are also common. Consider the PCBH mission closely when considering how to handle these situations.

14

COMMON ETHICAL ISSUES

"Do all the good you can, by all the means you can, in all the ways you can, in all the places you can, at all the times you can, to all the people you can, as long as ever you can."

—John Wesley

When thinking back to the beginning of our journey into primary care, we both remember all too keenly the sense of confusion that predominated. A flood of questions arose daily, and each day completed without a disaster seemed like a success. While sorting through issues of how to structure a PCBH service, how to perform the consultant function, and how to fit into the milieu, a number of questions surfaced about ethics.

Indeed, a new professional identity emerges in the transition to PCBH work, and this evolution requires attention to ethical principals. Situations often arise in primary care that are unique to this type of work and setting, and they are disconcerting until one finds an ethical solution. In this chapter we aim to help new BHCs avoid wandering into ethics landmines, by helping them recognize and address ethical issues before they become problems.

This chapter consists of manufactured case examples followed by analysis. We encourage the reader to try to identify the unique ethical issue(s) raised by each example before reading the subsequent analysis. Because we authors are psychologists, our reference point for the case analyses is the *Ethical Principles of Psychologists and Code of Conduct*, which can be perused and/or downloaded at http://www.apa.org/ethics/code2002.html (American Psychological Association, 2003). For each case we include relevant excerpts from the Code, though we have edited out parts not directly pertinent to the case example. We do recognize that other types of MH professionals, as well as colleagues from other countries, might have different ethical codes. In addition, the behavior of health professionals is governed by laws, and these laws vary from state to state and country to country. Clearly we cannot address here every issue that might come up for each of our companion fields in each state or each country, but instead we will highlight ethical issues that are likely to cut across these lines. Readers are strongly encouraged to consult the code from their governing professional organization and relevant laws as they think through the case examples that follow.

COMPETENCE: THE CASE OF DR. FEELGOOD

Dr. Feelgood, a clinical psychologist who had previously worked in specialty MH, was hired to develop a new primary care behavioral health service. Despite a reasonably strong health psychology background, Dr. Feelgood had never worked in a primary care clinic. Similarly, despite some experience with consultation-based work, this had never been the focus of Dr. Feelgood's work, and only rarely had he needed to make rapid decisions as a consultant. Most of his consultation experience involved doing traditional, lengthy psychological evaluations of medical patients and providing detailed reports to medical providers. Hallway or "curbside" consultations, a common primary care occurrence in which BHCs are asked for advice on patients they have never met or only barely know, had not previously been a part of Dr. Feelgood's clinical repertoire. Most of Dr. Feelgood's experiences in MH clinics had involved the usual combination of diagnostic assessments, hour-long therapy visits weekly or every other week, and psychoeducational groups. Before leaving his previous job, Dr. Feelgood had attended a workshop on PCBH consultation and had read a few journal articles about it, but this was the extent of his exposure to the field prior to beginning in primary care. Thus, Dr. Feelgood's specialty MH experiences hadn't prepared him too well for what he faced in his new job.

The characteristics of Dr. Feelgood's new patients also were quite a change from those with whom he had experience. Previously, in his private practice, Dr. Feelgood's typical clients were middle-class, English-speaking, and basically healthy. However, with the move to his new community health center job, Dr. Feelgood discovered an entirely different patient population. Suddenly he was presented with patients addicted to heroin and methamphetamine, psychotic patients unwilling or unable to get specialty care, and patients with multiple chronic and complex medical problems. He was often asked to help with problems with which he had little familiarity, such as diabetes and autism. The majority of patients in his clinic spoke primarily a language other than English, necessitating the use of interpreters and challenging his understanding of different cultures. For their part, PCPs weren't sure how to utilize Dr. Feelgood initially, and they peppered him with questions about medications. Questions such as, "How long should this patient stay on this medication?" and "Do you think a different medication might be warranted?" (and, "If so, which one?") were common.

In short, Dr. Feelgood was surprised by how different the challenges of his primary care job were from those of his private practice job. He faced a new and diverse patient population with many clinical problems he had not encountered before, and his new practice required that he respond to situations where his knowledge and training were lacking. Dr. Feelgood was surprised to find that the transition to primary care was more challenging than he had imagined it would be.

What Ethical Issues Can You Identify?

The case of Dr. Feelgood will probably sound very familiar to many readers. Most who enter a PCBH service will have had little if any experience with this type of work before starting. Further, given the incredible variety of behavioral problems encountered in primary care, no novice BHC could claim to be experienced in every clinical problem sent his or her way. Thus, the issues raised in this example and faced by many new BHCs pertain mostly to "Boundaries of Competence" (APA Ethics Standard 2.01).

In the case of Dr. Feelgood, he had very limited experience with brief consultation, especially primary care consultation, and very limited training in the primary BHC model. To add to his ethical concerns, this practice model is in many ways an emerging area that lacks recognized training standards or care guidelines. This makes for some difficulty defining "competent care," which Dr. Feelgood worried might leave him vulnerable to charges of incompetent care. Finally, Dr. Feelgood had not previously treated many of the problems and populations he was encountering in his new community health clinic job. His background with a mostly healthy, middle-class, English-speaking, American-born population included little of the diversity seen in his new clinic.

What Actions Should Dr. Feelgood Have Taken?

Certain parts of the Boundaries of Competence Standards are particularly relevant to Dr. Feelgood's situation. For example, Standard 2.01c says, *"Psychologists planning to provide services ... involving populations, areas, techniques or technologies new to them undertake relevant education, training, supervised experience, consultation or study."* Similarly, Standard 2.01e states, *"In those emerging areas in which generally recognized standards for preparatory training do not yet exist, psychologists nevertheless take reasonable steps to ensure the competence of their work and to protect client/patients ... from harm."* And Standard 2.01b states, *"Where ... an understanding of factors associated with ... race, ethnicity, culture, national origin ... disability, language, or socioeconomic status is essential for effective implementation of their services ... psychologists have or obtain the training, experience, consultation, or supervision necessary to ensure ... competence."*

The essence of these standards is the importance of obtaining as much training, consultation, and guidance as reasonably possible to ensure basic competence in areas that are new to the psychologist. As noted previously, most MH providers will have to attend to this to one extent or another when beginning work in primary care. It will probably be even more important for those working in community health centers, given the diversity of problems and populations encountered there.

After assessing his areas of knowledge and skill deficits, Dr. Feelgood took several steps to improve his competence. To improve his ability to work with persons of varying language, racial, ethnic, national origin, and cultural backgrounds, he attended workshops and conferences dealing with these issues. Because the majority of patients enrolled at his new clinic were Hispanic, he attended a conference on improving health care for Latino/a persons and used continuing education money to attend a weeklong course in basic "medical Spanish." He also attended a workshop on the use of interpreters, which included strategies for improving cultural sensitivity. To improve his understanding of the unique challenges facing persons with disabilities and lower socio-economic status, he visited numerous social service organizations in the area of his clinic and occasionally attended events and trainings they sponsored. This not only improved his awareness of the challenges faced by these populations but also improved his ability to advocate for his patients.

To improve his general clinical competence in this new field of PCBH consultation, Dr. Feelgood found a mentor and made a plan for regular consultation visits. He found this person by contacting professionals who had written articles and books on this model of care. Though not in his local area, the professional mentor was available via phone and email for occasional consultation. (Of note, Mountainview Consulting Group, run by one of the authors (PR) and Kirk Strosahl, PhD, regularly consults on-site and/or from a distance with new BHCs. They can be accessed via their website, www.behavioral-health-integration.com. Also at the site, new BHCs may indicate supervision needs and perhaps connect with other local BHCs.) To further his competence in the field, Dr. Feelgood contacted others employed in similar work in his local area. Most were not utilizing an integrated, consultative model, but they were at least MH providers working in a primary care setting and so provided some helpful insight. He visited some of these persons and talked over the phone with others, eventually establishing a network of persons with whom he could consult. A number of organizations now feature workshops on PCBH consultation at their annual conferences, and Dr. Feelgood also made a point of attending as many of these as possible. Finally, Dr. Feelgood read some of the growing collection of books being published on the PCBH model.

Beyond the specifics of this case example, some general points pertaining to competence should also be remembered. First, a BHC in primary care is not conducting psychotherapy or other traditional specialty MH services. The interventions taught to patients and PCPs in primary care are basic and often generalize across problems. As a result, many ethical dilemmas related to competence can be avoided. For example, a patient complaining of insomnia may be provided sleep hygiene ideas or taught to do stimulus control, which could be used regardless of whether the insomnia is the primary condition or is secondary to depression or some other problem. A patient presenting with anxiety could be taught the importance of reducing avoidance, again a strategy that will be helpful regardless of diagnosis (e.g., panic disorder, phobias, posttraumatic stress disorder, and others all benefit from reducing avoidance). In other words, in the PCBH model the BHC need not be an expert on every presenting problem in order to add to the treatment plan. As another example, a BHC with no specific training in the treatment of heroin dependence may nonetheless help treat the problem by providing a motivational intervention to a user or helping the user recall and implement strategies that have promoted abstinence in the past.

This focus on improving functioning rather than providing diagnosis-specific specialty therapy allows the BHC to ethically engage with almost any presenting problem. Incidentally, this is an important difference between the PCBH model and a non-integrated model. Because of the Competence Standards, a provider of specialty psychotherapy services co-located in primary care will be much more limited than a BHC in the problems with which he or she can help.

Nonetheless, a BHC does have boundaries to the services he or she can competently provide and must remain vigilant to them. One area where this often gets tested involves medications. PCPs have been trained mostly to dispense medicine, and patients often come to their PCP wanting medicine. Both will often ask the BHC for prescribing advice. The majority of BHCs are not prescribers, however, and must resist any temptation to pretend to be. Giving basic recommendations, such as whether a patient might benefit from medicine, or helping monitor a patient for medication response or side effects, are perfectly ethical practices for most BHCs. However, suggesting a certain medication to try, instructing a patient to increase or decrease a dose, or giving other specific medication advice is outside the competence boundaries of most BHCs.

Similarly, a BHC must be prepared to answer, "I don't know," when asked to comment on a problem outside of his or her range of knowledge. Because a BHC will often be working with medical problems (e.g., hypertension, diabetes, hyperlipidemia), patients often ask questions the

BHC cannot competently answer. If a patient recovering from a recent heart attack asks, "How much exercise am I supposed to be doing?" the answer for many BHCs should be, "I don't know, but I will find out right now from your PCP." For their part, PCPs will also ask questions the BHC cannot answer, or might ask for help with a problem with which the BHC is not familiar. In such cases, the BHC might need to defer on helping until he or she can do some background research, or some more information might need to be solicited from the PCP. For example, one of us (JR) was recently asked to design a behavior plan to help a patient with irritable bladder syndrome decrease her frequency of urination. This was a wonderful referral but JR knew nothing about that condition! The PCP, however, was happy to explain the condition to JR and even gave him some ideas of how to structure the behavior plan. In this case, asking the PCP about the presenting problem helped JR deliver more competent and effective care.

One last issue relevant to the Competence standards involves concerns about the brevity of BHC interventions. Clinicians who are learning the PCBH model often feel they will be vulnerable to lawsuits from dissatisfied patients alleging inadequate care. They also worry that the brevity of the intervention leaves them open to ethics complaints of incompetent care. Indeed, the interaction patients have with the BHC in this model is vastly different from what would occur in a specialty MH clinic. Consumers and MH providers alike have come to expect that a visit with an MH professional consists of fifty minutes, not twenty, and that treatment involves extended weekly follow-ups. Patients in primary care that have received specialty MH services are often surprised to learn that they will have a fifteen- or thirty-minute visit with the BHC, with limited or no follow-up (though most often they express simply surprise, not displeasure).

For BHCs concerned about these issues, distinguishing the role of a consultant from that of a specialty provider is helpful. Consultations are meant to provide recommendations to a treating provider, in this case the PCP, with the goal of improving treatment *relative to usual care*. In this sense, treatment that involves visits with both a PCP and a BHC is far from abbreviated. Compared to usual primary care practices, the BHC model results in greatly *expanded* treatment that should actually buffer providers and clinics against liability claims and incompetence charges. Care does need to be taken not to represent (or bill) BHC visits as therapy visits, because if viewed as such then different expectations will be warranted. (The Health and Behavior CPT codes discussed in Chapter 4, which distinguish brief consultative interventions from therapy interventions, were developed largely to help with this issue.) As a consultant the primary goal is to improve the PCP's ability to treat her/his patient, meaning the PCP maintains control of the patient's treatment plan and the BHC is not expected to provide therapy. All of this is not to discount the potentially beneficial effects stemming directly from a patient's interactions with a BHC, or to suggest that a BHC visit is not an intervention. Any type of patient visit, consultative or otherwise, can have beneficial effects; and a BHC clearly hopes to influence patient behavior directly as well as indirectly via the PCP. As long as one maintains the primary goal of improving the PCP's ability to treat the patient, it is hard to imagine how the legal or ethical risks of practicing this model would be any greater than those of specialty MH care.

INFORMED CONSENT: THE CASE OF MS. B. HEALTHY, M.S.W.

Amy L. was a fifty-two-year-old woman visiting her doctor for a routine diabetes check. She had not been into the clinic for almost a year, and her Hemoglobin A1c value showed that her diabetes was poorly controlled. PCPs use the A1c test to monitor the glucose control of diabetics, and the goal of diabetes management is keep blood glucose levels as close to normal as possible and thereby avoid complications. When the doctor notified her of the lab results, Amy confessed that she had a lot of difficulty adhering to dietary recommendations and rarely exercised. Amy's PCP knew that she had a history of depression and thus screened for depression. Her screen was positive, and her PCP felt certain that depression was interfering with Amy's diabetes self-care. However, in the past when the PCP suggested a referral to a MH clinic, Amy had refused to go. She had always insisted that she didn't believe in telling her problems to others and always promised her PCP that she would improve her self-management efforts on her own (though she clearly had not done so).

This time the PCP was determined to get better MH care for Amy, and fortunately the clinic had recently begun a PCBH service. Thus, before concluding her visit with Amy, the PCP sought out the BHC and brought her into the exam room. Amy was a bit perplexed when the PCP returned with Ms. B. Healthy, but the PCP quickly explained, "This is Ms. B. Healthy, our BHC. Before you go, I'd like you to have a visit with her. She helps me figure out how to help my patients make healthy lifestyle changes, and she just happens to be available for an appointment right now. So I'd like you to take this prescription, see Ms. B. Healthy now, and see me again in two weeks. Any questions?" Amy answered, "No," but looked quizzically at Ms. B. Healthy as she shook hands with her. The three then left the exam room and Amy followed Ms. B. Healthy back to her office for a visit.

What Ethical Issues Can You Identify?

The issue most recognizable in this case involves "Informed Consent" (APA Ethics Standard 3.10). Quite often when MH providers transition from specialty clinics to primary care consultation, they have questions about informed consent. Mental health professionals, like all health professionals, are trained to take informed consent very seriously, and thus they often feel uneasy with warm handoffs in primary care. For example, in this scenario, one might question whether Amy truly understood what she would be doing with Ms. B. Healthy, or even why her PCP wanted her to see her. Given Amy's history of refusing MH treatment, one might wonder if she would have even consented to seeing Ms. B. Healthy if her PCP had provided more detail about the referral. Yet, interactions like the one in this example are common in BHC work. To ensure that informed consent is obtained in this scenario, what obligations does Ms. B. Healthy have? Does she need to have Amy sign a consent form?

What Actions Should Ms. B. Healthy Have Taken?

There are a few ethics standards pertaining to informed consent, but the one most applicable to this case (Standard 3.10) states, "*When psychologists conduct ... consulting services ... or other forms of communication, they obtain the informed consent of the individual or individuals using language that is reasonably understandable to that person or persons ...*" This standard clearly applies to primary care consultation work. However, new BHCs are often surprised to learn that a separate consent form for BHC visits is not only unnecessary; it also is not recommended. Regarding the former, all primary care clinics have new patients read and sign consent forms before care can be delivered, just as MH clinics do. However, because patients contact so many health professionals in the course of a visit (e.g., nurses, lab technicians, medical assistants, providers), these forms cover most any care delivered in the clinic from any member of the care team. The forms also typically cover visits with ancillary providers (e.g., nutritionists, diabetes nurse educators) or visiting specialists. Thus, because in an integrated service the BHC is considered a primary care team member, consultations with him/her should be covered by a clinic's usual informed consent form. To be certain of this, though, Ms. B. Healthy had reviewed her clinic's consent form when she began her BHC job and asked for some changes to it. She also consulted with her organization's Risk Manager for help with this.

As mentioned previously, use of a separate consent form for visits with the BHC is strongly discouraged. Not only is a separate form typically redundant with the clinic's general consent form, it also becomes a barrier to care. Brief interventions with a patient who can only stay five or ten minutes after a warm handoff become more difficult if the patient first has to read and sign a separate consent form. Additionally and perhaps more importantly, use of a separate consent form suggests to patients that behavioral health is perceived differently from physical health. This message, though subtle, can contribute to the stigma of seeing a BH provider. When a BHC is truly integrated into the primary care team, a visit with him or her should be framed as a routine aspect of health care, similar to a visit with a nurse educator or nutritionist, rather than something unusual or distinct that requires a separate consent form. As we have noted throughout this text, the more a BH service looks like primary care, the more patients (and providers) consider the role of emotions in health and the less stigmatized patients feel about seeing a BH provider.

All of this is not to understate the importance of informed consent, however. Even in an integrated service, a BHC must take pains to ensure patients understand who he or she is and what his or her role is. Patients who are seeing the BHC for the first time should be told about the purpose of the visit, the collaborative nature of the BHC/PCP relationship, and what to expect in terms of visit length and follow-up. This can easily be done verbally in a minute or two at the outset of the visit. One can see in the current case example how Amy might be confused about the role of

Ms. B. Healthy and the purpose of seeing her, and might even refuse to see her once she understands these things. Thus, Ms. B. Healthy needs to make certain Amy is clear about what to expect upon sitting down with her. Chapter 7 offers a scripted statement for the BHC to use in introducing patients to BHC services before diving into a visit.

CONFIDENTIALITY: THE CASE OF MR. SUFFERLESS, M.F.T.

Mr. Sufferless, marriage and family therapist, was excited to be in his first week of work in an integrated PCBH service. Mr. Sufferless had previously worked in specialty MH but had an interest in health psychology and so had jumped at the chance to work in primary care. The service he joined had been in place for a few years and thus had protocols and procedures already established, and Mr. Sufferless started the process of learning them.

When he began to see patients, Mr. Sufferless experienced concerns about some of the practices that were expected of him. For starters, Mr. Sufferless was told to write his notes in the patient's medical chart, where anyone with access to the chart could also access his notes. Mr. Sufferless was accustomed to a very different record-keeping process in MH, one in which his notes were never available for others to read without first obtaining the written consent of the patient. He wondered to himself, "What if a patient divulges something extremely personal to me, like a history of sexual abuse or recent commission of a crime? Will I need to write that in the medical record, for any staff person to see?"

A second area of concern for Mr. Sufferless involved the frequent interruptions by staff during his patient visits. He was a bit uncomfortable with PCPs knocking on his door to consult with him, but this he could understand better than the other interruptions that occurred. For example, early in the week someone from the Records department intruded during a visit to look for a medical chart that was missing. Then, later in the week, a medical assistant knocked on his door and wanted to know if Mr. Sufferless was meeting with a patient who had met earlier with a PCP. Apparently the patient had left his PCP visit without taking his prescription, so the medical assistant was searching for him in order to return it. The most disconcerting part of these interruptions for Mr. Sufferless was that the patient in his office was visible to the person at the door. In his previous practice, interruptions during a therapy visit were almost unheard of, partly to avoid disturbing the therapy process but also partly to protect the privacy of the patient. In the primary care clinic interruptions seemed almost routine. He had a difficult enough time adjusting his treatment style to the intrusions, without also having to worry about patient confidentiality. Shouldn't he be taking steps to better protect the privacy of his patients?

To add to these concerns, Mr. Sufferless felt very uncomfortable talking with PCPs after visiting with a patient. Quite often PCPs would approach him after a visit and ask, "How did it go with the patient I sent you?" He sometimes came across sensitive information during his patient visits and felt especially awkward spilling that information right out to the PCP. In the specialty system to which he was accustomed, Mr. Sufferless would never talk with others about information divulged by a patient during a visit, unless that patient had given him written permission to do so. He even insisted on written permission before talking with another professional that provided care to the patient, such as the PCP. "How," he mused, "can I be expected to develop a trust-based relationship with my patients if I have to divulge to another person (the PCP) the information given to me?"

What Ethical Issues Can You Identify?

Once again, the unease experienced by Mr. Sufferless will sound familiar to many new BHCs or those remembering their first weeks as a BHC. The issues raised in this case center around Confidentiality (APA Ethics Standards 4.01, 4.02, and 4.04 primarily). Confidentiality has always been a cornerstone of the therapist–client relationship, and the processes involved in PCBH consultation may seem to intrude upon this and seem alarming to some new BHCs. Indeed, the environment in primary care is also very different from specialty MH, and getting used to this takes time. However, one need not (and certainly should not) sacrifice confidentiality to work in primary care consultation. Medical settings such as primary care take confidentiality every bit as seriously as does the MH sector, and they are governed by the same strict laws and regulations. Nonetheless, the ways in which confidentiality is managed do vary between primary care and MH, and the BHC must learn to navigate this ethically.

What Actions Should Mr. Sufferless Take?

The most relevant APA standards for this case and for BHCs in general are the following: (4.01) *"Psychologists have a primary obligation and take reasonable precautions to protect confidential information obtained through or stored in any medium ..."*; (4.02a) *"Psychologists discuss with persons ... with whom they establish a ... professional relationship (1) the relevant limits of confidentiality and (2) the foreseeable uses of the information generated through their psychological activities"*; (4.02b) *"Unless it is not feasible or is contraindicated, the discussion of confidentiality occurs at the outset of the relationship and thereafter as new circumstances may warrant"*; (4.04a) *"Psychologists include in written and oral reports and consultations, only information germane to the purpose for which communication is made"*; and finally, (4.04b) *"Psychologists discuss confidential information obtained in their work only for appropriate scientific or professional purposes and only with persons clearly concerned with such matters."*

Mr. Sufferless had a few concerns about confidentiality in the primary care consultation setting. One concern involved integrating his notes with the rest of the patient's medical record, given the access of many staff persons to that record. Indeed, records are viewed by providers, medical assistants, referral coordinators, lab technicians, and numerous other members of the primary care clinic as needed. Primary care tends to be team-based, whereas specialty MH care tends to be provided by one person. However, as with the prior discussion of informed consent issues, all primary care clinics have patients read and sign agreement with the record-keeping practices of the clinic before the patient receives care. Patients are informed prior to care that information disclosed to staff persons may be shared with other relevant staff, if for purposes of providing health care to the patient. Patients are also informed of the limits of confidentiality (i.e., problems a provider is mandated to report) because PCPs are usually bound to the same reporting laws as BHCs. If feasible, Mr. Sufferless should remind patients at the outset of an initial visit that the information provided to him may be shared with the PCP and others on his team as needed. But beyond that no special measures outside the clinic's usual ones are needed.

Mental health providers often want to safeguard information they obtain, as if it is more sensitive than information obtained by other health care providers. Yet, a quick review of most any patient's primary care records will reveal highly sensitive information gleaned from other members of the primary care staff as well. Psychosocial information is crucial to the provision of health care, and it needs to be available to PCPs, especially if it is sensitive or traumatic to the patient. Indeed, uncovering pertinent information that improves the PCP's ability to provide care is one of the goals for a consultative visit. Assuming patients are made aware up front of the consultative nature of a BHC visit, Mr. Sufferless need not worry about including relevant information from his visit in the medical record or discussing that information with the PCP.

Notwithstanding all of these issues, a BHC will definitely face challenges to the protection of confidential information in primary care. The frequent intrusions during patient visits, in which Mr. Sufferless's patients came into view of other staff persons, are an example of this. Of course, all primary care staff members are bound to the same confidentiality laws and standards, and we must trust that they will adhere to them. We must trust, for example, that the medical assistant who noticed the patient in Mr. Sufferless's office while searching for another patient will keep her observation of the patient confidential. Yet, certain practices can help to ensure that sensitive information is protected even in the chaotic environment of primary care. For example, if opening the door for an interruption during a patient visit, do not leave it open. Step outside the room to talk with the colleague who knocked (and close the door to allow privacy). Similarly, take care to never talk about a patient within earshot of another patient. If conducting a curbside consultation or a warm handoff with a PCP, duck into a private area for the discussion. If notes are dictated, the BHC should dictate only in his or her office or in an area away from patients. One of us had sometimes observed PCPs in the clinic dictating "on the fly"; i.e., as they hurried down the corridor after finishing a patient visit. This is a risky practice from a confidentiality standpoint and should never be done (it was addressed in the clinic and no longer occurs). Finally, discussions with PCPs and staff about patients should be held only for purposes of patient care. A BHC should not, for example, discuss details of a patient visit with a lab technician who plays no significant role in that patient's care. Such behavior amounts to gossip, which is a clear violation of confidentiality guidelines and laws.

Certainly the PC arena and PCBH work, present some unique challenges to confidentially ethics. However, by remaining mindful of these basic precautions, one can maintain a highly ethical practice in this new environment.

SUMMARY

1. BHCs need to be familiar with the code of ethics for the governing professional organization to which they belong. The American Psychological Association offers excellent materials with case-based examples, as well as guidelines for newer areas of service such as telephone and Internet communications with patients.
2. Identify and address ethical issues before problems arise. The areas most commonly of concern to new BHCs include competence, informed consent, and confidentiality. All can be successfully addressed in the PCBH model.

15

EVALUATING YOUR SERVICE

"Mountains cannot be surmounted except by winding paths."
—Johann Wolfgang Von Goethe

Clinicians reading this text may have waited as long as possible to read this chapter, not simply because it is at the end of the book but also because it is a topic that is often of lesser concern for BH providers. Clinicians, quite reasonably, are first and foremost concerned with the how-to practice segments of books such as this. They usually want to be introduced to the theoretical underpinnings of new treatment models first, then to the clinical applications of the model and then, finally, to questions about how to measure the effectiveness of their work. (And, let's be honest, some clinicians would rather not think about how to measure their effectiveness at all!) On the other hand, an administrator reading this text might start with this chapter. Administrators, again quite reasonably, are often the first ones to ask questions about measuring the value of a new service. They need to know that the money they are spending to develop a new treatment delivery model is well spent. Specifically, they may want to know whether the service is significantly benefiting their patients, their providers, some aspect of their health care system, or all of the above. They may also want to know if the new service is saving them money, for example via cost-offsets, or simply costing them money. One of us (JR) recalls being asked during an interview how he might measure the outcome of a BHC service if he were hired. The interview was with two administrators (the medical director and clinical programs manager), and there was a very pregnant pause as JR considered his answer. Apparently the answer he stumbled through was sufficient, as he was offered the job; however, the answer was probably sufficient simply because the administrators had even fewer ideas for how to measure outcome than he did! Owing to the newness of the BHC model, a program evaluation plan takes some thinking through and will be a bit different from evaluating a specialty service.

Yet, whatever one's position in the PCBH world, this chapter is both relevant and important. Outcome measurement can help or hinder the growth of a service, and thus one needs to think carefully about how to measure outcome, when to do it, and to whom to present the results. A case in point is the BHC service JR helped develop (after being hired despite his rather nebulous ideas about outcome measurement during the interview). After spending the better part of his first year attending to the basic setup of the service and clinical orientation to the BHC model, the attention of JR and his co-workers turned to outcome measurement. The creation and completion of an outcome assessment protocol took some time, but the results provided compelling support for the service. Surprised and pleased by the findings, JR and colleagues asked for time at a meeting of the organization's executive committee to review the results with them. At the time of the meeting, the organization had hired two psychologists (JR and one other) to establish a BHC service in two different clinics, but four of the organization's clinics had no BHC service and no clear plan to begin one. The two starter clinics were regarded as pilot projects that might or might not spur expansion to the other four clinics.

Being a relatively new program, many members of the executive committee had never met JR or the other BHC in the organization, and they had only a hazy notion of the work being done in the BHC service. During the meeting, JR and his colleagues were given just twenty minutes to review the goals and outcomes of the service, but that proved to be enough time. The executives were, it seemed, pleasantly surprised to learn that we had conducted such an extensive outcome evaluation without being asked to do so, and they clearly shared our enthusiasm for the results. One expressed, "I had no idea how much you folks actually are doing!" The CEO expressed his desire to find a way to expand the BHC service to the other clinics, and the Medical Director chimed in that the PCPs in the organization were clamoring for more BHC services. Two years later, we now have BHCs in four clinics, graduate student interns in two additional clinics, and a commitment from the CEO to hire two more full-time BHCs next year (meaning each clinic in the organization will have a full-time BHC). Although expansion of the service can be attributed to numerous factors, there is no doubt that the outcome evaluation was an important catalyst.

A thorough evaluation provides the BHCs themselves with helpful feedback and also can demonstrate how valuable a BHC service truly is. There are many ways to conduct a program evaluation, but in this chapter we will cover the most basic components. Our hope is that this may help others to grow their service, just as it did for JR and his colleagues. The topics we will discuss include productivity, model fidelity, end user satisfaction, and clinical effectiveness.

PRODUCTIVITY

One of the most frequent questions that comes up when we are talking to groups about this model of care is, "How many patients do you usually see in a day?" Productivity, as in the number of patients seen per day per BHC, is indeed an important performance measure to track. However, other aspects of productivity must be considered as well. These include the trends over time, the range of problems and populations seen, and the impact of BHC services on PCP services. We will explore each of these as a part of our discussion on productivity. Data for some productivity indices can usually be obtained from billing records, while surveys may be necessary in order to obtain other information.

Patients Seen Per Day

The most commonly tracked aspect of productivity is the number of patients seen per day. In PCBH, as in general medicine, BHCs may be compensated according to productivity, so a thoughtful approach that takes into account the consultative nature of the model is important. Establishing productivity standards can be difficult, and the solutions for unexpectedly low productivity will be different from clinic to clinic. A BHC service in a larger clinic might expect to be busier than one in a smaller clinic, and that is often the case. Much can also depend, though, on the PCPs in the clinic. A small clinic with mostly biopsychosocially-inclined PCPs might keep a BHC continuously busy, whereas a larger clinic with mostly biomedically-inclined PCPs might be slower for a BHC. Similarly, one might expect that a busier clinic that sees a higher than average number of patients per day would also keep a BHC busier. Yet, because such clinics are so busy, PCPs may be reluctant to take the time for a BHC referral (especially in the early months of a BHC service, when its value is not yet perceived). Clinics with a high turnover of PCPs or in a period of flux with their providers also typically produce fewer BHC referrals, because temporary providers have not developed practice habits that include utilization of a BHC. The schedule of the BHC provider can also influence referral rates. Full-time BHCs usually have much more of a presence in the clinic, with more opportunity to penetrate the practice habits of PCPs and to involve themselves in clinical pathways, whereas part-time BHCs might have a harder time establishing themselves.

Because of these sources of variability, we hesitate to suggest a certain number of patients per day as the "industry standard," but do note that the solutions for increasing productivity need to consider all of the factors that influence BHC productivity. One needs to consider the characteristics of his or her clinic, evaluate the competencies of the BHC, and set goals based on a plan to address clinic and BHC practice factors. As a starting point, one can calculate a maximum productivity level, assess current productivity levels, and then systematically address barriers to the BHC performing at the maximum productivity level. Begin with an assumption that BHCs need to engage in patient care and consultation 90 percent of the day, as is the standard for PCPs. For an eight-hour day, this is around seven hours per day (see Table 15.1). Ideally, about half of the BHC contacts on any given day will be initial contacts and half will be follow-up. This means that in a BHC service using thirty-minute initial visits and fifteen-minute follow-up visits (and seeing an equal number of new and follow-up patients), a high level of productivity for a seven-hour day would be fourteen patients. While difficult to measure, the BHC needs to also be providing approximately two seven-minute consultations per hour (written or oral) to PCPs in the remaining fifteen minutes of every hour, and this would result in fourteen PCP consultative interactions daily. Some of the consultations would of course be related to patients referred and seen that day; while others might concern patients seen previously who are following up with the PCP or patients the PCP is managing without BHC direct involvement. The grand total for direct service time for the average BHC should be around seven hours, and this should involve contact with twelve to sixteen patients and a similar number of contacts with PCPs on average. Table 15.1 offers a list of assumptions about BHC productivity in an eight-hour day. If using 40-minute (initial) and 20-minute (follow-up) visits, the same method can be applied by reserving five minutes each visit for consultation.

Tracking the number of patient visits that a BHC has on a monthly basis is helpful in evaluating the start of a BHC service and the impact of developments that occur in the service over time, such as implementation of clinical pathways that enhance the penetration of BHC services into the clinic population. Table 15.2 offers a method for calculating productivity scores, which can help BHCs and others, evaluate various programmatic efforts to improve patient access to BHC services. For example, assume that a half-time BHC saw 110 patients in August. His or her productivity score for August would be 71 percent (i.e., $110/(11 \times 14) = 0.71$). If the clinic implemented a pathway program for chronic pain or depression over the next three months, the expectation would be that the score would increase toward 100 percent. The value of a productivity score goes beyond what it contributes as one of several measures that are useful in evaluating the number of patients a BHC sees, as it also reflects the BHC's success in enhancing PCP motivation to participate in programs that increase BHC service penetration to members of the clinic population other than those referred for individual consultations.

Table 15.1. BHC productivity assumptions for an 8-hour day

Visit time	# per day	Time per visit type
Initial (assume 30 minutes)	7	3.5 hours
Follow-up (assume 15 minutes)	7	1.75 hours
Total Patient Care Time		5.25 hours
Direct Consultation with PCPs		
(assumes 7.5 minutes/consultation)	14	1.75 hours
Grand Total of Direct Service Time		7.00 hours

Table 15.2. A method for calculating a productivity score

1. Assume 22 days worked for a full-time BHC (prorate the number of days for part-time BHCs, for example 11 days for a half-time BHC)
2. Calculate the number of patient encounters the BHC completed for the month (available from billing data)
3. Multiply the number of days the BHC was employed to work (#1) by 14 to get the number of patient encounters the BHC would see if 100 percent productive
4. Divide 2 above by 3 above
5. This is a productivity score, with a range of 0 to 100 percent

Range of Problems and Populations

A strong approach to program evaluation also needs to include a plan for tracking the range of problems and populations seen. A healthy BHC service should capture a range of patient problems that go well beyond depression and anxiety. Included in a list of the most commonly referred problems should be chronic medical conditions, nonspecific somatic complaints, and preventative visits, as well as the full gamut of psychological conditions. The types of patients seen should also mirror the clinic's population demographics. For example, if a clinic sees many pediatric patients, so too should the BHC. In such a case, problems common to that population (e.g., ADHD or enuresis) should be among the most frequently referred problems. If patient race, ethnicity, and/or primary language can be tracked, these should also be represented similarly in the BHC and general clinic patient rosters.

BHC Impact on PCPs

Since the PCBH mission is to influence PCPs in their efforts to deliver care to patients with behavioral issues, assessing influence is an important part of program evaluation. PCPs should be surveyed annually as to their experience with the program and the impact of program services on their practice of medicine. Surveys should ask PCPs about their participation in learning activities related to BH issues (e.g., the percentage of learning experiences related to BH that come from interactions with the BHC, the percentage of continuing education funds spent on presentations related to BH issues, etc.). Other survey questions should address their perceived frequency of delivery of behavioral interventions versus prescribing and their overall confidence in evaluating and treating patient whose health is negatively impacted by behavioral problems. Finally, a checklist of specific techniques that the BHC targets for teaching in any given year (e.g., mindfulness, relaxation training, stress management training, etc.) is appropriate for an annual survey. Such a survey may also include questions from the Referral Barriers Questionnaire (see Chapter 8), as such will provide information about PCP perceptions of barriers to access, which will hopefully diminish as the BHC service matures.

MODEL FIDELITY

Model fidelity refers to the extent to which a BHC adheres to the PCBH model. In order to evaluate a model, day-to-day implementation needs to be consistent with implementation guidelines, many of which can be measured. The quantification of productivity by various means suggested in the previous section provides estimates of BHC penetration into the population, and a basic goal of the model is to have the BHC see at least 20 percent of patients attending a clinic on any given year. Also discussed previously, the BHC's influence on PCP practices can be estimated by data from annual surveys. There are other important aspects to program fidelity which we will examine in this section.

Ratio of BHC Hours to Patients

Measurement of fidelity needs to start with an assessment of the adequacy of BHC staffing. Strosahl (2006) recommends a minimum staffing ratio of between two and six hours of BHC time per week per 1,000 patients served by a clinic. For clinics that serve healthier populations, fewer hours are often adequate. In community health centers where the physical and psychological morbidity rate is much higher, more BHC hours are necessary. A community health center clinic that serves 10,000 patients would ideally have sixty hours of BHC service per week, while a clinic that serves 10,000 healthier patients (such as an HMO in an upscale suburban area) might need just twenty hours of BHC services. When the staffing ratio is inadequate, the BHC is likely to struggle with maintaining fidelity to the model, and, while creative solutions may be pursued, they will ultimately falter if staffing is inadequate to meet demand.

Ratio of New to Follow-up Patients

A BHC might be seeing an impressive number of patients each day but, if they come from the same small pool of patients seen week after week, the overall penetration into the population will be poor (i.e., far less than the 20 percent standard). In our experience, a good goal to aim for is a 1.0 ratio, meaning on any given day the BHC is seeing roughly an equal number of new and established patients. A ratio favoring new over follow-up patients (i.e., 2:1) suggests that the practice is receiving a healthy influx of new patients. When the ratio favors follow up visits (1:3), this could indicate that the BHC is sliding back into a therapy focus rather than a population health focus. The BHC that falls into a pattern of seeing patients for an excessive number of follow-ups quickly develops access problems, and PCPs will adjust by either slowing down or stopping new referrals.

Ratio of Same-Day to Scheduled Patients

A primary goal of the PCBH model is to improve access to BH services for both PCPs and patients. Patients and providers prefer same-day access, and the "warm handoff" approach capitalizes on the "teachable" moment that increases the likelihood of a real behavior change. Scheduling patients limits future access, and often results in no-shows. The goal is for the BHC to see at least as many same-day handoffs as scheduled new appointments.

There are a number of factors that affect progress toward this ideal, including the BHC's template and the adequacy of BHC time in the clinic. A template that is split equally between services for same-day and scheduled patients supports access for same-day patients. In addition, having a full-time BHC helps PCPs fully embrace the same-day access aspect of the PCBH model. If the BHC service is part-time, the PCP hesitates in pursuing the same-day option because it takes more time to find out if the BHC is around than it does to have an assistant schedule an appointment. Unless the PCP is particularly worried about the patient, the tendency is to be efficient, ask the assistant to help with the referral, and move to the next patient. This problem may be worsened by variation in hours by part-time BHC providers, as PCPs will eventually give up and say, "I never know when he (she) is going to be here—so I just have the patient schedule an appointment." The other factor that may have a negative impact on efforts to achieve fidelity in this important area is understaffing of BHC time. When a clinic is understaffed, PCPs see their BHC colleague struggle to meet the demand for patient care and take pity on him or her. They may develop a habit of having their assistants check the BHC schedule to see if there is room for a same-day patient. When they see he or she has twenty-two scheduled patients, they forget about the same-day option and simply schedule the patient (and thus probably contribute to her or his having twenty-two scheduled patients seven days into the future).

Days to Next Available

Another important way to assess model fidelity related to access goals is to look at the number of days until a scheduled appointment is available for the BHC. Hopefully, the BHC template will have stops, such that there is always a next day appointment available. If not, the BHC may find that it is difficult to maintain one week access for all referred patients that do not (or cannot) take advantage of the same-day visit option. This is particularly the case after the BHC takes any type of leave time. It is a problem that has no clear solution at this point in the model's development, other than using the advanced access strategy of closing the BHC's schedule in advance for the number of days he or she plans to be out of the clinic and then opening the blocked scheduled one week prior to BHC return.

Average Number of Visits Per Patient

Another indicator of fidelity is the average number of visits per patients (or encounters per unique user seen by the BHC). This measure needs to be defined in yearly increments. Evaluation efforts might include looking at the percentage of patients with one BHC visit, two to three BHC visits, four to five BHC visits, and more than five BHC visits. The BHC showing fidelity to the PCBH model would see only 10 to 15 percent of patients more than four times. If a large percentage of patients are seen only once, the average number of encounters will be about 2, a very appropriate number.

Another helpful strategy is to randomly sample from the patient group that a BHC is seeing more than three times per year in an effort to identify emerging patterns. Hopefully, one would find that patients seen more than four or five times in a year are those with the greatest risk (e.g., noncompliant diabetics who are changing levels of readiness for change, older patients with multiple medical problems for whom a rehospitalization might be avoided, patients with schizophrenia who have limited access to other services) rather than patients who could be expected to be successfully treated by their PCP with less than five BHC visits (e.g., patients with mild to moderate symptoms of depression, garden variety psychosocial stress, etc.). This analysis will reveal difficulties that the BHC is having in targeting patients for less and more intensive follow-up. As the BHC is more successful in returning patients to PCPs, he or she is able to see more patients, particularly for preventive visits. BHCs may also find that creating clinical pathways associated with group services for high impact patients is an effective alternative to seeing them one at a time for multiple visits in one year.

Other Fidelity Indicators

Reviews of BHC chart notes may provide helpful information about BHC fidelity to specific aspects of the PCBH model, such as ability to focus on the referral problem, conduct a functional analysis, use health-related quality of life measures to plan with patients and PCPs, suggest self-management strategies for patients, and make feasible, descriptive recommendations to PCPs. Review of chart notes also allows evaluators to know if the BHC is using the planned format and staying within the specified length for BHC notes (which is usually well under one page). Chapter 3 offers ideas for chart reviews.

Visit length and recommendation patterns involving referral are also indicators of model fidelity. The model requires that BHC visits be completed in less than thirty minutes. The model also specifies that most referred patients will be served in PC. Assessment of percentage of BHC patients referred for specialty treatment is an important indicator of the extent to which the BHC is attempting to meet patient needs by supplementing PCP treatment with consultation versus operating a "triage clinic" in the PC center. Our clinical experience suggests that BHCs are no more successful than PCPs in getting PC patients to go to a specialty setting and that most PC patients prefer to receive BH services in PC. Therefore, it is important that referring patients to specialists not become a dominant intervention for the BHC.

Finally, the model requires that the BHC practice in a population-based care model. The indication of fidelity to this aspect of the model can come from a brief review of narrative reports that the BHC writes on a monthly basis for the clinic manager and clinic medical director. These reports need to demonstrate sustained focus on development of programs that are a priority in the clinic. All of the measures of fidelity will be useful in helping BHCs shape their practice, and they may be particularly helpful to administrators in a large system with multiple clinics where there are significant differences in BHC productivity outcomes among the clinics.

CONSUMER (PCP AND PATIENT) SATISFACTION

As we have described in earlier chapters, there are two basic customers of the PCBH model: the consumer–patient and the referring medical provider. Thus, customer satisfaction assessment should be a cornerstone of any outcome evaluation. In our experience, positive consumer responses provide compelling support for a BHC service in the eyes of administrators. Unfavorable responses may help a BHC isolate potential service delivery problems. As mentioned in Chapter 8, the Referral Barrier's Questionnaire offers a brief assessment approach to provider satisfaction with BHC services. These satisfaction scores can be tracked from year to year. Of course, some clinics will want to obtain more detailed information from PCPs specific to satisfaction with BHC services, and hopefully PCPs can complete one survey that addresses satisfaction, as well as impact of BHC services on PCP practice (as suggested in the Productivity section of this chapter). Provider surveys are best distributed at a PCP meeting, with all PCPs present and away from the hustle and bustle of the clinic. (Surveys left on a PCP's desk for completion stand a slim chance of being returned.) If possible, secure time for PCPs to actually complete the survey during the meeting. This will maximize your return rate. To ensure anonymity, ask the clinic's lead provider or medical director to be in charge of collecting the surveys for the BHC.

The PCBH model, by design, should promote changes that improve patient experience in receiving PC services, and it is important to identify these specifically in program evaluation efforts. Contemporary directions for PC system improvement include use of teams in medicine, establishment of meaningful PC partnerships, and integration of care that lessens patient experience of fragmentation (Safran, 2003). When successful, implementation of the PCBH model should result in creation of more functional work teams that enhance patient experience of continuity. Additionally, patients treated in clinics where this model is practiced should report better communication with the PCP and superior whole-person care over time. Items of use in evaluating these hypothesized changes may include items that assess patient opinion concerning (1) PCP knowledge of the patient as a person (i.e., their values and beliefs), (2) PCP coordination between members of the PC treatment team, and (3) PCP skills in explaining health problems or treatments needed. The Primary Care Assessment Survey (Safran et al., 1998) offers examples of useful items.

In regards to patient satisfaction more specifically, we recommend at least annual assessments. While some systems or clinics will prefer to use the same patient satisfaction surveys for BHCs as used for other PCPs, we recommend that the BHC obtain feedback from patients annually using questions specific to BHC services. Table 15.3 provides items from a survey specific to BHC services developed by PR and her colleagues, Dr. Jenifer Schultz and Dennis Anderson. Patients respond to items on a scale ranging from 0 to 10, with 0 indicating "not true" and 10 indicating "completely true." As with PCP surveys, patient surveys need to be completed anonymously to help ensure candid responses. Patient surveys are probably best completed by randomly selecting a week each quarter and asking every patient seen by the BHC during that week to complete a survey. Patients can be given the survey and a stamped return envelope at the conclusion of a BHC visit, asked to complete it at home and drop it in any mail box. In addition, a collection box should be placed in the waiting room for patients who agree to complete their survey before leaving the clinic. It is also useful to develop specific patient satisfaction measures for patients in clinical pathways and group medical care programs. Patients

Table 15.3. Items for measuring patient satisfaction with BHC services

1.	The BHC seemed warm, supportive, and caring
2.	The BHC treated me with respect
3.	The BHC did a good job of listening
4.	I talked about the problems that bother me
5.	The approach we used made sense to me
6.	I learned new ways to deal with my problems
7.	I believe the BHC has good ideas for me and my PCP
8.	I intend to use what I learned in the visit

like to express their opinions, and their ideas can help BHCs make quick corrections in programmatic efforts, if needed.

CLINICAL EFFECTIVENESS

Those new to this model of care frequently ask about the model's effectiveness. At conference presentations, we frequently hear questions such as, "What good can you possibly do with one or two twenty-minute visits?" Indeed, considering the types of complex, chronic and often severe problems encountered in PC, twenty (or even forty) minutes does not seem like a lot of time to make a difference. Even if consumer satisfaction ratings are high and productivity is good, the question of clinical effectiveness still looms. Examining whether the patients receiving services are actually improving is therefore an important component of program evaluation.

Without conducting a randomized, controlled study (something few readers of this text will likely be able to do), scientifically "bullet proof" statements about clinical outcome are difficult to make. So many factors can help determine clinical outcomes that attributing clinical change to any one factor without accounting for other factors is risky business and poor science. The fact that a patient's functioning improves after a visit with the BHC does not necessarily demonstrate the effectiveness of the BHC. Perhaps the patient improved because of medications her or his PCP began, or perhaps the patient received good news or solved a problem that had been weighing him or her down. Nonetheless, measuring clinical change can be useful for guiding treatment and it can at least gauge whether patients are headed in a positive direction. Although one might not be able to state definitively the cause of a patient's improvement, demonstrating at least that patients *are* improving subsequent to a BHC visit is useful.

To this end, some sort of clinical measure should be used during every patient visit with the BHC. In Chapter 6 we discussed some of the more commonly used measures. Which to use depends mostly on the area of interest to the clinic. If, for example, a clinic wants to track outcome for patients with symptoms of depression, using the PHQ-9 with all patients would be helpful. If instead a clinic is more interested in global functioning changes, routine administration of the Duke Health Profile would be appropriate. Whatever the focus or the tool used, the BHC should maintain a secure database of scores so that analyses can be conducted as needed. Both of us use a simple Excel database, inputting scores of the Duke after each patient visit. When conducting program evaluations, this allows us to examine clinical change from visit one to visit two, from visit one to visit three, etc. As noted previously, showing significant improvement in functioning subsequent to a BHC visit(s) does not necessarily mean that change can be attributed to the BHC visit. However, it at least allows us to show that patients do improve (as opposed to being stagnant or deteriorating). This, combined with positive patient and provider satisfaction ratings and good productivity, makes a compelling case for the effectiveness of a BHC service.

SUGGESTIONS FOR FUTURE PROGRAM EVALUATION AND RESEARCH ACTIVITIES

Some may be interested in a more rigorous evaluation of the BHC model, and the field is greatly in need of such. Although impractical for the average BHC who is a full-time clinician, persons working in research settings or with some professional time available for research could make a significant contribution to the literature by evaluating this model more thoroughly. There are numerous questions that would be helpful to investigate in detail. One question is whether use of the BHC model improves the outcome of care for behaviorally based problems, relative to PC as usual. This is, after all, one of the core goals of a BHC service.

A number of randomized, controlled trials have evaluated models somewhat similar to the BHC model, and they have almost universally showed benefits of an augmented care system relative to PC as usual (for example, see Harpole et al., 2005; Katon et al., 1996; Mynors-Wallace, Gath, Lloyd-Thomas, & Tomlinson, 1995; Von Korff et al., 1998). Yet, more data are needed. In one type of study, patients with a given condition (e.g., depression) would be randomly assigned to receive usual PC or PC plus a BHC intervention. In addition to comparing the two approaches on functional improvement and consumer satisfaction, other meaningful comparisons might include primary health care utilization, emergency services utilization, and associated prescription medicine costs. This would allow for cost analyses on the two types of service delivery. Available information suggests that PCBH services would help save medical dollars but, again, much more data are needed (see Chiles, Lambert, & Hatch, 1999 for a discussion).

Other studies of value would compare a clinic with a BHC service to one without a BHC service. Assuming one controls for extraneous factors, a comparison of average appointment times and access to appointments would be interesting. One would anticipate that a clinic with a BHC service would have better access and shorter duration PCP visits, on average. Comparing outcome from a PCBH program to that of a specialty (tertiary) MH clinic would be interesting as well, though it would be mostly academic because of the realities of the health care system. That is, regardless of which approach yields better outcome, the realities outlined in Chapter 1 mean that most behavioral issues will continue to present in PC, not in specialty MH. Potentially more interesting would be a comparison of PC clinics using a BHC model versus some other model (e.g., a co-located specialty model).

SUMMARY

1. BHC productivity is a beginning point for evaluating the PCBH model. The average number of daily encounters is probably the single most important program measure. Productivity estimates need also to reflect BHC consistency in effort and success in impact on PCP knowledge, confidence, and practice patterns by whatever means, including creating pathways and group programs.

2. Appropriate implementation of the PCBH model involves several measurable practice parameters, including adequate BHC to patient

staffing ratios and balanced ratios on other practice indicators, including new to follow-up visits and same-day to scheduled visits. Consistent monitoring of days to next available BHC visits supports evaluation of several program fidelity measures, and exploration of average number of visits yields fruitful information about appropriate and inappropriate utilizers of BHC services. Other measures of fidelity are worthwhile when the purpose of program evaluation includes helping BHCs refine their skills, and we believe this must be a part of an evaluation plan.

3. Customer satisfaction assessment is a must, and this includes surveying both patients and referring medical providers. It's also a good idea to assess BHC job satisfaction and address problems early.

4. We strongly recommend using some type of functional status measure at every contact, including individual, class and group medical appointments. These data need to be explored in aggregate form. Only scientific studies beyond the scope of the typical BHC practice can demonstrate the efficacy of the PCBH model (e.g., randomized clinical trials), and we hope that this book in a small way promotes a better recognition of the need for such studies in academia.

REFERENCES

Aastopoulos, A. D., Barkley, R. A., & Shelton, T. L. (1996). Family-based treatment: Psychosocial intervention for children and adolescents with attention deficit hyperactivity disorder. In E. D. Hibbs & P. S. Jensen (Eds.), *Psychosocial treatment for child and adolescent disorders: Empirically based strategies for clinical practice.* Washington, DC: American Psychological Association.

Agency for healthcare research and quality. (2003a). *Screening for dementia. Recommendations and rationale.* AHRQ Publication Number 03–520A. www.preventiveservices.ahrq.gov.

Agency for healthcare research and quality. (2003b). http://www.ncbi.nlm.nih.gov/books/bv.fcgi?rid=hstat3.section.28274.

American Academy of Pain Medicine. (2005). *Sample agreement: Long-term controlled substances therapy for chronic pain.* Available at http://www.painmed.org/productpub/statements/sample.html.

American Academy of Pediatrics. (1991). American academy of pediatrics committee on child abuse and neglect: Guidelines for the evaluation of sexual abuse of children. *Pediatrics, 87*(2), 254–260.

American Academy of Pediatrics. (1997). *Guidelines for health supervision III.* Elk Grove, IL: Committee on Psychosocial Aspects of Child and Family Health.

American Academy of Pediatrics. (2000). Suicide and suicide attempts in adolescents. *Pediatrics, 105,* 871–874.

American Medical Association. (1997). *Guidelines for adolescent preventive services.* Chicago: AMA.

American Medical Association. (1992a). American medical association diagnostic and treatment guidelines on child physical abuse and neglect. *Archives of Family Medicine, 1*(2), 187–197.

American Medical Association. (1992b). *AMA Council on scientific affairs: Diagnostic and treatment guidelines on elder abuse and neglect.* Chicago: American Medical Association.

American Medical Association. (1992c). *Diagnostic and treatment guidelines on domestic violence.* Chicago: American Medical Association.

American Medical Association. (1993). American medical association diagnostic and treatment guidelines on child sexual abuse. *Archives of Family Medicine, 2*(1), 19–27.

American Medical Association Council on Scientific Affairs. (1987). Elder abuse and neglect. *Journal of the American Medical Association, 257*(7), 966–971.

American Psychiatric Association. (1994). *Diagnostic and statistical manual of mental disorders* (4th ed.) (DSM-IV). Washington, DC: American Psychological Association.

American Psychological Association. (1989). *Ethical principles of psychologist sand code of conduct.* Washington, DC: American Psychological Association.

American Psychological Association. (2003). *Ethical principles of psychologist sand code of conduct.* http:// www.apa.org/ethics/ code2002. html.

American Psychological Association Government Relations Staff. (2004). FAQs on the Health and behavior CPT codes 2002, February 27, 2004. http://www.apapractice.org/apo/pracorg/ new_cpt_codes.html#.

Ash, P. (1949). The reliability of psychiatric diagnoses. *Journal of Abnormal and Social Psychology, 44,* 272–277.

Asher, S. R., & Paquette, J. A. (2003). Loneliness and peer relations in childhood. *Current Directions in Psychological Science, 12*(3), 75.

Badamgarav, E., Weingarten, S. R., Henning, J. M., Knight, K., Hasselblad, V., Gano, A., Ofman, J. J. (2003). Effectiveness of disease management programs in depression: A systematic review. *American Journal of Psychology, 160,* 2080–2090.

Barlow, D., O'Leary, T. A., & Craske, M. G. (1992). *Mastery of your anxiety and worry: Client workbook.* Albany, New York: Graywind Publications.

Barry, C. A., Stevenson, F. A., Britten, N., Barber, N., & Bradley, C. P. (2001). Giving voice to the lifeworld: More humane, more effective medical care? A qualitative study of doctor–patient communication in general practice. *Social Science and Medicine, 53,* 487–505.

Beardsley, R., Gardocki, G., Larson, D., & Hidalgo, J. (1988). Prescribing of psychotropic medication by primary care physicians and psychiatrists. *Archives of General Psychiatry, 45,* 1117–1119.

Beck, A. (1962). Reliability of psychiatric diagnoses. I. A critique of systematic studies. *American Journal of Psychiatry, 119,* 210–216.

Beck, A., Scott, J., Williams, P., Robertson, B., Jackson, D., Gade, G., Cowan, P. (1997). A randomized trial of group outpatient visits for chronically ill older HMO members: The cooperative health care clinic. *Journal of the American Geriatric Society, 45,* 543–549.

Becvar, D. S. (2001). *In the presence of grief: Helping family members resolve death, dying, and bereavement issues.* New York: Guilford.

Biglan, A. (1995). *Changing cultural practices: A contextualist framework for intervention research.* Reno, NV: Context Press.

Blount, A. (1998). *Integrated primary care: The future of medical and mental health collaboration.* New York: Norton.

Bodenheimer, T., Lorig, K., Holman, H., & Grumbach, K. (2002). Patient self-management of chronic disease in primary care *Journal of the American Medical Association, 288,* 2469–2475.

Bodenheimer, T., Wagner, E. H., & Grumbach, K. (2002a). Improving primary care for patients with chronic illness. *Journal of the American Medical Association, 288*(14), 1775–1779.

Bodenheimer, T., Wagner, E. H., & Grumbach, K. (2002b). Improving primary care for patients with chronic illness. The chronic care model. Part 2. *Journal of the American Medical Association, 288*(15), 1909–1914.

Bolls, T. J. Introduction to the Series. (2004). In Handbook of clinical health psychology. In R. G. Frank, A. Baum, & J. L. Wallander (Eds.), *Models and perspectives in health psychology* (Vol. 3). Washington, DC: American Psychological Association.

Borson, S., Brush, M., Gil, E., Scanlan, J., Vitaliano, P., Chen, J., et al. (1999). The clock drawing test: Utility for dementia detection in multiethnic elders. *Journal of Gerontology and Biological Science and Medical Science, 54*(11), M534–M540.

Boustani, M., Peterson, B., Hanson, L., Harris, R., & Lohr, K. N. (2003). Screening for dementia in primary care: A summary of the evidence for the U. S. preventive services task force, *Clinical Guidelines, 138*(11), 927–937. http://www.annals.org/cgi/content/full/138/11/927.

Bray, J. H., Frank, R. G., McDaniel, S. H., & Heldring, M. H. (2004). Education, practice, and research opportunities for psychologists in primary care. In R. G. Frank, S. H. McDaniel, J. H. Bray, & M. Heldring (Eds.), *Primary care psychology*. Washington, DC: American Psychological Association.

Brock, H. (2005). Personal phone communication.

Brown, A. (1993). Violence against women by male partners: Prevalence, outcomes, and policy implications. *American Psychologist, 48*, 1077–1087.

Brown, R. (2002). *Roadmaps for clinical practice: Case studies in disease prevention and health promotion–intimate partner violence*. Chicago: AMA.

Brown, R. L., & Rounds, L. A. (1995). Conjoint screening questionnaires for alcohol and drug abuse. *Wisconsin Medical Journal, 94*, 135–140.

Brownell, K. D. (1997). *The LEARN program for weight control* (7th ed.). Texas: American Health Publishing Company.

Burke, B. L., Arkowitz, H., & Menchola, M. (2003). The efficacy of motivational interviewing: A meta-analysis of controlled clinical trials. *Journal of Consulting and Clinical Psychology, 71*, 843–861.

Burns, D. D. (1980). *Feeling good: The new mood therapy*. New York: Avon Books.

Butler, S. F., Budman, S. H., Fernandez, K., & Jamison, R. N. (2004). Validation of a screener and opioid assessment measure for patients with chronic pain. *Pain, 112*, 65–75.

Cappeliez, P., O'Rourke, N., & Chaudhury, H. (2005). Functions of reminiscence and mental health in later life. *Aging and Mental Health, 9*(4), 295–301.

Chabal, C., Miklavz, E., Jacobson, L., Mariano, A., & Chaney, E. (1997). Prescription opiate abuse in chronic pain patients: Clinical criteria, incidence, and predictors. *Clinical Journal of Pain, 13*, 150–155.

Chang, G. (2001). Alcohol-screening instruments for pregnant women. *Alcohol Research, 25*(3), 204–209.

Chelminski, P. R., Ives, T. J., Felix, K. M., Prakken, S. D., Filler, T. M., Perhac, J. S., et al. (2005). A primary care, multi-disciplinary disease management program for opioid-treated patients with chronic non-cancer pain and a high burden of psychiatric comorbidity. *BMC health services research, 5.* http://www.biomedcentral.com/1472–6963–5–3.

Cherpitel, C. J. (2002). Screening for alcohol problems in the U.S. general population: Comparison of the CAGE, RAPS4, and RAPS4-QF by gender, ethnicity, and service utilization. Rapid alcohol problems screen. *Alcoholism, Clinical and Experimental Research, 26*(11), 1686–1691.

Chiles, J., Lambert, M., & Hatch, A. (1999). The impact of psychological interventions on medical cost offset: A meta-analytic review. *Clinical Psychology: Science and Practice, 6,* 204–220.

Chiles, J. A., & Strosahl, K. D. (2005). *Clinical manual for assessment and treatment of suicidal patients.* Washington, DC: American Psychiatric Publishing, Inc.

Christophersen, E. R., & Mortweet, S. L. (2003). *Treatments that work with children: Empirically supported strategies for managing childhood problems.* Washington, DC: American Psychological Association.

Clark, H. W., & Sees, K. L. (1993). Opioids, chronic pain, and the law. *Journal of Pain Symptom Management, 8*(5), 297–305.

Coleman, E. A., Smith, J D., Frank, J. C., Min, S-J., Parry, C., & Kramer, A. M. (2004). Preparing patients and caregivers to participate in care delivered across settings: The care transitions intervention. *Journal of the American Geriatrics Society, 52*(11), 1817–1825.

Commonwealth Department of Health and Ageing. (2002). Medicare benefits schedule book: Operating from 1 November 2002. Canberra: Commonwealth of Australia. Available at http://www.health.gov. au/pubs/mbs/mbs/css/ mbs_book_nov_02?cata.pdf.

Commonwealth Fund. (1999). *Health concerns across a woman's lifespan: The commonwealth fund 1998 survey of women's health.* New York: The Commonwealth Fund.

Cooper, B., Bickel, H., & Schaufele, M. (1996). Early development and progression of dementing illness in the elderly: A general-practice based study. *Psychological Medicine, 26,* 411–419.

Corrigan, P. (2004). How stigma interferes with mental health care. *American Psychologist, 59*(7), 614–625.

Costello, E. J., Burns, B. J., Costello, A. J., Edelbrock, C., Dulcan, M., & Brent, D. (1988). Service utilization and psychiatric diagnosis in pediatric primary care: The role of the gatekeeper. *Pediatrics, 82*, 415–424.

Craske, M. G., & Barlow, D. H. (2000). *Mastery of your anxiety and panic* (3rd ed.) (MAP-3): Client Workbook. The psychological corporation (800–211–8378; Fax: 800–232–1223; www.PsychCorp.com/).

Craske, M. G., Barlow, D. H., & Meadows, E. A. (2000). *Mastery of your anxiety and panic* (3rd ed.) (MAP-3): Therapist Guide. The psychological corporation (800–211–8378; Fax: 800–232–1223; www.PsychCorp.com/).

Cummings, N. A., & Follette, W. T. (1968). Psychiatric services and medical utilization in a prepaid health plan setting: Part II. *Medical Care, 6*, 31–41.

Currey, S. S., Rao, J. K., Winfield, J. B., & Callahan, L. F. (10-7-2003). Performance of a generic health-related quality of life measure in a clinic population with rheumatic disease. American College of Rheumatology. (http://www3.interscience.wiley.com/cgi-bin/abstract/105561268)

Das, A. K., Olfson, M., Gameroff, M. J., Pilowsky, D. J., Blanco, C., Feder, A., et al. (2005). Screening for bipolar disorder in a primary care practice. *Journal of the American Medical Association, 293*, 956–963.

DeLeon, P. H., Giesting, B., & Kenkel, M. B. (2003). Community health centers: Exciting opportunities for the 21st century. *Professional Psychology: Research and Practice, 34*(6), 579–585.

Dickinson, J. C., Evans, K. L., Carter, J., & Burke, K. (2004). Task force report 4. Report of the task force on marketing and communications. *Annals of Family Medicine, 2*, S75–S87.

Dittmann, K. (2004). CPT codes: Use them or lose them. *APA Monitor, 35*(9), 58–59.

Dodson, W. W. (2005). Pharmacotherapy of adult ADHD. *Journal of Clinical Psychology*. Published online at www.interscience.wiley.com.

Doleys, D. M., & Rickman, L. (2003). Other benefits of an "Opioid" agreement, *Journal of Pain and Symptom Management, 25*(5), 402–403.

Doody, R. S., Stevens, J. C., Beck, C., Dubinsky, R. M., Kaye, J. A., Gwyther, L., et al. (2001). Practice parameter: Management of dementia (an evidence-based review). *Neurology, 56*, 1154–1166.

Dunbar-Jacob, J., & Mortimer-Stephens, M. K. (2001). Treatment adherence in chronic disease. *Journal of Clinical Epidemiology, 54*, 857–860.

Elliott, L., Nerney, M., Jones, T., & Friedmann, P. D. (2002). Barriers to screening for domestic violence. *Journal of General Internal Medicine, 17*, 112–116.

Engel, G. (1977). The need for a new medical model: A challenge for biomedicine. *Science, 196*, 129–136.

Ewart, C. K. (2004). How integrative behavioral theory can improve health promotion and disease prevention. In R. G. Frank, A. Baum, & J. L. Wallander (Vol. Eds.), *Handbook of clinical health psychology, Vol. 3: Models and Perspectives in Health Psychology.* Washington, DC: American Psychological Association.

Ewing, J. A. (1984). Detecting alcoholism. The CAGE questionnaire. *Journal of the American Medical Association, 252*(14), 1905–1907.

Fadiman, A. (1997). *The spirit catches you and you fall down: a Hmong child, her American doctors, and the collision of two cultures.* New York: Garrar, Straus and Giroux.

Faraone, S. V., & Wilens, T. E. (2003). Does stimulant treatment lead to substance use disorder? *Journal of Clinical Psychiatry, 64*(11), 9–13.

Felitti, V. J. (2002). The relationship between adverse childhood experiences and adult health: Turning gold into lead. *The Permanente Journal, Winter, 6*(1), 44–47. http://xnet.kp.org/permanentejournal/winter02/goldtolead.pdf.

Felitti, V. J., Anda, R. F., Nordenberg, D., Williamson, D. F., Spitz, A. M., Edwards, V., et al. (1998). Relationship of childhood abuse and household dysfunction to many of the leading causes of death in adults. The adverse childhood experiences (ACE) study. *American Journal of Prevention Medicine, 14*(4), 245–258. http://www.meddevel.com/site.mash?left=/library.exe&m1=4&m2=1&right=/library.exe&action= search_form&search. mode=simple&site=AJPM&jcode=AMEPRE.

Fendrich, M., Weissman, M. M., & Warner, V. (1990). Screening for depressive disorder in children and adolescents: Validating the center for epidemiologic studies depression scale for children. *American Journal of Epidemiology, 131*(3), 538–551.

Fergusson, D. M., Horwood, L. J., & Woodward, L. J. (2000). The stability of child abuse reports: A longitudinal study of the reporting behaviour of young adults. *Psychological Medicine, 30*(3), 529–544.

Fishman, S. M., & Kreis, P. G. (2002). The opioid contract. *Clinical Journal of Pain, 18*, 70–75.

Follette, W. T., & Cummings, N. A. (1967). Psychiatric services and medical utilization in a prepaid health plan setting. *Medical Care, 5*, 25–35.

Folstein, M. F., Folstein, S. E., & McHugh P. R. (1975). "Mini-mental state". A practical method for grading the cognitive state of patients for the clinician. *Journal of Psychiatric Research, 12*, 189–198.

Fordyce, W. W. (1976). *Behavioral methods for chronic pain and illness.* St Louis: Mosby.

Fortrin, A., Robinson, P., & Walsh, K. (in preparation). Using the bull's eyeprescription pad to prevent onset of chronic pain.

Fraser, A. D. (1998). Use and abuse of the benzodiazepines. *Therapeutic Drug Monitoring, 20*(5), 481–9.

Friedman, B., Heisel, M. J., & Delavan, R. L. (2005). Psychometric properties of the 15-item geriatric depression scale in functionally impaired, cognitively intact, community-dwelling elderly primary care patients. *Journal of the American Geriatric Society, 53*(9), 1570–1576.

Friedman, R., Sobel, D., Myers, P., Caudill, M., & Benson, H. (1995). Behavioral medicine, clinical health psychology, and cost offset. *Health Psychology, 14*(6), 509–518.

Gardner, W., Murphy, M., Childs, G., Kelleher, K., Pagano, M., Jellinek, M., et al. (1999). The PSC-17: A brief pediatric symptom checklist with psychosocial problem subscales. A report from PROS and ASPN. *Ambulatory Child Health, 5*, 225–236.

Garretty, D. J., Wolff, K., Hay, A. W. M., & Raistrick, D. (1997). Benzodiazepine misuse by drug addicts. *Annals of Clinical Biochemistry, 34*, 68–73.

Gatchel, R. J., & Oordt, M. S. (2003). *Clinical health psychology and primary care: Practical advice and clinical guidance for successful collaboration.* Washington, DC: American Psychological Association.

Gilden, J. L., Hendryx, M. S., Clar, S., Casia, C., & Singh, S. P. (1992). Diabetes support groups improve health care of older diabetic patients. *Journal of American Geriatric Society, 40*(2), 147–150.

Gielen, A. C., O'Campo, P. J., Campbell, J. C., Schollenberger, J., Woods, A. B., Jones, A. S., et al. (2000). Women's opinions about domestic violence screening and mandatory reporting. *American Journal of Preventive Medicine, 19*, 279–285.

Giler, J. Z. (1998). *Socially ADDept: A manual for parents of children with ADHD and/or learning disabilities.* Santa Barbara, CA: CES Publications.

Goldfried, M. R., & Davison, G. C. (1994). *Clinical behavior therapy.* New York: Wiley & Sons, Inc.

Gray, G. V., Brody, D. S., & Johnson, D. (2005). The evolution of behavioral primary care. *Professional Psychology, Research and Practice, 36*(2), 123–129.

Greco, L. A., & Dew, S. E. (2005). PAACT-friendly reading list for children and families, ACT Summer Institute 2005, Philadelphia, Pennsylvania.

Gregg, J. (2004). Personal communication. National Centers for Post Traumatic Stress Disorder, Veterans' Administration Hospital, Palo Alto, CA.

Halverson, J., & Chan, C. (2004). Screening for psychiatric disorders in primary care. *Wisconsin Medical Journal, 103*(6), 46–51.

Hamberger, L. K., Saunders, D. G., & Hovey, M. (1992). Prevalence of domestic violence in community practice and rate of physician inquiry. *Family Medicine, 24,* 283–287.

Harpole, L. H., Williams, J. W., Olsen, M. K., Stechuchak, K. M., Oddone, E., Callahan, C. M., et al. (2005). Improving depression outcomes in older adults with comorbid medical illness. *General Hospital Psychiatry, 27*(1), 4–12.

Hayes, S. C. (2004). Acceptance and commitment therapy, relational frame theory, and the third wave of behavioral and cognitive therapies. *Behavior Therapy, 35*(4), 639–665.

Hayes, S. C., & Smith, S. (2005). *Get out of your mind and into your life.* Oakland, CA: New Harbinger.

Hayes, S. C. ACT List Serve.

Hayes, S., Strosahl, K., & Wilson, K. (1999). *Acceptance and commitment therapy: An experiential approach to behavior change.* New York: Guilford Press.

Hayes, S. C., & Strosahl, K. D. (2004). *A practical guide to acceptance and commitment therapy.* New York: Springer.

Health Care Financing Administration, www.hcfa.gov, Bio-medical.com

Hermos, J. A., Young, M. M., Gagnon, D. R., & Fiore, L. D. (2004). Characterizations of long-term oxycodone/acetaminophen prescriptions in veteran patients. *Archives of Internal Medicine, 164,* 2361–2366.

Hibbs, E. D., & Jensen, P. S. (1996). Attention deficit hyperactivity disorder: Introduction. In E. D. Hibbs, & P. S. Jensen (Eds.), *Psychosocial treatments for child and adolescent disorders: empirically based strategies for clinic practice* (pp. 263–266). Washington, DC: American Psychological Association.

Hickie, I., & Groom, G. (2002). Primary care-led mental health service reform: An outline of the better outcomes in mental health care initiative. *Australas Psychiatry, 10,* 376–382.

Hirschfeld, R. M., Williams, J. B., Spitzer, R. L., Calabrese, J. R., Flynn, L., Keck, P. E., et al. (2000). Development and validation of a screening instrument for bipolar spectrum disorder: The mood disorder questionnaire. *American Journal of Psychiatry, 157*(11), 1873–1875.

Horwitz, S. M., Leaf, P. J., Leventhal, J. M., Forsyth, B., & Speechley, K. N. (1992). Identification and management of psychosocial and developmental problems in community-based primary care clinics. *Pediatrics, 89,* 480–485.

Inouye, S. K., van Dyck, C. H., Alessi, C. A., Balkin, S., Siegal, A. P., & Horwitz, R. I. (1990). Clarifying confusion: The confusion assessment method. A new method for detection of delirium. *Annals of Internal Medicine, 113*(12), 941–948.

Institute of Medicine of the National Academies. (1996). Primary care: America's health in a new era. Washington, DC: Institute of Medicine. Available at http://www.iom.edu/CMS/3809/27706.aspx.

Jackson-Bowers, E. H. C., & McCabe, D. (2002). Primary mental health care Australian resource centre online: http:// som.flinders.edu.au/ FUSA/PARC.

Jacobson, P. L., & Mann, J. D. (2004). The valid informed consent-treatment contract in chronic non-cancer pain: Its role in reducing barriers to effective pain management. *Comprehensive Therapy, 30*(2), 101–104.

Jacobson, N. S., & Margolin, G. (1979). *Marital therapy: Strategies based on social learning and behavioral exchange principles.* New York: Brunner/Mazel, Inc.

Jellinek, M. S., Murphy, J. M., Little, M., Pagano, M. E., Comer, D. M., & Kelleher, K. F. (1999). Use of the pediatric symptom checklist to screen for psychosocial problems in pediatric primary care: A national feasibility study. *Archives of Pediatric and Adolescent Medicine, 153*(3), 254–260.

Johnson, S. B. (2001). Integrating behavior into health research and health care: One psychologist's journey. *Journal of Clinical Psychology in Medical Settings, 11*(2), 91–99.

Kabat-Zinn, J. (1994). *Wherever you go there you are: Mindfulness meditation in everyday life.* New York: Hyperion.

Kaplan, S. H., Gandek, B., Greenfield, S., Rogers, W., & Ware, J. E. (1995). Patient and visit characteristics related to physicians' participatory decision-making style: Results from the medical outcomes study. *Medical Care, 33,* 1176–1187.

Katon, W., Robinson, P., Von Korff, M., Lin, E., Bush, T., Ludman, E., et al. (1996). A multifaceted intervention to improve treatment of depression in primary care. *Archives of General Psychiatry, 53,* 924–932.

Katon, W., Von Korff, M., Lin, E., Lipscomb, P., Russo, J., Wagner, E., et al. (1990). Distressed high utilizers of medical care. DSM-III-R diagnoses and treatment needs. *General Hospital Psychiatry, 12*(6), 355–362.

Katon, W., Von Korff, M., Lin, E., Walker, E., Simmon, G. E., Bush, T., et al. (1995). Collaborative management to achieve treatment guidelines: Impact on depression in primary care. *Journal of the American Medical Association, 273*(13), 1026–1031.

Kazdin, A. (2001). *Behavior modification in applied settings.* New York: Wadsworth.

Kilpatrick, D., Edmunds, C., & Seymour, A. (1992). Rape in America: A report to the nation. Washington, D. C.: National Institute of Drug Abuse, the National Victim Center and the National Crime Victims Research and Treatment Center at the Medical University of South Carolina.

Kohlenberg, R. J., Kanter, J. W., Bolling, M., Wexnes, R., Parker, C., & Mavis, T. (2004). Functional analytic psychotherapy, cognitive therapy, and acceptance. In S. Hayes, V. Follette, & M. Linehan (Eds.), *Mindfulness and acceptance: Expanding the cognitive-behavioral tradition.* New York: Guilford Press.

Knight, J., Shrier, L., Bravender, T., Farrell, M., VanderBilt, J., & Shaffer, H. (1999). A new brief screen for adolescent substance abuse. *Archives of Pediatric and Adolescent Medicine, 153,* 591–596.

Knight, J. R., Sherritt, L., Harris, S. K., Gates, E. C., & Chang, G. (2003). Validity of brief alcohol screening tests among adolescents: A comparison of the AUDIT, POSIT, CAGE, and CRAFFT. *Alcoholism, Clinical and Experimental Research, 27,* 67–73.

Koss, M. P., Woodruff, W. J., & Koss, P. G. (1990). Relation of criminal victimization to health perceptions among women medical patients. *Journal of Clinical and Consulting Psychology, 58,* 147–152.

Kroenke, K., & Mangelsdorff, A. (1989). Common symptoms in primary care: Incidence, evaluation, therapy and outcome. *American Journal of Medicine, 86,* 262–266.

Kroenke, K., Spitzer, R. L., deGruy, F. V., Hahn, S. R., Linzer, M., Williams, J. B. W., et al. (1997). Multisomatoform disorder. An alternative to undifferentiated somatoform disorder for the somatizing patient in primary care. *Archives of General Psychiatry, 54,* 52–8.

Lang, A. J., & Stein, M. B. (2002). Generalized screening for anxiety in primary care: Why bother? *General Hospital Psychiatry, 24,* 365–366.

Last, J. M. (1988). *A dictionary of epidemiology.* Oxford: Oxford University Press.

Lewinsohn, P. M. (1984). *The coping with depression course: A psychoeducational intervention for unipolar depression.* Eugene, OR: Castalia Publishing Company.

Lewinsohn, P. M., Hops, H., Roberts, R. E., Seeley, J. R., & Andrews, J. A. (1993). Prevalence and incidence of depression and other DSM-III-R disorders in high school students. *Journal of Abnormal Psychology, 102*(1), 133–44.

Linehan, M. M. (1993). *Skills training manual for treating borderline personality disorder.* New York: Guilford Press.

Lipkin, M., & Lybrand, W. A. (Eds.). (1982). *Population-based medicine.* New York: Praeger.

Lundren, T., & Robinson, P. (in preparation). The BULLI-PC: Bringing value-driven behavior change to primary care patient education materials.

Lynn, J. (2001). Serving patients who may die soon and their families: The role of hospice and other services. *Journal of the American Medical Association, 285*(7). Downloaded from www.jama.com.

Marlatt, A. (2001). *Master clinician presentation on substance abuse.* Reno, NV: American Association for Behavior Therapy.

Maxwell, A. E., Hunt, I. F., & Bush, M. A. (1992). Effects of a social support group, as an adjunct to diabetes training, on metabolic control and psychosocial outcomes. *Diabetes Education, 18*(4), 303–309.

McGinnis, J. M., & Foege, W. H. (1993). Actual causes of death in the United States. *Journal of the American Medical Association, 270*(18), 2207–2212.

Meier, B. (2002). Oxycontin prescribers face charges in fatal overdoses. *New York Times,* section A, column 1:14.

Meresman, J. F., Hunkeler, E. M., Hargreaves, W. A., Kirsch, A. J., Robinson, P., Green, A., et al. (2003). A case report: Implementing a nurse telecare program for treating depression in primary care. *Psychiatric Quarterly, 74*(1), 61–73.

Miller, W. R., Rollnick, S., & Conforti, K. (2002). *Motivational interviewing, second edition: Preparing people for change,* NY: Guilford.

Mishra, R. (2001). Painkiller tears through Maine. *Boston Globe*

Molinari, V., Karel, M., Jones, S., Zeiss, A., Cooley, S. G., Wray, L., et al. (2003). Recommendations about the knowledge and skills required of psychologists working with older adults. *Professional Psychology, Research and Practice, 34*(4), 435–443.

Morgan, J. R., Reid, F., & Lacey, J. H. (1999). The SCOFF questionnaire: Assessment of a new screening tool for eating disorders. *British Medical Journal, 319,* 1467.

Moriarty, D. G., Zack, M. M., & Kobau, R. (2003). The centers for disease control and prevention's healthy days measures -population tracking of perceived physical and mental health over time. health quality life outcomes, Published online 2003 September 2. DOI: 10.1186/1477– 7525–1–37. See http://www.hqlo.com/content/1/1/37.

Motarazzo, J. D. (1982). Behavioral health's challenge to academic, scientific, and professional psychology. *American Psychologist, 37,* 1–14.

Mountainview Consulting Group. See www.behavioral-health-integration.com.

Muelleman, R. L., Lenaghan, P. A., & Pakieser, R. A. (1996). Battered women: Injury locations and types. *Annals of Emergency Medicine, 28*(5), 486–492.

Murray, M., & Berwick, D. M. (2003). Advanced access: Reducing waiting and delays in primary care. *Journal of the American Medical Association, 289*(8), 1035–1040.

Mynors-Wallace, L., Gath, D. H., Lloyd-Thomas, A. R., & Tomlinson, D. (1995). Randomized controlled trial comparing problem solving treatment with amitriptyline and placebo for major depression in primary care. *British Medical Journal, 310,* 441–446.

Narrow, W. E., Regier, D. A., Rae, D. S., Manderscheid, R. W., & Locke, B. Z. (1993). Use of services by persons with mental and addictive disorders. *Archives of General Psychiatry, 50,* 95–107.

Nathan, P. E., & Gorman, J. M. (2002). *A guide to treatments that work* (2nd ed.). New York: Oxford University Press.

National Council on the Aging, Complete Toolkits (Healthy Moves for Aging Well, Healthy IDEAS for a Better Life, Healthy Changes/ Diabetes Self-management, Healthy Eating for Successful Living) available from NCOA, PO Box 411, Annapolis Junction, MD 20701 (Phone: 800–373–4906).

National Institute on Drug Abuse. (2005). See http://www.nida.nih.gov/.

National Institute of Health Consensus Statement. (1998). Diagnosis and treatment of attention deficit hyperactivity disorder (ADHD). *NIH Consensus Statement, 16,* 1–37.

National Institute of Mental Health. (1990). *National plan for research on child and adolescent mental disorders.* Rockville, MD: Author.

Nelson, H. D., Nygren, P., McInerney, Y., & Klein, J. (2004). Screening women and elderly adults for family and intimate partner violence: A review of the evidence for the U.S. Preventive Services Task Force. *Annals of Internal Medicine, 140*(5), 387–396.

Newacheck, P. W., & Taylor, W. R. (1992). Childhood chronic illness: Prevalence, severity, and impact. *American Journal of Public Health, 82,* 364–371.

Nezu, A. M. (1986). Efficacy of a social problem-solving therapy approach to unipolar depression. *Journal of Consulting and Clinical Psychology, 54*(2), 196–202.

Nezu, A. M., Nezu, C. M., Felgoise, S. H., McClure, K. S., & Houts, P. S. (2003). Project genesis: Assessing the efficacy of problem-solving therapy for distressed adult cancer patients. *Journal of Consulting and Clinical Psychology, 71*(6), 1036–1048.

Nicolaidis, C. (2002). The voices of survivors documentary: Using patient narrative to educate physicians about domestic violence. *Journal of General Internal Medicine, 17,* 117–124.

Noffsinger, E. B. (1999). Increasing quality of care and access while reducing costs through Droup-In Group Medical Appointments (DIGMAs), *Group Practice Journal, 48(1),* 12–18.

Norris, F. H. (1992). Epidemiology of trauma: Frequency and impact of different potentially traumatic events on different demographic groups. *Journal of Consulting and Clinical Psychology, 60,* 409–418.

Novack, D. H., Volk, G., Drossman, D. A., & Lipkin, M. (1993). Medical interviewing and interpersonal skills teaching in US medical schools. *Journal of the American Medical Association, 269,* 2101–2105.

Nygren, P., Nelson, H. D., & Klein, J. (2004). Screening children for family violence: A review of the evidence for the U.S. Preventive Services Task Force. *Annals of Family Medicine, 2*(1), 161–169.

O'Donohue, W. T., Byrd, M. R., Cummings, N. A., & Henderson, D. A. (Eds.). (2005). *Behavioral integrative care: Treatments that work in the primary care setting.* New York: Brunner-Routledge.

Ogden, C. L., Flegal, K. M., Carroll, M. G., & Johnson, C. L. (2002). Prevalence and trends in overweight among US children and adolescents, 1999–2000. *Journal of the American Medical Association, 288,* 1728–1732.

Olfson, M., Marcus, S. C., & Druss, B. (2002). National trends in the outpatient treatment of depression. *Journal of the American Medical Association, 287,* 203–209.

Olfson, M., Shea, S., Feder, A., Fuentes, M., Nomura, Y., Gameroff, M., et al. (2000). Prevalence of anxiety, depression, and substance use disorders in an urban general medicine practice. *Archives of Family Medicine, 9,* 876–883.

Olsen, Y., & Daumit, G. L. (2004). Opioid prescribing for chronic nonmalignant pain in primary care: Challenges and solutions. *Advances in Psychosomatic Medicine, 25,* 138–150.

Pagano, M. E., Cassidy, L. J., Little, M., Murphy, J. M., & Jellinek, M. S. (2000). Identifying psychosocial dysfunction in school-age children: The pediatric symptom checklist as a self-report measure. *Psychology in Schools, 37,* 91–105.

Parker, R. S., & Pettijohn, C. E. (2003). Ethical considerations in the use of direct-to-consumer advertising and pharmaceutical promotions:

The impact on pharmaceutical sales and physicians. *Journal of Business Ethics, 48*(3), 279–290.

Parkcrson, G. (1996). *User's guide for the Duke health profile (Duke).* Manual available from author at dept. of community and family medicine, Box 3886, Duke University Medical Center, Durham, North Carolina, 27710.

Patterson, J., Peek, C. J., Heinrich, R. L., Bischoff, R. J., & Scherger, J. (2002). *Mental health professionals in medical settings: A primer.* New York: W.W. Norton.

Pfeffer, R. I., Kurosaki, T. T., Harrah, C. H. Jr., Chance, J. M., & Filos, S. (1982). Measurement of functional activities in older adults in the community. *Journal of Gerontology, 37,* 323–329.

Pignone, M. P., Gaynes, B. N., Rushton, J. L., Burchell, C. M., Orleans, T., Mulrow, C. D., et al. (2002). Screening for depression in adults: A summary of the evidence for the U.S. preventive services task force. *Annals of Internal Medicine, 136*(10), 760–764.

Piette, J. D., Heisler, M., & Wagner, T. H. (2004). Do patients with chronic illnesses tell their doctors? *Achieves of Internal Medicine, 164,* 1749–1755.

Piette, J. D., Heisler, M., Krein, S., & Kerr, E. A. (2005). The role of patient-physician trust in moderating medication nonadherence due to cost pressures. *Achieves of Internal Medicine, 165,* 1749–1755.

Pincus, H. A., Tanielian, M. A., Marcus, S. C., Olfson, M., Zarin, D. A., Thompson, J., et al. (1998). Prescribing trends in psychotropic medications. *Journal of the American Medical Association, 79*(7), 526–531.

Pinquart, M., & Sorensen, S. (2002). Preparation for death and preparation for care in older community-dwelling. *The Journal of Death and Dying, 45*(1), 69–88.

Pinto-Meza, A., Serrano-Blanco, A., Penarrubia, M. T., Blanco, E., & Haro, J. M. (2005). Assessing depression in primary care with the PHQ-9: Can it be carried out over the telephone? *Journal of General Internal Medicine, 20*(8), 738–742.

Pliszka, S. R., Carlson, C. L., & Swanson, J. M. (1999). Disruptive behavior disorders and substance abuse. In S. R. Pliszka, Carlson, & Swanson (Eds.), *ADHD with comorbid disorders: Clinical assessment and management.* New York: Guilford.

Portenoy, R. K., & Foley, K. M. (1986). Chronic use of opioid analgesics in nonmalignant pain: Report of 38 cases. *Pain, 25,* 171–186.

Pruitt, S. D., Klapow, J. C., Epping-Jordan, J. E., & Dresselhaus, T. R. (1998). Moving behavioral medicine to the front line: A model for the integration of behavioral and medical sciences in primary care. *Professional Psychology: Research and Practice, 29*(3), 230–236.

Rabin, D. L. (1998). Adapting an effective primary care provider STD/HIV prevention training programme. *AIDS Care, 10*(2), 75–82.

Radlof, L. S. (1991). The use of the center for epidemiologic studies depression scale in adolescents and young adults. *Journal of Youth and Adolescence, 20*(2), 149–166.

Ratey, J., Greenberg, M. S., Bemporad, J. R., & Lindem, K. (1992). Unrecognized attention-deficit hyperactivity disorder in adults presenting for outpatient psychotherapy. *Journal of Child and Adolescent Psychopharmacology, 2,* 267–275.

Ravens-Sieberer, U., & Bullinger, M. (1998). Assessing health-related quality of life in chronically ill children with the German KINDL: First psychometric and content analytical results. *Quality of Life Research, 7,* 399–407.

Regier, D. A., Narrow, W. E., Rae, D. S., Manderscheid, R. W., Locke, B. Z., & Goodwin, F. K. (1993). The de facto U.S. mental and addictive disorders service system. *Archives of General Psychiatry, 50,* 85–94.

Reid, G., Engles-Horton, L. L., Weber, M. B., Kerns, R. D., Rogers, E. L., & O'Connor, P. G. (2002). Use of opioid medications for chronic noncancer pain syndromes in primary care. *Journal of General Internal Medicine, 17,* 173–179.

Reid, M. C., Fiellin, D. A., & O'Connor, P. G. (1999). Hazardous and harmful alcohol consumption in primary care. *Archives of Internal Medicine, 159*(15), 1681–1689.

Reiter, J., Berghuis, J., & Robinson, P. (in preparation). Overcoming referral barriers in primary care. *The Behavior Therapist.*

Reynolds, C. F., Miller, M. D., Pasternak, R. E., Frank, E., Perel, J. M., Cornes, C., et al. (1999). Treatment of bereavement-related major depressive episodes in later life: A controlled study of acute and continuation treatment with nortriptyline and interpersonal psychotherapy. *American Journal of Psychiatry, 156,* 202–208.

Rickard, J. (2005). Personal communication.

Robinson, P. (1996). *Living life well: New strategies for hard times.* Reno, NV: Context Press.

Robinson, P. (2002). Treating depression in primary care: What are the cost-offset opportunities? In N. Cummings, W. O'Donohoe, & K. Ferguson (Eds.), *The impact of medical cost offset on practice and research: Making it work for you* (pp. 145–166). Reno, NV: Context Press.

Robinson, P. (2003). Implementing a primary care depression critical pathway. In N. Cummings, W. O'Donohoe, & K. Ferguson (Eds.), *Behavioral health as primary care: Beyond efficacy to effectiveness* (pp. 69–94). Reno, NV: Context Press.

Robinson, P. (2005a). Adapting empirically supported treatments to the primary care setting: A template for success. In W. T. O'Donohue, M. R. Byrd, N. A. Cummings, & D. A. Henderson (Eds.). (2005). *Behavioral integrative care: Treatments that work in the primary care setting* (pp. 53–72). New York: Brunner-Routledge.

Robinson, P. (2005b). Survivors of suicide. In J. A. Chiles & K. D. Strosahl (Eds.), *Clinical manual for assessment and treatment of suicidal patients.* Washington, DC: American Psychiatric Publishing, Inc.

Robinson, P., Bush, T., Von Korff, M., Katon, W., Lin, E., Simon, G. E., et al. (1995). Primary care physician use of cognitive behavioral techniques with depressed patients. *Journal of Family Practice, 40*(4), 352–357.

Robinson, P., Bush, T., Von Korff, M., Katon, W., Lin, E., Simon, G. E., et al. (1997). Primary care physician use of cognitive behavioral techniques with depressed patients. *Journal of Family Practice, 40*(4), 352–357.

Robinson, P., Del Vento, A., & Wischman, C. (1998). Integrated treatment of the frail elderly: The group care clinic. In S. Blount (Ed.), *Integrated care: The future of medical and mental health collaboration.* New York: Norton.

Robinson, P., Wicksell, R. K., & Olsson, G. L. (2004). ACT with chronic pain patients. In Hayes, S., & Strosahl, K. (Eds.), *A practical guide to acceptance and commitment therapy.* NY: Springer Science+Business Media, Inc.

Robinson, P., Wischman, C., & Del Vento, A. (1996). *Treating depression in primary care: A manual for primary care and mental health providers.* Reno, NV: Context Press.

Roche, B., Barnes-Holmes, Y., Barnes-Holmes, D., Steward, I., & O'Hora, D. (2002). Relational frame theory: A new paradigm for the analysis of social behavior. *Behavior Analyst, 25*(1), 75–91.

Rose, S. Bisson, J., Churchill, & Wessely, S. (2005). Psychological debriefing for preventing post traumatic stress disorder (PTSD). (Cochrane Review). *The cochrane library* (Vol. 2). Chichester, UK: John Wiley & Sons, Ltd. http://www.cochrane.org/cochrane/revabstr/AB000560.htm.

Sadur, C. N., Moline, N., Costa, M., Michalik, D., Mendlowitz, D., Roller, S., et al. (1999). Diabetes management in a health maintenance organization: Efficacy of care management using cluster visits. *Diabetes Care, 22*(12), 2011–2017.

Safran, D. G. (2003). Defining the future of primary care: What can we learn from patients? *Annals of Internal Medicine, 138*, 248–255.

Safran, D. G., Kosinski, M., Tarlov, A. R., Rogers, W. H., Taira, D. H., Lieberman, N., et al. (1998). The primary care assessment survey: Tests of data quality and measurement performance. *Medical Care, 36*(5), 728–739.

Saunders, J. B., Aasland, O. G., Babor, T. F., De la Fuente, J. R., & Grant, M. (1993). Development of the alcohol use disorders identification test (AUDIT): WHO Collaborative project on early detection of persons with harmful alcohol consultation - II. *Addiction, 88*(6), 791–804.

Savage, S. R. (1996). Long-term opioid therapy: Assessment of consequences and risks. *Journal of Pain Symptom Management, 11*, 274–286.

Schuurmans, M. J., Deschamps, P. I., Markham, S. W., Shortridge-Baggett, L. M., & Duursma, S. A. (2003). The measurement of delirium: Review of scales. *Research and Theory in Nursing Practice, 17*(3), 207–224.

Schwartz, L., Woloshin, S., Wasson, J. Renfrew, R. A., & Welch, G. (1999). Setting the revisit interval in primary care. *Journal of General Internal Medicine, 14*(4), 230–235.

Scodol, A., Dohrenwend, B., Link, B., & Shout, P. (1990). The nature of stress: Problems of measurement (pp. 3–20). In J. Noshpitz & R. Coddington (Eds.), *Stressors and the adjustment disorders.* New York: Wiley.

Scott, J. C., Douglas, A. C., Venohr, I., Gade, G., McKenzie, M., Kramer, A. M., Bryant, L., & Beck, A. (2004). Effectiveness of a group outpatient visit model for chronically ill older health maintenance organization members: A 2-year randomized trail of the cooperative health care clinic. *Journal of the American Geriatrics Society, 52(9)*, 1463.

Searight, H. R. Burke, J. M., & Rottnek, F. (2000). Adult ADHD: Evaluation and treatment in family medicine. *American Family Physician, 62*, 2077–2086, 2091–2092.

Segal, Z. V., Williams, M. G., & Teasdale, J. D. (2002). *Mindfulness-based cognitive therapy for depression: A new approach to preventing relapse,* New York: Guilford.

Sherbourne, C. D., Wells, K. B., Meridith, L. S., Jackson, C. A., & Camp, P. (1996). Comorbid anxiety disorder and the functioning and well being of chronically ill patients of general medical providers. *Archives of General Psychiatry, 53*, 889–895.

Shulman, K. (2000). Clock-drawing: Is it the ideal cognitive screening test? *International Journal of Psychiatry, 15*, 548–561.

Siften, D. W. (Ed.). (2002). *PDR Drug guide for mental health professionals* (1st ed.). Montvale, NJ: Thompson Medical Economics.

Simon, G., Von Korff, M., & Barlow, W. (1995). Health care costs associated with depressive and anxiety disorders in primary care. *Archives of General Psychiatry, 52*, 850–856.

Sloane, H. N. (1976). *The good kid book: How to solve the 16 most common behavior problems.* Champaign, IL: Research Press.

Smyth, A., Haas, E. M., & Jones, H. (1995). *The complete home healer: Your guide to every treatment available for over 300 of the most common health problems.* New York: HarperPrism.

Snugg, N. K., & Inui, T. (1992). Primary care physicians' response to domestic violence: Opening pandora's box. *Journal of the American Medical Association, 267*, 3157–3193.

Spiegel, A. (2005, January 3). The dictionary of disorder: How one man revolutioned psychiatry. *The New Yorker*, 58–59.

Spitzer, R. L., Kroenke, K., & Williams, J. B. (1999). Validation and utility of a self-report version of PRIME-MD: The PHQ primary care study Primary care evaluation of mental disorders. Patient health questionnaire. *Journal of the American Medical Association, 282*(18), 1737–1744.

Steer, R. A., Cavalieri, T. A., Leonard, D. M., & Beck, A. T. (1999). Use of the beck depression inventory for primary care to screen for major depression disorders. *General Hospital Psychiatry, 21*(2), 106–111.

Strosahl, K. (1996a). Primary mental health care: A new paradigm for achieving health and behavioral health integration. *Behavioral Healthcare Tomorrow, 5,* 93–96.

Strosahl, K. (1996b). Confessions of a behavior therapist in primary care: The odyssey and the ecstasy. *Cognitive and Behavioral Practice, 3,* 1–28.

Strosahl, K. (1997). Building primary care behavioral health systems that work: A compass and a horizon. In N. Cummings, J. Cummings & J. Johnson (Eds.), *Behavioral health in primary care: A guide for clinical integration* (pp. 37–68). Madison, CN: Psychosocial Press.

Strosahl, K. (1998). Integrating behavioral health and primary care services: The primary mental health model. In A. Blount (Ed.), *Integrated primary care: The future of medical and mental health collaboration* (pp. 139–166). New York: W.W. Norton.

Strosahl, K. D. (2005). Training behavioral health and PCPs for integrated care: A core competencies approach. In W. T. O'Donohue, M. R. Byrd, N. A. Cummings, & D. A. Henderson (Eds.). (2005). *Behavioral integrative care: Treatments that work in the primary care setting.* New York: Brunner-Routledge, 15–52.

Strosahl, K. D. (2006). Personal communication.

Strosahl, K., Baker, N., Braddick, M., Stuart, M., & Handley, M. (1997). Integration of behavioral health and primary care services: The group health cooperative model. In N. Cummings, J. Cummings & J. Johnson (Eds.), *Behavioral health in primary care: A guide for clinical integration* (pp. 61–86). Madison, CN: Psychosocial Press.

Strosahl, K. D., & Robinson, P. J. (unpublished). The behavioral health consultant core competency tool.

Sugg, N. K., & Inui, T. (1992). Primary care physicians' response to domestic violence: Opening pandora's box. *Journal of the American Medical Association, 267*(23), 3157–3160.

Taplin, S., Galvin, M. S., Payne, T., Coole, D., & Wagner, E. (1998). Putting population-based care into practice: Real option or rhetoric. *Journal of the American Board of Family Practice, 11*(2), 116–126.

Thompson, L. W., Gallagher, D., & Breckenridge, J. S. (1987). Comparative effectiveness of psychotherapies for depressed elders. *Journal of Consulting and Clinical Psychology, 55*(3), 385–390.

Trevino, R. P., Pugh, J. A., Hernandez, A. E., Menchaca, V. D., Ramirez, R. R., & Mendoza, M. (1998). Bienestar: A diabetes risk-factor prevention program. *Journal of School Health, 68*(2), 62–67.

Turk, D. C. (1996). Clinicians' attitudes about prolonged use of opioids and the issue of patient heterogeneity. *Journal of Pain Symptom Management, 11*, 218–230.

United States Department of Health & Human Services. (2000). *Healthy people 2010: Understanding and improving health* (2nd ed.). Washington, DC: U.S. Government Printing Office.

United States Preventive Services Task Force. (2002). Screening for depression: Recommendations and rationale. *Annals of Internal Medicine, 136*, 765–776.

United States Preventive Services Task Force. (2004). Behavioral counseling interventions in primary care to reduce alcohol misuse: Recommendation statement. *Annals of Internal Medicine, 140*, 554–556.

United States Preventive Services Task Force (USPSTF). (2004). Screening and behavioral counseling interventions in primary care to reduce alcohol misuse: Recommendation statement. *Annals of Internal Medicine, 140*(7), 554–556.

United States Public Health Service. (2000). *Report of the surgeon general's conference on children's mental health: A national action agenda.* Washington, DC: Department of Health and Human Services.

Unutzer, J., Patrick, D. L., Simon, G., Grembowski, D., Walker, E., Ruter, C., et al. (1997). Depressive symptoms and the cost of health services in HMO patients age 65 years and older: A 4-year prospective study. *Journal of the American Medical Association, 277*, 1618–1623.

Valcour, V., Masaki, K., Curb, J., & Blanchette, P. (2000). The detection of dementia in the primary care setting. *Archives of Internal Medicine, 160*, 2964–2968.

Von Korff, M., Katon, W., Bush, T., Lin, E., Simon, G. E., Saunders, K., et al. (1998). Treatment costs, cost offset, and cost-effectiveness of collaborative management of depression. *Psychosomatic Medicine, 60*, 143–149.

Von Korff, M., Ustun, T. B., Ormel, J., Kaplan, I., & Simon, G. (1996). Self-report disability in an international primary care study of psychological illness. *Journal of Clinical Epdemiology, 49(3)*, 297–303.

Von Korff, M., & Myers, L. (1987). The primary care physician and psychiatric services. *General Hospital Psychiatry, 9*, 235–240.

Walsh. J. M., Wheat, M. E., & Freund K. (2000). Detection, evaluation, and treatment of eating disorders: The role of the primary care physician. *Journal of General Internal Medicine, 15*, 577–590.

Waltner-Toews, D. (2001). An ecosystem approach to health and its applications to tropical and emerging diseases. Cad. Saude Publica, 17, 7–36; ISSN 0102. http://www.scielo.br/pdf/csp/v17s0/3878.pdf-311X.

Ware, J. E., Kosinski, M., & Keller, S. D. (1996). A 12-item short-form health survey: Construction of scales and preliminary tests of reliability and validity. *Medical Care, 34*(3), 220–233.

Weaver, M. F., Jarvis, M. A., & Schnoll, S. H. (1999). Role of the primary care physician in problems of substance abuse. *Archives of Internal Medicine, 159*(9), 913–924.

Webster-Stratton, C. (2001). *Dina dinosaur's classroom-based social skills, problem solving and anger management curriculum.*

Webster-Stratton, C., & Reid, M. J. (2004). Strengthening social and emotional competence in young children -the foundation for early school readiness and success: Incredible years classroom social skills and problem-solving curriculum. *Infants and Children, 17*(2), 96–113.

Whooley, M. A., Avins, A. L., Miranda, J., & Browner, W. S. (1997). Case-finding instruments for depression. Two questions are as good as many. *Journal of General Internal Medicine, 12*(7), 439–445.

Wilens, T. E. (2003). Drug therapy for adults with attention-deficit/hyperactivity disorder. *Drugs, 63*, 2395–2411.

Williams, R., & Vinson, D. C. (2001). Validation of a single screening question for problem drinking. *Journal of Family Practice, 50*(4), 307–312.

World Health Organization. (1946). Preamble to the Constitution of the World Health Organization as adopted by the International Health Conference, New York, 19–22, June.

World Health Organization. (1996). *International classification of diseases, 9th revision, clinical modification* (ICD-9-CM) (6th ed.). Geneva.

Issued for use beginning October 1, 2003 for federal fiscal year 2004 (FY04).

Working party concerning general practice and victorian mental health services. (1995). *All things to all people. The general practitioner as provider of mental health care. Role. Benefits. Problems. Some solutions.* Melbourne: The Royal Australian College of General Practitioners Victorian Faculty.

Zarowitz, B. J., Muma, B., Coggan, P., Davis, G., & Barkely, G. L. (2001). Managing the pharmaceutical industry-health system interface. *The Annals of Pharmacotherapy, 35*(12), 1661–1668.

Zenz, M., Strumpf, M., & Tryba, M. (1992). Long-term oral opioid therapy in patients with chronic nonmalignant pain. *Journal of Pain Symptom Management, 7,* 69–77.

Zuckerman, B., Stevenson, J., & Bailey, V. (1987). Stomachaches and headaches in a community sample of preschool children. *Pediatrics, 79,* 677–682.

Note: HCFA is now named Center for Medicare Medicaid Services or CMS.

APPENDIX A

THEORIES AND THERAPIES: RECOMMENDED READING FOR THE BHC

Stress-coping-vulnerability Model, Coping Styles

Davis, M., Robbins-Eshelman, E., & McKay, M. (1995). *The stress reduction and relaxation workbook*. Oakland, CA: New Harbinger Publications.

Glasser, R., & Kiecolt-Glaser, J. K. (Eds.). (1994). *Handbook of human stress and immunity*. San Diego: Academic Press.

Mauck, S. B., Jennings, R., Rabin, B. S., & Baum, A. (Eds.). (2000). *Behavior, health, and aging*. Mahwah, NJ: Erlbaum.

Talmon, M. (1990). *Single-session therapy: Maximizing the effect of the first (and often only) therapeutic encounter*. San Francisco: Jossey-Bass.

Zeidner, M., & Endler, N. S. (Eds.). (1996). *Handbook of coping: Theory, research and applications*. New York: John Wiley.

Motivational Interviewing and Brief Interventions

Cox, W. M., Klinger, E. (Ed). (2004). *Handbook of motivational counseling: Concepts, approaches, and assessment*. New York: John Wiley & Sons Ltd.

Resnicow, K., Baskin, M., Rahotep, Simone, S., Periasamy, S., Rollnick, S. C., Miles, W. M., Klinger, E. (Ed.). (2004). *Handbook of motivational counseling: Concepts, approaches, and assessment*. New York: John Wiley & Sons Ltd.

Rollnick, S., Allison, J., Heather, N., Peters, T. J. (Eds.). (2001). *International handbook of alcohol dependence and problems*. New York: John Wiley & Sons, Ltd.

Rollnick, S., Morgan, M., Washton, A. M. (Ed.). (1996). *Psychotherapy and substance abuse: A practitioner's handbook. Guilford substance abuse series.* New York: Guilford Press.

Second and Third-Wave Behavior Therapies

Baucum, D. H., Epstein, N., LaTaillade, & J. J., Jaslean (2002). Cognitive behavioral couple therapy. In Gurman, A. S., & Jacobson, N. S. (Eds.), *Clinical handbook of couple therapy* (3rd ed., pp. 26–58), New York: Guilford Press.

D'Zurilla, T. J., Nezu, A. M., Dobson, K. S. (Eds). (2001). *Handbook of cognitive-behavioral therapies* (2nd ed.). New York: Guilford Press.

Eifert, G., Forsyth, J. P., & Hayes, S. C. (2005). *Acceptance and commitment therapy for anxiety disorders.* Oakland, CA: New Harbinger.

Hayes, S. C. (2005). *Get out of your mind and into your life.* Oakland, CA: New Harbinger.

Hayes, S. C. (2004). Acceptance and commitment therapy, relational frame theory, and the third wave of behavioral and cognitive therapies. *Behavior Therapy, 35*(4), 639–665.

Hayes, S., Fischer, J., & O'Donohoe, W. (Eds.). (2002). Integrated behavioral health treatments, University of Reno, NV.

Hayes, S. C., Follette, V. M., & Linehan, M. M. (Eds.). (2004). *Mindfulness and acceptance: Expanding the cognitive-behavioral tradition.* New York: Guilford Press.

Hayes, S. C., & Strosahl, K. D. (2004). *A practical guide to acceptance and commitment therapy.* New York: Springer.

Hayes, S., Strosahl, K., & Wilson, K. (1998). *Acceptance and commitment therapy: An experiential approach to behavior change.* New York: The Guilford Press.

Holman, H., Sobel, D., Laurent, D., Gonzalez, V., Minor, M., & Lorig, K. (Eds.). (2000). *Living a healthy life with chronic conditions: Self-management of heart disease, arthritis, diabetes, asthma, bronchitis, emphysema & others.* Palo Alto, CA: Bull Publishing Company.

Kohlenberg, R. J., Kanter, J. W., Bolling, M., Wexnes, R., Parker, C., & Mavis, T. (2004). Functional analytic psychotherapy, cognitive therapy, and acceptance. In S. Hayes, V. Follette, & M. Linehan (Eds.),

Mindfulness and acceptance: Expanding the cognitive-behavioral tradition. New York: Guilford Press.

Rose, S. D. (1999). Group therapy: A cognitive-behavioral approach. In J. R. Price, D. R. Hescheles, & A. R. Price (Eds.), *A guide to starting psychotherapy groups* (pp. 99–113). San Diego, CA: Academic Press, Inc.

Teasdale, J. D. (2004). Mindfulness-based cognitive therapy. In J. Yiend, & T. D. Borkovec (Eds.), *Cognition, emotion and psychopathology: Theoretical, empirical and clinical directions* (pp. 270–289), Cambridge, UK: Cambridge University Press.

Watson, D. L., Tharp, R. G. (1997). *Self-directed behavior: Self-modification for personal adjustment* (7th ed.). New York: Brooks/Cole Publishing Co.

APPENDIX B

RECOMMENDED READING FOR CHILDREN, PARENTS, PCPS, AND BHCS

Books for Children

Lovell, C. M. (2005). *The star: A story to help young children understand foster care*. Battlecreek, MI: Roger Owen Rossman.

Mack, A. (1978). *The toilet learning: The picture book technique for children and parents*. Canada: Little, Brown, and Company Limited.

Webster-Stratton, C. (1998). *Wally learns a lesson from Tiny Turtle. Parents, teachers, and children training series*. Seattle, WA: Seth Enterprises.

Webster-Stratton, C. (1998). *Wally meets Dina Dinosaur. Parents, teachers, and children training series*. Seattle, WA: Seth Enterprises.

Webster-Stratton, C. (1998). *Wally's detective manual for solving problems at home. Parents, teachers, and children training series*. Seattle, WA: Seth Enterprises.

Webster-Stratton, C. (1998). *Wally's detective manual for solving problems at school. Parents, teachers, and children training series*. Seattle, WA: Seth Enterprises.

Act-friendly Books for Children and Parents*

Andreae, G. (1999). *Love is a handful of honey*. London: Orchard Books.

Bottner, B. (2003). *The scaredy cats*. New York: Simon & Schuster.

Cave, K. (2003). *You've got dragons*. Atlanta, GA: Peachtree

Costellow, J., & Haver, J. (2004). *Zen parenting: The art of learning what you already know*. Beltsville, MD. Robins Lane Press.

Deprau, J. (2003). *The city of Ember*. New York: Random House

MacLean, K. L. (2004). *Peaceful piggy meditation*. Morton Grove, IL: Albert Whitman & Company.

Parr, T. (2001). *It's okay to be different*. New York: Little, Brown & Co.

Rosman, D. (2002). *Meditating with children: The art of concentrating and centering*. Virginia: Integral Yoga Publications.

Schuurmans, H. (2001). *Sidney won't swim*. New York: Scholastic.

Viorst, J. (1972). *Alexander and the terrible, horrible, no good, very bad day*. New York: Macmillan.

*We acknowledge Laurie Greco, PhD and her students at Vanderbilt University for compiling this list of delightful books.

Books for Parents

Forgatch, M., & Patterson, G. R. (1989). *Parents and adolescents living together*. Part 2: *Family problem solving*. Eugene, OR: Castillia Publishing Company.

Giler, J. Z. (1998). *Socially ADDept: A manual for parents of children with ADHD and/or learning disabilities*. Santa Barbara, CA: CES Publications.

Hirschmann, J. R., & Zaphiropoulos, L. (1993). *Preventing childhood eating problems: A practical, positive approach to raising children free of food and weight conflicts*. Carlsbad, CA: Gurtz Books.

Lee, S. (2004). *It worked for me! Parents reveal their secrets to solving the everyday problems of raising kids -from thumb sucking to schoolyard fights!*. New York: St Martins.

Patterson, G. R. (1976). *Living with children: New methods for parents and teachers*. Champaign, IL: Research Press.

Patterson, G. R., & Forgatch, M. (1987). *Parents and adolescents living together: The basics*. Eugene, OR: Castillia Publishing Company.

Sloane, H. W. (1979). *The good kid book: A manual for parents*. Champaign, IL: Research Press.

Webster-Stratton, C. (1992). *The incredible years: A trouble-shooting guide for parents of children ages 3–8 years*. Toronto: Umbrella Press.

Books for BHCS and PCPS

Christophersen, E. R., & Mortweet, S. L. (2003). *Treatments that work with children: Empirically supported strategies for managing childhood problems*. Washington, DC: American Psychological Association. (See Appendix A: The Home Chip System).

Hayes, S., & Strosahl, K. (Eds.). (2004). *Acceptance and commitment therapy: A practitioner's guide.* New York: Plenum Kleuwer.

Miller, W. R., Rollnick, S., & Conforti, K. (2002). *Motivational interviewing: Preparing people for change* (2nd ed.). New York: Guilford.

O'Donohoe, W., & Hayes, S. (Eds.). (2004). *Empirical treatments in primary care,* University of Reno, NV.

Webster-Stratton, C. (2001). *Dina dinosaur's classroom-based social skills, problem solving and anger management curriculum.* (Contact author at UW, Seattle, WA).

Webster-Stratton, C. (2000). *How to promote social and academic competence in young children.* London, England: Sage Publications.

Webster-Stratton, C., & Herbert, M. (1994). *Troubled families – Problem children: Working with parents: A collaborative process.* New York: Wiley & Sons.

APPENDIX C

RECOMMENDED READING FOR BHCS AND PCPS CONCERNING ADULT PATIENTS

Blount, A. (1998). *Integrated primary care: The future of medical and mental health collaboration.* New York: Norton.

Chiles, J. A., & Strosahl, K. D. (2005). *Clinical manual for assessment and treatment of suicidal patients.* Washington, DC: American Psychiatric Publishing, Inc.

Cummings, N., Cummings, J., & Johnson, J. (1997). *Behavioral health in primary care: A guide for clinical integration.* Madison, CN: Psychosocial Press.

Eifert, G. H., & Forsyth, J. P. (2005). *Acceptance and commitment therapy for anxiety disorders: A practitioner's treatment guide to using mindfulness, acceptance, and values-based behavior change strategies.* Oakland, CA: New Harbinger Publications, Inc.

Gatchel, R. J., & Oordt, M. S. (2003). *Clinical health psychology and primary care: Practical advice and clinical guidance for successful collaboration.* Washington, DC: American Psychological Association.

Hayes, S. C. (2005). *Get out of your mind and into your life.* Oakland, CA: New Harbinger.

Hayes, S., Fischer, J., & O'Donohoe, W. (Eds.). (2002). *Integrated behavioral health treatments,* University of Reno, NV: Context Press.

Hayes, S. C., & Strosahl, K. D. (2004). *A practical guide to acceptance and commitment therapy.* New York: Springer.

Hayes, S. C., Strosahl, K. D., & Wilson, K. G. (1999). *Acceptance and commitment therapy: An experiential approach to behavior change.* New York: Guilford Press.

Hendricks, G. (1995). *Conscious breathing: Breathwork for health, stress release, and personal mastery*. New York: Bantam.

James, L. C., & Folen, R. A. (2005). *The primary care consultant: The next frontier for psychologists in hospitals and clinics*. Washington, DC: APA Press.

Jamison, R. N. (1996). *Learning to master your chronic pain*. Sarasota, Florida: Professional Resource Press.

Johnson, S. B., Perry, N. W., & Rozensky, R. H. (2002). *Handbook of clinical health psychology*. (Vols. 1–3). Washington, DC: American Psychological Association.

Kabat-Zinn, J. (2005). *Coming to our senses: Healing ourselves and the world through mindfulness*. New York: Hyperion.

Kabat-Zinn, J. (1990). *Full catastrophe living: Using the wisdom of your body and mind to face stress, pain, and illness*. New York: Delta.

Kabat-Zinn, J. (1994). *Wherever you go there you are: Mindfulness meditation in everyday life*. New York: Hyperion.

Lazarus, A., & Fay, A. (1975). *I can if I want to: Change your thinking, change your behavior, change your life*. New York: William Morrow and Company, Inc.

Lewinsohn, P. M., Munoz, R. F., Youngren, M. A., & Zeiss, A. M. (1986). *Control your depression*. New York: Prentice Hall Press.

Miller, W. R., & Rollnick, S. (2002). *Motivational interviewing: Preparing people for change* (2nd ed.). New York: Guilford.

Molinari, V., Karel, M., Jones, S., Zeiss, A., Cooley, S. G., Wray, L., et al. (2003). Recommendations about the knowledge and skills required of psychologists working with older adults. *Professional Psychology: Research and practice, 34*(4), 435–443.

Nathan, P. E., & Gorman, J. M. (2002). *A Guide to treatments that work* (2nd ed.). New York: Oxford University Press.

O'Donohue, W. T., Byrd, M. R., Cummings, N. A., & Henderson, D. A. (Eds.). (2005). *Behavioral integrative care: Treatments that work in the primary care setting*. New York: Brunner-Routledge

Parkerson, G. (1996). *User's guide for the Duke Health Profile (Duke)*. Manual available from author at Dept. of Community and Family Medicine, Box 3886, Duke University Medical Center, Durham, North Carolina, 27710.

Patterson, J., Peek, C. J., Heinrich, R. L., Bischoff, R. J., & Scherger, J. (2002). *Mental health professionals in medical settings: A primer.* New York: W.W. Norton.

Robinson, P. (2005). Understanding and providing care to the survivors of suicide. In J. A. Chiles, & K. D. Strosahl (Eds.), *Clinical manual for assessment and treatment of suicidal patients.* Washington, DC: American Psychiatric Publishing, Inc.

Robinson, P. (1996). *Living life well: New strategies for hard times.* Reno, NV: Context Press.

Robinson, P., Wischman, C., & Del Vento, A. (1996). *Treating depression in primary care: A manual for primary care and mental health providers.* Reno, NV: Context Press.

Roth, A., & Fonagy, P. (2005). *What works for whom: A critical review of psychotherapy research* (2nd ed.). New York: Guilford Publications, Inc.

Siften, D. W. (Ed.). (2002). *PDR drug guide for mental health professionals* (1st ed.). Montvale, NJ: Thompson Medical Economics.

Watson, D. L., & Tharp, D. L. (1972). *Self-directed behavior: Self-modification for personal adjustment.* Belmont, CA: Wadsworth Publishing Company, Inc.

APPENDIX D

PATIENT EDUCATION HANDOUTS AND PRACTICE TOOLS (SEE ALSO ACCOMPANYING CD)

1. TOOLS FOR BHCS AND PCPS TO USE IN INTERVENTIONS WITH PATIENTS
   A. The ACT Behavioral Health Prescription Pad
   B. Primary Care Patient Values Plan
   C. BHC Diabetes Screener
2. PATIENT EDUCATION HANDOUTS FOR ADULT PATIENTS
   D. Beating Insomnia
   E. CALM Exercise
   F. Change Plan Worksheet
   G. Diaphragmatic Breathing Tips
   H. The ABCs of Habit Change
   I. Healthy Sleeping Tips
   J. Managing Chronic Pain
   K. Progressive Muscle Relaxation
   L. Premature Ejaculation
   M. Stress Awareness
3. PATIENT EDUCATION HANDOUTS FOR PARENTS
   N. Enuresis Plan
   O. Great Reward Ideas
   P. Designing Reward Plans
   Q. Using Time Out with Your Child
4. HANDOUTS FOR BHCS TO USE TO INFLUENCE AND SUPPORT PCPS
   R. HO for PCPs: BHC Referrals
   S. Staff Overview (Handout for Introducing new BHC)

TOOLS FOR BHCS AND PCPS TO USE
IN INTERVENTIONS WITH PATIENTS

Acceptance and Commitment Therapy
Behavioral Health Prescription Pad*

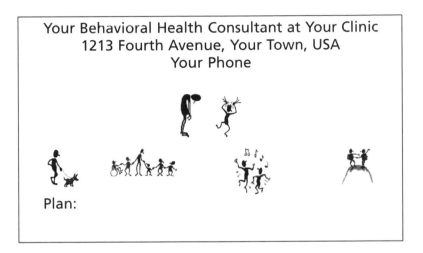

Your Behavioral Health Consultant at Your Clinic
1213 Fourth Avenue, Your Town, USA
Your Phone

Plan:

*This format is useful with patients who are struggling with emotions, such as sadness and fear. The BHC or PCP can explain that the figures at the top represent people experiencing negative thoughts and emotions, as most people do from time to time. Then, he or she can ask the patient if he or she would like to learn ways to have these emotions without giving up on the things most people enjoy and value (represented by figures at the bottom of the pad). The BHC or PCP can teach mindfulness strategies to help the patient be present with the unwanted feelings at the top of the pad and help the patient plan specific activities related to the patient's values represented by figures at the bottom of the pad (e.g., enjoying the outdoors, caring for his or her body, caring for animals, being a part of a family/community/strong work group, being able to dance/have fun/enjoy music, working hard/being a team player/getting to the top, etc.). To complete the visit, the BHC or PCP can jot down the behavior change plan on the pad. We often have these pads made with pressure sensitive copies, so that the BHC or PCP has a copy for reference when charting or dictating after the visit. This supports more specificity in behavioral planning and in questioning in follow-up visits.

Note: We provide another version of a Behavioral Health Prescription Pad (the Bull's Eye) in Chapter 10, along with instructions for using it.

Primary Care Patient Values Plan

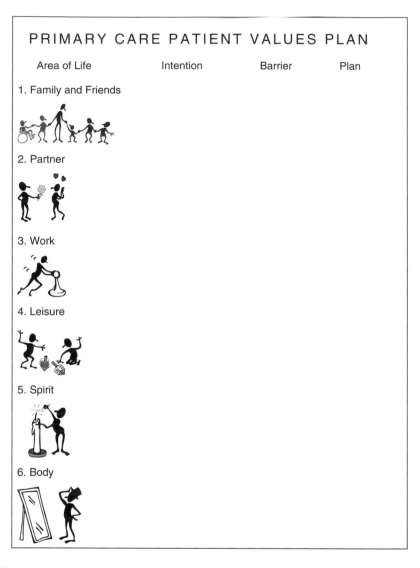

There are a variety of ways that the BHC or PCP can use the Primary Care Values Plan (PCV Plan). Its general purpose is to bring the patient's values into the process of planning long-term lifestyle changes to improve quality of life.

Prior to starting the planning process, the provider (whether BHC or PCP) needs to explain the difference between a goal and a value. Goals are specific, objective plans (e.g., walk outdoors twenty minutes daily), while values are global and abstract (e.g., treat my body well so that it treats me well).

Here are two possible ways for a provider to use the PCV Plan in visits with patients.

1. The provider may simply ask the patient to talk about his or her values in one or more of the six areas/dimensions. This lays the groundwork for future discussions. The provider can begin by suggesting, "In a world where anything was possible, what would your intention be in regards to _____ (your family and friends / partner / work / leisure time / spirituality / body)?" As the patient talks, the provider can make a few notes and conclude the visit by summarizing what he or she has heard. The provider should express appreciation to the patient for the discussion and suggest spending more time discussing the patient's values in future visits.

2. The provider may also use the form to establish a behavioral plan. This begins by asking the patient to select one value dimension that is of importance in their lives at the present moment. The provider can then listen and make notes on the form as the patient explains his or her value and intention. Next, the provider can ask the patient to explain which of his or her behaviors in the past week has reflected the stated value or intention. As the patient talks, the provider can reinforce value-based actions and/or record perceived barriers to action on the form. The provider might then ask the patient to generate ideas for feasible behavioral experiments that could be performed over the subsequent few weeks. The goal of the experiments are to see if they bring the patient closer to his or her stated values. The pros and cons of each experiment can be discussed to produce a specific plan that can be charted.

The provider can use a PCV Plan over multiple visits, and more than one provider can facilitate a patient's work on the plan.

BHC Diabetes Screener

1. How much do you know about how to manage your diabetes?

   1   2   3   4   5   6   7   8   9   10
   Nothing   A lot

2. How much do your friends and family know about your diabetes?

   1   2   3   4   5   6   7   8   9   10

Nothing   A lot

3. How much do family/friends support you in managing your diabetes?

   1   2   3   4   5   6   7   8   9   10

Not at all   A lot

4. Please list dietary changes you need to make for your diabetes:

_____

_____

5. How motivated are you to make these dietary changes?

   1   2   3   4   5   6   7   8   9   10

Not at all   Very

6. How confident are you that you can make the necessary dietary changes?

   1   2   3   4   5   6   7   8   9   10

Not at all   Very

7. How motivated are you to make changes in exercise to help your diabetes?

   1   2   3   4   5   6   7   8   9   10

Not at all   Very

8. How confident are you that you can make the necessary changes in exercise?

   1   2   3   4   5   6   7   8   9   10

Not at all   Very

9. How motivated are you to begin testing your glucose regularly?

   1   2   3   4   5   6   7   8   9   10

Not at all   Very

10. How confident are you that you will test your glucose regularly?

   1   2   3   4   5   6   7   8   9   10

Not at all   Very

11. How motivated are you to take your medicines as prescribed?

    1   2   3   4   5   6   7   8   9   10

    Not at all   Very

12. How confident are you that you will take your medicines as prescribed?

    1   2   3   4   5   6   7   8   9   10

    Not at all   Very

13. How much control do you think you can have over diabetes?

    1   2   3   4   5   6   7   8   9   10

    None at all   Complete Control

14. How often do you worry about your diabetes?

    1   2   3   4   5   6   7   8   9   10

    Never   Constantly

15. How much will your work (or housework) or school schedule interfere with your diabetes self-care?

    1   2   3   4   5   6   7   8   9   10

    Not at all   A lot

16. How much stress do you have in your daily life?

    1   2   3   4   5   6   7   8   9   10

    None at all   A lot

17. How much will stress interfere with your diabetes self-care?

    1   2   3   4   5   6   7   8   9   10

    Not at all   A lot

18. Please list below any other concerns you have about managing your diabetes.

19. Please list below any questions you have about your diabetes.

20. Please list any mental health diagnoses you have had:

    _____

PATIENT EDUCATION HANDOUTS FOR ADULT PATIENTS
Beating Insomnia

For many people, insomnia is a learned problem. Repeated nights spent worrying or tossing and turning in bed teaches the body to associate the bed with arousal and alertness, when instead we want the body to associate the bed with relaxation and drowsiness. In order to break this problem we need to help the body "relearn" to associate the bed with sleepiness. The steps below will do this. Read them carefully, follow them closely, and call the clinic if you have any questions. You can sleep better!

STEP 1: DO NOT GO TO BED UNTIL YOU ARE VERY DROWSY (NO MATTER WHAT TIME IT IS!).
Do not go to bed according to the clock. Instead, go to bed only when you are so drowsy you can barely stay awake. You might end up getting in bed long after your usual bed time if you do this, but that's okay. With time, you will get drowsy earlier in the night.

STEP 2: IF YOU ARE AWAKE IN BED MORE THAN TWENTY MINUTES, GET OUT OF BED AND DO SOMETHING RELAXING.
This is very important! Remember that by lying in bed a long time awake, you are teaching your body to associate the bed with wakefulness. We want the opposite to happen, so you must leave the bed if you're not sleeping. When you get out of bed, avoid doing activities that excite you or make you tense. Instead, do something relaxing.

STEP 3: WHEN YOU BEGIN TO FEEL DROWSY AGAIN, TRY GOING TO BED AGAIN.
If you again lie awake in bed for twenty minutes, it's important to go back to Step 2 by getting out of bed. Repeat Steps 2 and 3 until you eventually fall asleep. When you start this program, you might need to repeat these steps several times until you fall asleep, but this will improve after 1 week for most people.

STEP 4: GET OUT OF BED AT THE SAME TIME EACH DAY.
No matter what time you fall asleep during the night, make sure to get up at about the same time each day (even weekends). Do not stay in bed more than 1 hour later than your usual waking time.

STEP 5: DO NOT NAP DURING THE DAY.
If you absolutely must nap, limit the nap to twenty minutes. You might want to set a timer to make sure you don't sleep longer.

MOST IMPORTANTLY: HAVE PATIENCE!
Chronic insomnia doesn't develop overnight and it doesn't go away overnight. In fact, most people who follow these steps find their sleep gets worse before it gets better. However, in one to two weeks, you should notice significant improvement in your sleep if you follow these steps closely.

SWEET DREAMS!

The "CALM" Exercise

This relaxation strategy is designed to help you relax muscles that have become tense due to stress. Because you have immediate and direct control over your muscles, you can learn to relax them on command. However, this is a skill that requires practice.

As the word "CALM" is used here, each letter stands for a particular muscle group to relax. The "C" stands for chest, "A" stands for arms (including hands and shoulders), "L" stands for legs (including feet), and "M" stands for mouth (including the jaw).

For this exercise, say the word "CALM" to yourself. If you are able, close your eyes so you can concentrate better. As you repeat the word to yourself, scan each of the four areas for muscle tension, then relax that area. Move from the Chest to the Arms to the Legs to the Mouth, scanning for tension and releasing any that exists, as you rehearse the word "CALM".

Repeat this as long as needed, but at least thirty to sixty seconds. If you are using a particular muscle group and so cannot relax it (e.g., if you are walking down the street), simply focus on the other muscle groups.

The CALM Exercise

Chest: Chest/torso sinks back into the chair
Arms: Shoulders and arms sag, hands rest in lap
Legs: Loose and flexible, not crossed
Mouth: Jaw drops slightly

Change Plan Worksheet

Here's a way to think about making some changes. . . .

1. The changes I want to make are (right now or in the future):

2. The steps I plan to take in changing are:

3. The ways other people can help me are:
   Person   Possible ways to help

4. Some things that could interfere with my plan are (e.g., boredom):

5. How realistic is this plan? How likely are you to follow through with it?

YOUR CONFIDENCE IN SUCCESSFULLY MAKING THIS CHANGE

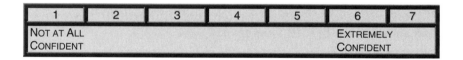

1	2	3	4	5	6	7
NOT AT ALL CONFIDENT					EXTREMELY CONFIDENT	

Diaphragmatic Breathing Tips

If you've taken Lamaze classes before, you might have been taught diaphragmatic breathing. This relaxation strategy involves breathing in a slow and deep fashion using your diaphragm, which is a muscle that separates your abdominal and chest cavities. Breathing with the help of the diaphragm is the most natural way for your body to breathe (as opposed to using your upper chest).

You can tell you are using your diaphragm to breathe if your stomach expands as you breathe in (like a balloon filling up with air). You can check for this during breathing by placing one hand on your stomach and one on your chest, then watching them as you breathe deeply. The hand on your stomach should be moving up and down more than the one on your chest. Check for this when you practice diaphragmatic breathing until you are certain you're doing it correctly.

Here's the basic breathing procedure:

(1) Breathe in deeply and slowly (about four seconds) through your nose.
(2) Breathe out deeply and slowly (again about four seconds) through your mouth, allowing the air to fully escape.
(3) Repeat this procedure for thirty to sixty seconds, or as long as needed.

Keep in mind that diaphragmatic breathing is a skill that requires practice. Like all skills, some people will have more trouble learning it than others. For most people, diaphragmatic breathing feels awkward initially. Stick with it! With practice, you will begin to feel more comfortable with it and will be able to use it more effectively.

The ABC's of Habit Change

Are you hoping to change your diet; exercise more; stop smoking; eliminate caffeine or alcohol from your diet; or make some other change in behavior? If so, you are trying to develop a new habit. The steps below can guide you through this process...give them a try!

STEP 1: PRIORITIZE
If you have more than one habit to change, don't try to change them all at the same time. Start with the most important or, alternatively, the easiest.

STEP 2: CHOOSE SPECIFIC AND MEASURABLE GOALS

GOOD:	NOT AS GOOD:
walking/swimming/tennis regularly	getting into shape
eat less fatty food/cholesterol	change my diet
schedule more relaxation, call friends more	manage my stress better

STEP 3: BREAK YOUR OVERALL GOAL INTO SMALLER PIECES
WALKING REGULARLY: Buy walking shoes; walk ten minutes three days/week; increase as able

454 • PATRICIA J. ROBINSON AND JEFFREY T. REITER

EAT LESS FAT/CHOLESTEROL: Buy new cookbook; buy low-fat/cholesterol foods; reduce intake by 1/4 for two weeks

MORE RELAXATION/FRIENDS: Call two friends this week; go bowling this week

STEP 4: MAKE SURE EACH PIECE IS REALISTIC

REALISTIC:	UNREALISTIC:
Walk for ten minutes	Walk for an hour everyday, rain or shine!
Count calories, cut back as needed	Never eat junk food again
Call one friend I've been out of touch with	Re-connect with all my friends
Schedule fifteen minutes of relaxation daily	Take an hour to myself everyday

STEP 5: SET A DATE FOR COMPLETING EACH PIECE

Examples: I'll buy my walking shoes by Tuesday
            I'll call my friend this weekend
            I'll buy different food on tomorrow's grocery trip

STEP 6: MAKE IT FUN—REWARD YOURSELF; PICK A FUN WAY TO CHANGE THE BEHAVIOR

STEP 7: HAVE A RELAPSE PLAN

- Don't panic! Problems/slips happen, you can get back on track
- Revise your goal (is it unrealistic? no fun? not clear?)
- Review your reasons for wanting to change
- Enlist someone for support

Healthy Sleeping Tips

If you've been having trouble sleeping, check out the suggestions below. Sometimes making just a few adjustments in your lifestyle can help sleep a lot.

1. AVOID ALCOHOL WITHIN TWO HOURS OF BEDTIME. Although alcohol may help you fall asleep faster, it will also lead to broken, lighter sleep. You don't have to stop alcohol completely, but do not drink close to bedtime.

2. AVOID SMOKING/DIPPING WITHIN TWO HOURS OF BED-TIME. Many people feel smoking/dipping is relaxing, but actually nicotine is a stimulant that may make it harder to sleep. If you must smoke/dip at night, be sure not to do so close to bedtime.

3. DO NOT EXERCISE OR TAKE A HOT BATH WITHIN TWO HOURS OF BEDTIME. Either of these activities will help if done earlier in the day or evening, but anything that raises your body temperature close to bedtime will hurt your sleep.

4. AVOID CAFFEINE IN THE EVENINGS. Some people are very sensitive to caffeine, so be sure to avoid it at night. Remember that tea, chocolate and colas, as well as coffee have a lot of caffeine.

5. KEEP SNACKS LIGHT. If you snack before bed, avoid heavy, greasy foods or anything you know might upset your stomach. If you wake during the night, try not to snack.

6. MAKE SURE YOUR BEDROOM HELPS YOUR SLEEP! Make sure your mattress is comfortable, the temperature is right in the room, and there is not too much noise. Sometimes just adding another blanket, playing soft music, or wearing ear plugs can make a big difference.

7. USE YOUR BED FOR WHAT IT'S BEST FOR: SLEEPING (NOT WATCHING TV!). Avoid worrying, arguing, watching TV, or reading in bed. If you do these activities, try to do them outside the bedroom. Also, avoid tossing and turning for more than twenty minutes. If you can't sleep, leave the bed to do something relaxing until you are tired again.

8. HAVE A PRE-BEDTIME ROUTINE. Prepare your body for sleep by keeping the same routine each night close to bedtime. After a short time, your body will start to expect sleep when you start your routine.

If your sleep continues to be a problem after trying these suggestions, be sure to mention it to your primary care provider. He or she can refer you to the Behavioral Health Consultant, who may have additional suggestions.

Managing Chronic Pain: The Basics

FIRST, A LITTLE BACKGROUND: "Chronic pain" is pain that lasts longer than three months. This can be very frustrating because there might be no quick fix and doctors might not even be able to explain the cause of the pain. As a result, it is extremely important for people with chronic pain to begin thinking about how to live a healthy, satisfying lifestyle despite the pain. What follows are some tips for making this happen. Give 'em a try!

1. ACCEPT THE PAIN: It might sound odd, but people actually do best when they accept that they have pain that might not go away. "Accepting the pain" means realizing your doctor can't cure the pain. It means you begin to work on living life again, despite the pain. Try to focus on improving your functioning rather than decreasing your pain.

2. UNDERSTAND THE DIFFERENCE BETWEEN "ACUTE" AND "CHRONIC" PAIN: Acute pain is that which usually results from an injury (for example a sprain or cut or broken bone). Treatment for this often involves resting the injured area to allow it to heal. However, with chronic pain, the original cause of the pain has usually healed. As a result, resting is not likely to help. In fact, it often makes the problem worse.

3. BEGIN TO EXERCISE: The decrease in activity that often occurs with chronic pain can make the pain worse. When you are less active, you lose muscle strength and flexibility. This means that an activity that caused pain before might cause even more pain after a period of rest. To avoid the cycle this can produce, ask your doctor or physical therapist for some simple stretching and strengthening exercises to try.

4. PACE YOUR ACTIVITIES: People with chronic pain often avoid chores or other activities on "bad pain days" and then try to make up for this by doing a lot on "good pain days". Unfortunately, this usually produces a flare-up in pain after a good pain day, which results in more rest and inactivity. This back-and-forth worsens the pain problem. To avoid this, try to do the same amount of activity on good days as you do on bad ones. Do not do less activity on bad days and do not do more on good days.

5. PRACTICE RELAXATION: Have you noticed that your pain worsens when you are stressed or upset? Stress naturally produces muscle tension, which can worsen pain. Ask your doctor about ways to relax your muscles when you feel tense, then practice these at the first signs of stress or increased pain.

6. DISTRACT YOURSELF WHEN YOU HAVE PAIN: We have all heard stories of athletes who get injured but continue to play. When focused on the game an athlete doesn't notice pain as much. Try this yourself: When you feel pain, find something to distract yourself. The less you think about your pain, the less it will bother you.

7. TRY NOT TO WORRY ABOUT THE PAIN. Remember that for chronic pain, pain is not the same as injury. Worry increases muscle tension which increases pain.

Progressive Muscle Relaxation

Both diaphragmatic breathing and the CALM exercise are helpful for breaking up stress when it starts to occur. Sometimes, though, they do not produce the deep level of relaxation that is desired. Other times, they are not enough to break up stress (for example, when it is very intense). For such times, progressive muscle relaxation (PMR) can be very helpful. It requires more time and a quiet environment, but the results can be very worthwhile!

PMR involves tensing one muscle group to about 1/3–2/3 maximum tension for four to five seconds, followed by a complete release of tension for forty-five to sixty seconds. The muscle group is then tensed again and given a second release period. After completing both cycles, the next muscle group is used. The muscles used and the positions for tensing them are presented below:

1. BOTH LEGS: Lift both legs off the ground, straighten your knees and point your toes toward your head.
2. CHEST: Take a very deep breath (through the upper chest, not the diaphragm) and hold it.
3. BOTH ARMS: Turn your palms up and then make a fist. Bring your fists up to your shoulders while tensing the biceps.
4. ABDOMEN: Tighten these muscles as if you were about to be elbowed in the stomach.
5. SHOULDERS: Lift both shoulders up toward your ears.
6. BACK OF NECK: Tuck in and lower your chin toward your chest.
7. FOREHEAD: Raise your eyebrows.
8. EYES: Squint.

Help for Premature Ejaculation

Premature ejaculation is a common condition in which orgasm occurs before or shortly after intercourse begins. It is a harmless condition but can cause stress in the relationship.

Your partner's help will be important for overcoming premature ejaculation. One way she or he can help is to work with you on becoming more aware of each other's bodies. Practice caressing each other's body without intercourse. When doing this, focus on the pleasures of touch and don't worry about having intercourse. In fact, do not plan intercourse during these interactions.

Another way your partner can help is called the "squeeze technique". For this, engage in sexual activity (including penile stimulation) without intercourse until you are almost ready to ejaculate. At that time, have your partner squeeze the head of your penis for several seconds. After the pressure has decreased, wait about thirty seconds. After waiting, you may continue foreplay. Repeat this process until both you and your partner are ready to climax. The goal of this technique is for the man to become accustomed to the feeling of delayed ejaculation. After several sessions, regular intercourse may be tried without the squeeze technique. This can also be practiced during masturbation.

Remember that the most common problem related to premature ejaculation is relationship stress. A partner might feel frustrated and need to talk about the problem. Enlisting his or her help (using the squeeze technique or perhaps just being patient) can take some pressure off the sexual act. Remember also that premature ejaculation has nothing to do with masculinity or "weakness" and that it can be overcome.

STRESS: WHAT IT IS AND HOW TO RECOGNIZE IT

"Stress" is defined as a change in emotions, behavior, and/or physical functioning resulting from a perceived threat. Emotional changes include how you feel "on the inside" (your mood, for example). Behavioral changes include changes in what you do or how you act. Physical changes include actual changes in how your body functions or feels.

The first step to managing stress is to notice how it affects you. Once you recognize stress, you can catch it early and work on managing it. Stress affects us all differently, but most people experience the same effects over time.

How to Use This Handout

(1) Review the list below and circle those things that usually happen to you when you feel stressed.

(2) Watch for these changes in your daily life.

(3) When you notice one or more of these changes, use relaxation or some other stress management technique to break up the stress.

If you catch stress early and often, you can prevent it from becoming a problem!

Physical	Emotional	Behavioral
Headaches Stomach problems	Sad Angry	Increased substance use (cigarettes alcohol, drugs, caffeine)
Muscle aches/tension	Impatient, irritable	Isolate/withdraw from people
Flushed/warm face Increased heart rate	Feeling guilty Nervous/ anxious	More aggressive (yelling, swearing, throwing things, fighting)
Decreased/increased appetite	Lose interest in things	Increased/decreased eating
Decreased/increased sleep	Hard to concentrate	Decreased activity level
Increased muscle/ joint pain	Hopelessness	Talking more/less
Being ill more than usual	Thoughts of suicide/ homicide	Arguing more/snapping at people

(Note: There are other physical, emotional, and behavioral changes that can occur with stress. You might notice some in yourself that are not on this list. Some of these changes can also result from a medical condition. Talk to your doctor about these problems.)

See your Behavioral Health Consultant if you would like more information on stress.

PATIENT EDUCATION HANDOUTS FOR PARENTS
Treatment Routine for Nocturnal Enuresis

This procedure will help you help your child with the problem of bedwetting. When a good behavior plan is followed consistently, results are usually positive. Follow these steps carefully and call if you have questions.

1. Use either a pad or sensor that attaches to underwear (see your provider about this). This device will sound as soon as your child begins to urinate.
2. Follow the routine below when the alarm sounds on the pad or sensor:
   a. Ensure the child goes to the bathroom. There may only be a couple of drops left in the bladder but s/he must still go to the bathroom.
   b. Have your child remove soiled clothing and dispose of them in the proper place.
   c. Have your child clean his or her body with soap and water.
   d. Have the child put on clean underwear/clothing.
   e. Have the child put on clean bed sheets and reattach the alarm.
3. Avoid scolding your child, putting him/her down, or penalizing him/her in anyway. Instead, simply follow the above steps and act in a supportive manner.
4. Reward dry nights. Usually this can be done by granting a sticker for each dry night, and arranging ahead of time for stickers to be turned in for rewards. This part of the plan should be discussed with the Behavioral Health Consultant before starting.
5. Be patient! Most cases will resolve in two to three months if the above plan is followed consistently.

Ideas for Great Rewards

(See Also the "USING REWARDS WITH YOUR CHILD" Handout)
Many parents use rewards to try to change a child's behavior. For example, you've probably said, "If you clean your room today, you can have pizza for dinner!" or "When you finish your homework, then you can visit your friend." There are many things you can use for rewards, and most don't cost any money. The best rewards are probably the things your child likes

to do in his or her spare time. The list below contains many examples. Check it out and see if they might work for your child.

Having a friend stay overnight
Choosing what is for dinner
Staying up fifteen minutes later than usual
Going on a walk with Mom or Dad
Having a friend over to play
Selecting a movie to rent
Fifteen minutes of "special time" with Mom or Dad
Having a friend over for dinner
Mom or Dad does one of the child's chores for the day
Getting to pick a favorite food on the next grocery trip
Going to visit a friend during the day
Rental of a video game
Going to a friend's house for the night
One penny (or nickel or dime, etc.)
A smiley sticker (or some other sticker that s/he likes)
Having Mom or Dad read to him or her fifteen minutes
Going to the pet store to look at pets
Choosing the screensaver for the family computer
Buying a small toy

If you'd like more information on how to use rewards effectively to improve your child's behavior, ask to see the Behavioral Health Consultant in the clinic. A second handout titled, "Using Rewards with Your Child," might also be helpful for you to read. Good luck!!

Using Rewards with Your Child

Many parents try at one time or another to manage a child's behavior by providing rewards. The good news is that reward plans can work great. The bad news is that developing a good reward plan can be tricky. Many times when parents get frustrated with a reward plan it's because the plan wasn't developed quite right. If you're using rewards with your kids, check out the ideas below. If you'd like more information or help, ask your provider about seeing the clinic's Behavioral Health Consultant. Good luck!

Be Specific About What Behaviors Earn the Reward

Asking a child to "clean your room" to get a reward might cause problems because your idea of "clean" probably differs from your child's. Instead, you might say, "Putting away all of your clothes and making your bed" earns the reward. (You might also make the bed yourself once to show your child exactly what "making the bed" means.)

Don't Try to Work on Too Many Behaviors At Once

Select one or two behaviors that concern you the most and focus on these. Choose your battles carefully!

Involve Your Child in Choosing Rewards

Of course, you're the final authority on what rewards are possible, but ask your child for ideas. (S/He'll have plenty!) The key is to find rewards that your child gets excited about. Also think about what activities your child chooses to do during free time. Those activities will probably make great rewards. And remember, rewards don't have to cost money. (See the "Great Rewards Ideas" handout for ideas).

Make it Easy for Your Child to Get the Reward

We want your child to get the reward, because that means s/he is behaving appropriately. Also, in order for the appropriate behavior to occur again it needs to be rewarded. Thus, make it easy for your child to earn a reward at the beginning. As his/her behavior improves, you may gradually make it harder to get a reward.

Explain the Plan to Your Child

Before starting, take a few minutes to sit down with your child and explain exactly what behaviors will be rewarded, what rewards are possible, and when the plan will start. Your time will be well spent!

Be Consistent

Using rewards one day but not the next, or failing to give rewards that have been earned, will almost surely prevent the rewards from being successful.

(Think of it this way...would you go to work everyday and work hard if your employer only paid you some of the time?)

Develop New Rewards as Needed

Rewards often lose their power over time. This doesn't mean the plan stopped working, it simply means you might need to find some new rewards that will excite your child again.

Remember to Praise Your Child, Too!

Every time you give a reward, give lots of praise, too. Praise is a reward, and will also increase the positive feelings between you and your child.

USING TIME-OUT WITH YOUR CHILD

WHAT IS TIME-OUT? Time-Out is a punishment given to children when they act inappropriately. It involves sending the child to a specific chair or room if he or she refuses to stop acting out. She or he stays in the room/chair for a set amount of time. However, he or she is not released from Time-Out unless calm (see "General Guidelines" below).

WHEN SHOULD I USE TIME-OUT? Parents might use this if a child is yelling, whining, being aggressive, refusing to listen, or in other situations where the child's behavior is a problem. Time-Out should NOT be used for sadness or nervousness; only use it for disruptive behavior.

HOW DOES TIME-OUT WORK? By removing the child when he or she acts out, you remove any possibility that the behavior will be rewarded. Also, the child learns that acting out has a cost. Together, this makes the child less likely to act out again in the future.

General Guidelines for Using Time-Out

SELECT A TIME-OUT SPOT AHEAD OF TIME

Your Time-Out spot can be a chair placed in the corner of the room you're in; or it can be a separate room. Choose your spot ahead of time and use the same spot for each Time-Out. If you decide to use a room that will be out of your sight (for example, the child's bedroom), make sure there is nothing fun for the child to do in the room.

WARN YOUR CHILD BEFORE SENDING HIM OR HER TO TIME-OUT

First, use a simple statement to ask your child to stop the behavior (for example: "Please stop changing the channels on the TV").

Wait 10 seconds. If the behavior doesn't stop, warn the child about Time-Out:

"If you don't stop changing the TV channels, it will be a Time-Out."

Wait 10 seconds again. If the behavior doesn't stop, give the Time-Out.

"You didn't stop changing the channels. That's a Time-Out."

DO NOT INTERACT AT ALL WITH YOUR CHILD DURING TIME-OUT

Do not check on, talk to, or comfort your child during Time-Out. Ignore any of his or her comments.

USE THE CORRECT AMOUNT OF TIME

Time-Out should last less than five minutes if your child is age 5 or younger. Add one minute for each year over 5 (for example, an 8-year-old would need eight-minute Time-Outs). Use a timer if possible.

WHAT IF MY CHILD WON'T GO??

For every ten seconds that your child refuses to go to Time-Out, add one minute. For example, if your 5 year-old child refuses to go for twenty seconds, he or she must stay in Time-Out for seven minutes (five minutes plus two extra minutes for the two ten-second delays). Announce the extra minutes every ten seconds (for example, after the first ten seconds of delay say, "Okay, that's six minutes.") Do not use Time-Out for longer than ten minutes, however.

STAY CALM WHEN SENDING THE CHILD TO TIME-OUT

Keep a neutral and calm appearance, and do not yell. However, be firm.

DO NOT TALK ABOUT THE PROBLEM AFTERWARD

Do not make your child apologize after the Time-Out; praise for calming down is okay.

THE CHILD MUST BE CALM AT THE END OF THE TIME-OUT

If the time is up and the child is still acting-out, add one more minute. If he or she is not calm at the end of that minute, add one more. Continue this as needed, but do not use more than ten minutes total time. Tell the child each time you add one minute ("You're still yelling, so that's one more minute.")

BHC Referrals

Common Referrals

✓ Typical psych complaints (anxiety and mood disorders, grief, stress, ADHD, substance abuse, etc.)

✓ Tension or Migraine HA

✓ Hypertension

✓ Diabetes

✓ Back pain, headaches, or other chronic pain

✓ Fatigue without medical etiology

✓ Hyperlipidemia

✓ Obesity

✓ Smoking cessation

✓ Parenting and behavioral problems in kids

Other Appropriate but Less Common Referrals

✓ Temporomandibular Disorder (TMD)
  ○ often successfully treated with habit-reversal and stress management education

✓ Habit-reversal (Thumbsucking, fingernail-biting, hair-pulling)

✓ Acute post-trauma problems
  ○ recent evidence that early behavioral intervention can prevent PTSD

✓ Irritable Bowel Syndrome w/o clear psychiatric comorbidity
  ○ behavioral interventions can reduce IBS symptoms

✓ Some dermatological problems (urticarias, alopecia, hyperhydrosis)
  ○ often worsened by stress

✓ Chronic nonspecific dizziness
  ○ 2001 study showed 2/3 of chronic dizziness patients had panic attacks

✓ Irritable Bladder Syndrome
  ○ patients may need a behavioral plan to gradually increase time between voids

✓ Patients currently doing well, but w/ a history of chronic problems or high relapse risk
  ○ patients often utilize BHC instead of PCP in a future crisis or for case management needs (thus decreasing the load on PCP)

✓ Every newly diagnosed diabetes patient
  ○ BHC will screen for potential problems, intervene before problem develops

BHC Uses You Might not Have Thought Of

✓ Information-gathering calls (e.g., to school, other health care providers)
  ○ such persons often will call BHC for future needs because of easier access, thus decreasing your phone call load
✓ Complete medication contracts with patients
✓ Gather history on a work-in (same-day)with acute psychiatric symptoms
✓ Gather history on a scheduled patient with psychiatric problems when you are behind
✓ Return phone call to patient with psychiatric complaints

YOUR NEW BEHAVIORAL HEALTH CONSULTANT: WHO I AM AND WHAT I'M DOING HERE

WHO IS THIS GUY (GAL)? Your consultant, _____, is a _____ who has recently moved to the area. I am not a physician and do not prescribe medications. Instead, I use "talk" interventions with patients.

WHAT DOES A BEHAVIORAL HEALTH CONSULTANT DO? My role here is to provide CONSULTATION TO THE PHYSICIANS when they have patients whose problem is at least partly psychosocial. This includes patients whose stress is affecting their medical condition, as well as patients whose primary problem is psychiatric. Thus, I'm just as likely to see patients with headaches or insomnia or gastrointestinal problems as I am to see patients with depression or anxiety.

WHAT WILL YOU ACTUALLY DO WITH PATIENTS? It might be easier to describe what I *won't* be doing. As a consultant, I won't be doing traditional "therapy" with patients. When a physician identifies an acute problem that needs my attention, I will see the patient briefly to help the patient and physician figure out a treatment plan. I will often only see the patient once or twice, and for brief visits. The goal is to teach the patient some self-management techniques, which their physician can support and monitor. I'll focus on small changes with patients, not broad or major life changes. If patients need more than I can offer, we will still try to refer them to a specialty mental health service.

HOW DO PATIENTS GET SCHEDULED WITH YOU? Because I am a consultant, patients must be referred to me by their physician. If the patient can stay, I will typically see him/her right after they see the physician, then I might schedule him/her for follow-up appointments.

HOW WILL YOU DOCUMENT PATIENT VISITS? I will chart in the medical records, just like a regular medical visit. I'll dictate my notes.

WHAT WILL YOU DO WHEN NOT SEEING PATIENTS? This is a very new way of delivering mental health care to patients, and has never been done at this organization. Thus, I will initially be getting the service organized and educating staff about the service. I'll also work on developing patient education handouts, group medical visits and other special services.

If you've read to here, congratulations! Thanks for reading, and please feel free to discuss with me any questions you have. I look forward to working with you all!

Dr. / Ms. / Mr. _____, BHC ext. _____

INDEX

Page numbers followed by f and t indicate figures and tables, respectively.

Printed in the United States of America